'*Communicating Pain* is a situated first-person narrative of author Stephanie de Montalk's quest for ways to manage, live with, and articulate extreme chronic pain, undergirded by the authority of experience as a patient and a nurse. Engaging historical and literary others who have trod similar paths, this brilliant cross-genre work interweaves narrative with poetry with history. The book contributes both to the expressive history of disability/chronic illness and also to the cultural analysis of the aesthetics that emerges from distinctive lives lived with pain. It is a wonderful reminder that some of the most notable and innovative intellectual and artistic figures were people with disabilities – and that the history of creativity and the history of living with suffering are inextricably intertwined. Boasting an impressive base of practical and scholarly knowledge, *Communicating Pain* is a gorgeously written, poetic book that makes reading about pain surprisingly pleasurable.'

Professor Martha Stoddard Holmes, *California State University, USA*

'Stephanie de Montalk, writing under a hostile and capricious force, not just *about* pain but in pain, through pain, has produced a work already recognised by health professionals as ground-breaking and riveting and beautiful. Her book is political, fierce, open, buzzing with ideas about how the body treats the mind and vice versa. It's an unflinching account, terrifying and bleak in its tracing of nerve pain's unpredictable torture methods. If the defeating of a narrative pattern –its lack of a progress – is one of chronic pain's cruel manoeuvres, this book is itself a triumph of patterning. It does two things at the same time: it practices an extraordinary embrace, making us come closer and closer, while at the same time reminding us of the arm's length of suffering. We feel the pull of the writer's terrible plight, but we also experience the necessarily harsh corrective of de Montalk's exclusivity, since it is, according to this powerfully argued text, only the fellow sufferer who can connect finally. Everyone else is just a literary tourist. Books like this one remind us we should never get used to anything.'

Professor Damien Wilkins, *Victoria University of Wellington, New Zealand*

'*Communicating Pain* is a wonderfully powerful, important, and beautiful piece of work which makes a major contribution to the understanding of the subject of pain. The success of the project lies in the fact that Stephanie de Montalk illuminates the ugly problem of pain, from so many angles, using so many light sources, with such beauty.'

Professor Michael Hanne, *University of Auckland, New Zealand*

Communicating Pain

Combining critical research with memoir, essay, poetry and creative biography, this insightful volume sensitively explores the lived experience of chronic pain.

Confronting the language of pain and the paradox of writing about personal pain, *Communicating Pain* is a personal response to the avoidance, dismissal and isolation experienced by the author after developing intractable pelvic pain in 2003. The volume focuses on pain's infamous resistance to verbal expression, the sense of exile experienced by sufferers and the under-recognised distinction between acute and chronic pain. In doing so, it creates a platform upon which scholarly, imaginative and emotional quotients round out pain as the sum of physical actualities, mental challenges and psychosocial interactions. Additionally, this work creates a dialogue between medicine and literature. Considering the works of writers such as Harriet Martineau, Alphonse Daudet and Aleksander Wat, it enables a multi-genre narrative heightened by poetry, fictional storytelling and life-writing.

Coupled with academic rigour, this compelling monograph constitutes a persuasive and unique exploration of pain and the communication of suffering. It will appeal to students and researchers interested in fields such as Medical Humanities, Autobiography Studies and Sociology of Health and Illness.

Stephanie de Montalk worked as a nurse and documentary film maker before becoming a writer in 1996. She is the author of four collections of poems, a literary novel, a memoir-biography and the award-winning memoir-study of pain: *How Does It Hurt?*; adapted from her PhD thesis in Creative Writing. Since an accident in 2003, she has been constrained by pain.

Routledge Advances in the Medical Humanities

Collaborative Arts-based Research for Social Justice
Victoria Foster

Person-centred Health Care
Balancing the Welfare of Clinicians and Patients
Stephen Buetow

Digital Storytelling in Health and Social Policy
Listening to Marginalized Voices
Nicole Matthews and Naomi Sunderland

Bodies and Suffering
Emotions and Relations of Care
Ana Dragojlovic and Alex Broom

Thinking with Metaphors in Medicine
The State of the Art
Alan Bleakley

Medicine, Health and Being Human
Edited by Lesa Scholl

Meaning-making Methods for Coping with Serious Illness
Fereshteh Ahmadi and Nader Ahmadi

A Visual History of HIV/AIDS
Exploring the Face of AIDS Film Archive
Edited by Elisabet Björklund and Mariah Larsson

Communicating Pain
Exploring Suffering through Language, Literature and Creative Writing
Stephanie de Montalk

www.routledge.com/Routledge-Advances-in-Disability-Studies/book-series/RADS

Communicating Pain

Exploring Suffering through Language, Literature and Creative Writing

Stephanie de Montalk

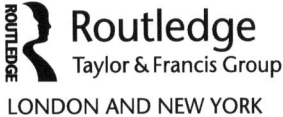

Routledge
Taylor & Francis Group

LONDON AND NEW YORK

First published 2019
by Routledge
4 Park Square, Milton Park, Abingdon, Oxon OX14 4RN
605 Third Avenue, New York, NY 10017

First issued in paperback 2023

Routledge is an imprint of the Taylor & Francis Group, an informa business

British Library Cataloguing-in-Publication Data
A catalogue record for this book is available from the British Library

Library of Congress Cataloging-in-Publication Data
A catalog record has been requested for this book

ISBN: 978-1-03-257043-3 (pbk)
ISBN: 978-1-138-61105-4 (hbk)
ISBN: 978-0-429-46545-1 (ebk)

DOI: 10.4324/9780429465451

Typeset in Times New Roman
by Wearset Ltd, Boldon, Tyne and Wear

Publisher's Note
The publisher has gone to great lengths to ensure the quality of this reprint but
points out that some imperfections in the original copies may be apparent.

For John,
Til a' the seas gang dry

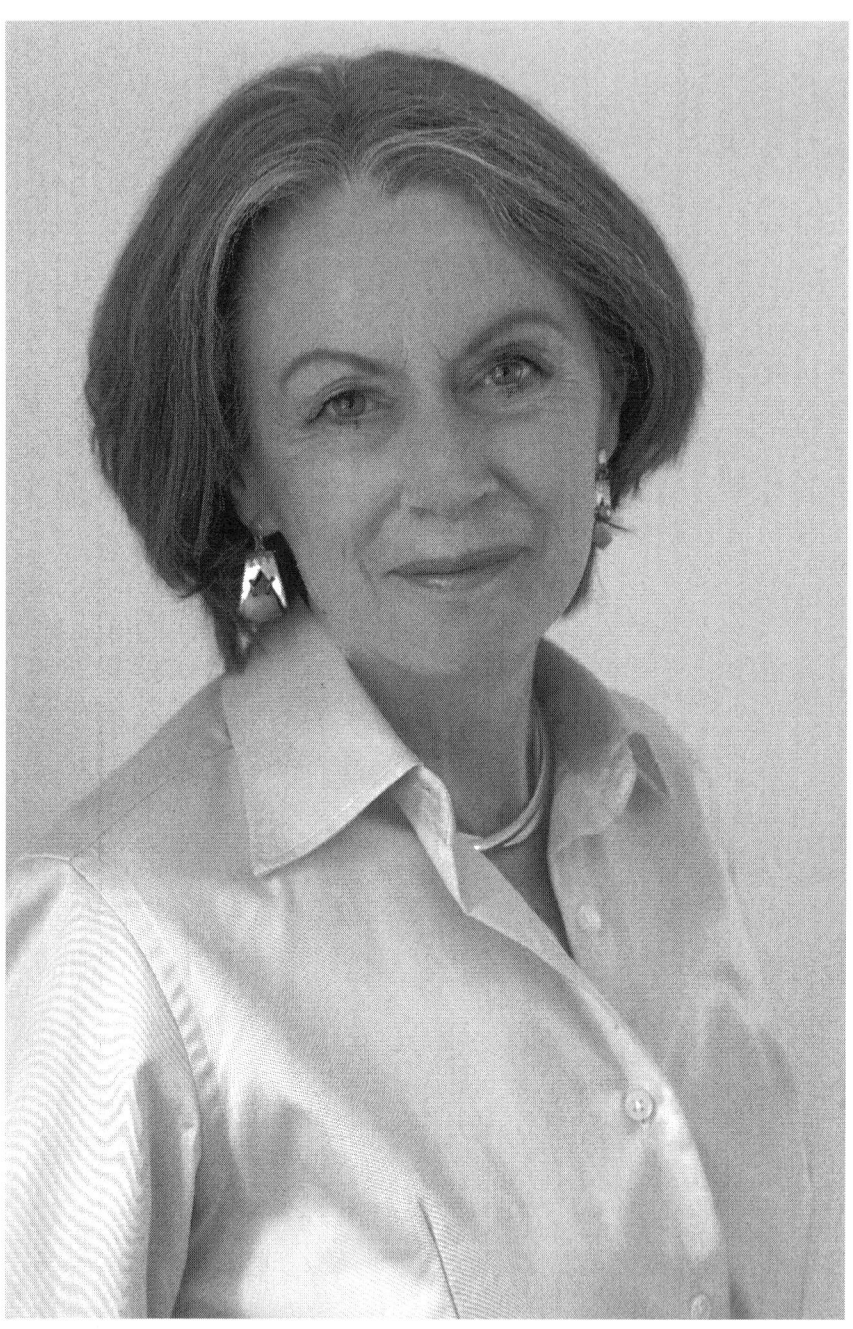

Photo credit: Sabrina Hyde

Contents

Acknowledgements

The understanding and encouragement of many people made the doctoral dissertation from which this book has been adapted, possible.

I am deeply indebted to my PhD supervisors, Professor Bill Manhire, Professor Kathryn Walls and Professor Damien Wilkins of Victoria University of Wellington, for their insight and invaluable guidance, and for awakening my interest in the absorbing, rewarding world of scholarship.

I am additionally grateful to the members of the PhD workshops, 2010–2013, including: Pip Adam, Maxine Alterio, Angela Andrews, Michalia Arathimos, Arini Beautris, Laurence Fearnley, David Fleming, Helen Heath, Christine Leunens, Lynn Jenner, Tina Makareti, Gavin McGibbon, Lawrence Patchett and Steven Toussaint.

Warmest thanks are also due to Fergus Barrowman of Victoria University Press for his awareness and support during publication of the 2014 adaptation of the thesis, *How Does It Hurt?*

To Tordis Flath: Thank you for your superb, interpretive indexing, and your invaluable editorial assistance.

To Lindsay Manning: Thank you for being an enduring companion and source of strength on The Glass Mountain.

To my children, Donovan Miller, Dylan Miller, Jonathon Miller and Melissa Moon: Thank you for your humour, practical help, computer wizardry and spirit-lifting animal postcards – of which there are dozens and the panda still reigns supreme!

To my husband, John Miller: Your patience and empathy sustain me. Your faith in my ability to undertake a study and memoir of pain, and your active interest in the work in progress, made this book attainable. I cannot count the ways in which you are here for me.

1   The shirt of Nessos[1]

An essay on the experience of writing about pain

> Pain is an unpleasant sensory and emotional experience with actual or potential tissue damage, or described in terms of such damage.
>
> The International Association for the Study of Pain (1979)[2]

> We don't like to talk about pain – are somehow ashamed by it and try to shrug it off. Well, enough with that. Pain is a crucial part of our medical tales. It needs to be articulated, then confronted – even if, sometimes, the pain is beyond words.
>
> Dana Jennings, *New York Times* (2009)[3]

> We are determined to raise the profile of pain. […] There is a lack of awareness that pain brings side effects and mortality. It reduces life expectancy. To do nothing is not an option.
>
> Professor Richard Langford,[4] President of the British Pain Society (2012)

A necessary preface

In 2003, I slipped and fell heavily on a marble bathroom floor in Warsaw, injuring my pelvis. As the acute pain of that accident turned first into the severe chronic pain of an obscure nerve entrapment, and then into the intractable neuropathic pain[5] of nerve damage, I became aware of much awkwardness around, and reluctance to speak plainly about, physical pain – continuing pain, in particular.

Initially, there were commiserations – pain after an accident is expected. The expressions of interest and sympathy were followed by appreciative assumptions that the trauma, having been treated, had healed, leaving an inconsequential degree of discomfort. However, as the pain persisted, the sense of solidarity turned to inklings of disbelief and dismissal. I found myself struggling to describe the pain, and even to speak of it. Increasingly, I felt emotionally isolated – exiled in the realisation that pain's forestalling of language was limiting understanding, fellow feeling and also, it seemed, compassion. I could admit that I, too, might once have been dubious about the severity of another's invisible, ongoing pain. Although I had personally experienced a range of acute or temporary pain, and as a former nurse had cared for patients in pain, a state of non-cancer pain, for which strong narcotics were taken daily for years outside hospital settings, had rarely occurred to me. Neither had I registered the disparity between palliative end-of-life relief and control of unbearable pain when life must continue.

I encountered others whose chronic pain – that is, a continuous pain lasting six months or longer – was doubted. I read their anonymous blogs and postings – sufferer to sufferer – on Internet forums. I observed them in pain specialists' clinics reading magazines and walking to and from the consulting rooms without obvious signs of physical distress. I saw them, uncomplaining, in the wider community, struggling to adopt the roles of supportive partner, attentive parent, sharing friend. And I perceived that, beyond the online listings of symptoms and the advent of storytelling as therapy, despite the prevalence of self-help texts and the growing interest of scholars, the 'patient voice' as a source of empathic disclosure – as, wrote nineteenth-century French author and sufferer Alphonse Daudet, a 'solace and relief [...] a mirror and a guide' – remained in relatively short supply.

Why the inability, or unwillingness, to acknowledge continuing pain? Was it initiated because for many people, including those afflicted by pain, physical distress, like death, is threatening, beyond understanding?

Emily Dickinson wrote:

> Pain has but one Acquaintance
> And that is Death –
> Each one unto the other
> Society enough.

> Pain is the Junior Party
> By just a second's right –
> Death tenderly assists Him
> And then absconds from Sight.[6]

Did the origins of this hesitance to speak about pain also lie in primitive mistrust of weakened 'tribe' members; societal expectations of stoicism; the paucity of reflection on bodily torment in literature? Was the linguistic derivation of 'pain', from the Ancient Greek *poine*, meaning 'penalty', and the Latin *poena*, meaning 'punishment', relevant? In which case, had a primal part of the public mind remembered that to be in pain was to have incurred suffering sent by the gods for wrongdoing? (I had not forgotten my mother's accusatory, 'I wonder what you were doing to deserve that' when, as a child, I fell ill or had an accident.) How about the riddling nature of pain as unequivocally present for the sufferer, yet a cause for doubt in a bystander for whom another's pain cannot be shared or confirmed? Or was the evasion principally related to a one-dimensional interpretation of pain based on the long-held model of acute pain – a response evident, I noted, even among health professionals?

'The act of verbally expressing pain,' said Elaine Scarry in *The Body in Pain* (1985),[7] 'is a necessary prelude to the collective task of diminishing pain.'

In 2010, I set myself the task of examining the lived reality of chronic physical pain as a PhD in Creative Writing entitled *How Does It Hurt?: Narrating Pain*. I hoped to bring visibility and a measure of clarity to the condition – to break the cycle of misunderstanding, silence, isolation. In particular, I wanted to confront the paradox of writing about personal pain, notwithstanding physical pain's resistance to verbal expression; and to determine where the greater challenge lay: in finding descriptors for the 'raw sensation' of pain; or in communicating the emotional and mental implications that constitute suffering.

I stalled. Could I round out this complex and intensely personal territory and identify it as the sum of its physical sensations and psychosocial interactions? Could I research and write against continuous pain, lying down? What form should my thesis take?

'The artist is extremely lucky,' said John Berryman in a *Paris Review* interview, 'who is presented with the worst possible ordeal which will not actually kill him. At that point he's in business.'[8]

Should I write a novel or a pathography? Would the flexibility of a memoir or personal essay be most appropriate, as pain pushed me this way and that?

Difficulties and mysteries

Amorphous and abstruse, physical pain flickers at the edges of thought, communication and medical science, defying description and, when extreme, reducing verbal expression to a pre-language of moans and cries. Hidden deep within a network of cells and synapses, it can only be independently verified by a functional MRI (fMRI) of the brain, in which it may be seen as flares of light as it occurs. In an absence of precision treatments capable of targeting its transmission symptoms, it resists complete and enduring relief. When it does desist, it is likely to be recalled less for its sensory actuality than for the psychological response engendered by that actuality. 'The mind is its own place,' wrote Milton in *Paradise Lost* (speaking for Satan), 'and in itself/Can make a Heaven of Hell, a Hell of heaven.'

The link between mind and body in the pain experience – a relationship surely integral to the understanding and verbal communication of pain – has proved as elusive as the parameters of consciousness. A key to uncovering this connection appears to lie not only in knowledge of the way in which pain-activated neurons, viewable on fMRI, connect with the felt and perceived experience of pain, but also the understanding of 'the complex nuances of [the neurons'] language'.[9] To date, as *New York Times* journalist and chronic pain sufferer Melanie Thernstrom pointed out in her work of personal narrative and reportage *The Pain Chronicles* (2010), all these scans offer is 'a silent film of a concert':[10] a performance in which the musicians' movements are seen, but the components of the music they are playing – the melody, harmony and balance, the contours, tensions and resolutions – are unknowable.

Increasingly, the inexpressibility of pain is seen to hinder medicine's inability to manage it. In order to render a rounded account of physical pain, it may be necessary to 'test' ourselves, in the words of Michel de Montaigne, 'in the thickest of pain'.[11] Yet, of such testing, Montaigne – born in 1533 and generally viewed as one of the first writers to fully explore pain autobiographically[12] – admitted that although when experiencing pain he remained 'capable of speaking, thinking, and answering as sanely as at any other time', he found that his abilities became less steady, 'being troubled and distracted'. Consequently, and given the inconsistencies of his symptoms and the interruptions of his imagination, Montaigne found himself limited to assessing his pain state 'only by actual sensation, not by reasoning'.[13]

The challenges of rationally and analytically communicating physical pain persist, notwithstanding advances in neurobiological pain research and the inroads scholars have made into the nature and meaning of pain: pursuits which demonstrate connections between the anatomical, physiological and psychological vocabularies of pain, and those of history, philosophy and culture.[14] Despite, too, our current public preoccupation with wellness, and, in the thrall of the Internet's encouragement of confession and storytelling, an unprecedented outpouring of the difficulties and mysteries of being in pain – the latter supplementing, even replacing, the face-to-face assistance of medical professionals, family and friends.

It is particularly striking that, by comparison with the reflections on the psychological anguish of mental and emotional distress that have played central roles in poetry, non-fiction and drama, literature's contemplation of sustained physical pain has been marginal. While feelings of isolation, loss, grief and despair are an integral part of severe and chronic bodily suffering, non-scientific writers (autobiographers in particular) have focused on the transient effects of acute pain.

As I have found, it is impossible to share fully the sensory and emotional impact of chronic pain with anyone but a fellow sufferer. In this respect, the difference between acute pain and chronic pain is worth reiterating – for, regardless of significant developments in the science of pain since the mid-1960s, much societal, and even medical, understanding of pain remains based on what it is to be in acute pain.

Acute pain, the purpose of which is protective, is temporary: it warns of harm, attends healing and passes, having run a largely predictable course of hours, days, weeks or even months. It ranges from the mundane to the unbearable: from the discomfort of a sprained ankle to the agony of the rack. It is depicted in literature, dramatised in films, reported in the media. For sufferers who cannot articulate the acute pain of their injury, illness, surgery or childbirth, the failure of language, although perturbing, is transient.

Chronic pain, as we know, serves no obvious beneficial biological function. In *The Culture of Pain* (1993), David B. Morris characterised chronic pain as a state as different from acute pain as is cancer from the common cold.[15] In *The Pain Chronicles*, Dr Clifford Woolf, a Harvard professor of neurobiology, described chronic pain as 'a terrible, abnormal sensory experience, pathological activity in the nervous system'[16] – confirming that chronic pain not only defies pain's evolutionary warning and protective mechanisms, but also, in outliving its original function, becomes a pathological condition of itself. Unlike acute pain, writes Morris, the wearying constancy of chronic pain, upon both the sufferer and the 'patience and goodwill' of friends and carers, 'constitutes a radical assault on language and on human communication'.[17] This is a complex pain, personally, medically, socially. It wears on long after an injury or disease has been treated or has apparently healed, with no end in sight. It is, therefore, life changing: a debilitating state of elusive diagnosis, failed intervention and irreversible tissue impairment. At its most consuming, it is akin to the pain of terminal disease, without the heroic 'combative image' and prospect of final easement. An authority on pain research, James L. Henry, has reported analysis that shows chronic pain as second only to bipolar disorder as a cause of suicide.[18]

As control over once fatal injuries and medical conditions is asserted, and despite advances in the science of pain and the alleviation of acute pain, the incidence of chronic pain reaches epidemic proportions.[19] Today, advises Canadian education professor and chronic pain sufferer Lous Heshusius, there is a greater number of chronic pain patients than the combined total of those living with diabetes, heart disease, obesity and cancer.[20]

One in six New Zealanders[21] (around 700,000) suffer from varying degrees of chronic pain. In America, 100 million people (one-third of the country's population) live with unrelieved pain; of this number, some 10 million are significantly disabled.

I imagined, as I began to explore chronic pain, that all the untold stories of sufferers were surrounding me, pressing in on me, reinforcing the importance of telling my own story within a broad study of the state of being that is pain and the imaginative framework of literature.

Why, I wondered, given the heightened profile of pain in medical research, scholarship and via the worldwide web, is chronic bodily distress, and in particular the 'patient voice', still sparingly mirrored in literature? Is the disparity between the outpourings online and the paucity of personal pain narratives in literary form related to the respective readerships' understandings of chronic pain? Could it be attributable to the fact that Internet communication can become a spontaneous and heartfelt exchange between anonymous sufferers, in a language 'ready-made', while literature requires a writer to distil '[t]he dialect of a village high upon inaccessible mountains'[22] into local, approachable images, rhythms and sounds? William Carlos Williams observed that the greatest challenge to 'really good writing'[23] is that of transferring to the imagination 'those things that lie under the direct scrutiny of the senses'. How then is one to bring the intense sensory scrutiny of persistent bodily pain to a visible and persuasive reality?

Moreover, why does social and even medical misunderstanding of chronic pain remain commonplace?[24] To what extent is sufferer *isolation* significant? Once chronic pain takes over, not only do all parts of a patient's life become challenging, but many relinquish their relationships rather than attempt to 'incorporate them into their altered lives', as one authority in pain management,

Scott M. Fishman, has observed.[25] The lived experience of chronic pain is 'not well tolerated. It's naturally uncomfortable for people who aren't suffering to be in that place.'

Settings

When considering the verbalisation of pain, antiquity (as with most things!) is the place to start. In *The History of Pain* (1993), Roselyne Rey explained that not only do the texts of Ancient Greece, like the *Iliad* and the *Odyssey*, 'make up part of a common Western cultural identity which has continued to the present day', they also place 'much emphasis on pain'.[26]

The ancients were aware of the differences in the communication of acute as opposed to chronic pain. Acute pain was the pain of the epic genre – of heroic battle and wounds and exhaustion. It was described in terms of 'the extent to which the subject is engrossed in pain, and how he or she perceives it with respect to time and to its origin: long-lasting and fast, sharp or cutting'; importantly, it referenced the causative instrument and its simultaneous definition of the received sensation.[27] Chronic pain, as the pain of the tragic genre, assumed a quality 'radically different' from those found in the epics.[28] This is a pain that 'teaches us not only about pain but also about suffering in the most physical, tangible and blunt way'.[29] Physical distress of this nature was perceived as 'consuming', as 'devouring', as a 'being which takes possession of the subject, invades it and takes over': the sufferer is fed upon by pain, which gradually strengthens as the victim weakens. Only the cry survives. Wrote Rey of such pain, 'the Greek texts simply say that it is unapproachable, ἀποτίβατος (*apotibatos*) and intractable.'[30]

The inability to communicate chronic pain and the isolation that results were addressed by Sophocles in *Philoctetes*,[31] in the plight of Philoctetes abandoned on the island of Lemnos with a festering – possibly gangrenous – leg. The play is a sustained depiction of the toll of unrelieved pain on the sufferer's language, emotions and spirit. But, as Sophocles made clear, there is more to Philoctetes' anguish than the agony of a pain that he describes as 'beyond words': there is the additional trauma of suffering in exile.[32] 'I looked everywhere/but all I found around me was my pain,' Philoctetes cries. There was no one, the chorus sings, 'to answer him with sympathy/when he cried out against the plague/that ate his flesh and made him bleed'.[33] Sophocles further suggested, in the scorn and desertion of Philoctetes' compatriots, that the utterance of pain does not necessarily engender the fellow feeling and compassion that would lessen the sufferer's isolation.

In the poem 'Surgical Ward'[34] – an exploration of the collective silence imbued by post-operative pain – W.H. Auden acknowledged the way in which pain diminishes the function of language as a means of personal expression and a carrier of social narrative. Here, in a mood of subdued suffering, hospital patients are exposed to degrees of pain and 'isolation' that cannot be imagined by those who inhabit 'the common world of the uninjured' – where, although happiness and anger and 'the idea of love' can be shared, physical pain cannot.

'They are and suffer; that is all they do,' Auden told us. They 'lie apart like epochs from each other'. They are 'remote as plants'. All the while, the 'healthy' cannot recall an everyday 'scratch' beyond its healing.

The way in which we use language, suggested immunologist and poet Miroslav Holub in his poem 'Brief reflection on the word Pain',[35] is integral to our understanding of pain – a proposition which acknowledges that the word *pain*, as 'a pretence of silence', both expresses and suppresses the existence it describes:

> Wittgenstein says: the words 'It hurts' have replaced
> tears and cries of pain. The word 'Pain'
> does not describe the expression of pain but
> replaces it.
> Thus it creates a new behaviour pattern
> in the case of pain.
>
> The word enters between us and the pain
> like a pretence of silence.
> It is a silencing. It is a needle
> unpicking the stitch
> between blood and clay.
>
> The word is the first small step
> to freedom
> from oneself.
>
> In case others
> are present.

The context for Holub's poem was Ludwig Wittgenstein's discussion of 'private language' in his posthumously published *Philosophical Investigations* (1953) – in which, having pondered the possibility of communicating the most private parts of our lives, Wittgenstein decided that communication is possible, as long as we can locate the experience in its societal, and therefore shared, dimension.

> Imagine a language in which a person could write down or give vocal expression to his inner experiences – his feeling, moods, and the rest – for his private use? – Well, can't we do so in our ordinary language? – But that is not what I mean. The individual words of this language are to refer to what can only be known to the person speaking: to his immediate private sensations. So another person cannot understand the language.[36]

Wittgenstein asked, 'How do words *refer* to sensations?', answering that 'verbal expression of pain replaces crying and does not describe it'.[37] He further enquired, 'In what sense are my sensations private?' before deciding 'I know I am in pain', and concluding this means nothing more than 'I am in pain'.

He finally wondered whether a word or sign associated with a private sensation would have a grammatical structure, and concluded that words privately defined in one's mind lack the 'stage setting' that allows language to make sense, or carry meaning:

> When one says, 'He gave a name to his sensation' one forgets that a great deal of stage setting in language is presupposed if the mere act of naming is to make sense. And when we speak of someone's having given a name to pain, what is presupposed is the existence of the grammar of the word pain; it shews the post where the new word is stationed.

This resistance to language

Literature as a potential 'setting' in which to make sense of and share physical distress was addressed by Virginia Woolf in her 1926 essay 'On Being Ill'.[38] Pondering the 'spiritual change' and potential for self-reflection when health fades, Woolf,[39,40] herself recovering at the time from an influenza-like malaise, asked why, 'considering how common illness is [...] it has not taken its place with love and battle and jealousy among the prime themes of literature'?[41] She suggested that the reason could lie primarily with literature's preoccupation with the mind and ideas – with the notion 'that the body is a sheet of plain glass through which the soul looks straight and clear, and save for one or two passions such as [the physical manifestations of] desire or greed, is null, and negligible and non-existent'.[42] She found that a significant factor in the hindrance of literary description is the 'poverty of the language'. 'English,' she famously said, 'which can express the thoughts of Hamlet and the tragedy of Lear, has no words for the shiver and the headache.'[43]

> It has all grown one way. The merest schoolgirl, when she falls in love, has Shakespeare or Keats to speak her mind for her; but let a sufferer try to describe a pain in his head to a doctor and language at once runs dry. There is nothing ready-made for him.

Perhaps an inability to describe pain is underpinned, she deliberated, by reluctance to tamper with the 'sacred' English language – to introduce speech 'more primitive, more sensual, more obscene'.[44] Maybe the sufferer's impaired concentration, memory and reasoning is a bar to literary expression. Possibly, the isolating effects of illness are also in some measure responsible: the hesitance of the healthy to engage with the unwell, to add other people's burdens into their busy working and personal lives; reluctance to consider pain part of the 'daily drama of the body';[45] the sufferer's preference for solitude in an absence of empathy in the 'army of the upright'?[46] The invalid's need for fellow feeling can never be met, Woolf decided – in which case, 'Here we go alone, and like it better so.'[47]

In her seminal 1985 meditation *The Body in Pain*, Elaine Scarry considered Woolf's statement about the 'poverty' of the language of pain: 'True of the headache, Woolf's account is of course more radically true of [...] severe and prolonged pain.'[48] Scarry, whose work arose out of the shift in thinking about pain that started with developments in the science of pain in the mid-1960s – when the perception of pain as a symptom of illness was tempered by the possibility that the symptom *was* the illness – concluded that pain 'does not simply resist language but actively destroys it'.[49] This resistance to language, suggested Scarry, is not limited to English: its origins are less in linguistic inflexibility and cultural difference than in the 'utter rigidity' that is physical pain's essential characteristic – a distinction marked by pain's inability to relate to an external object.[50] Examining pain's 'shattering of language' – an attribute 'essential to what [pain] is' – Scarry decided that bodily pain is an interior state of consciousness that 'unlike all our other interior states' lacks a 'referential content', or object, 'in the external world'.[51] In short, she said, 'we do not simply "have feelings" but have feelings for somebody or something', meaning that 'love is love of x, fear is fear of y, ambivalence is ambivalence about z'. Physical pain, however, is 'not *of* or *for* anything. It is precisely because it takes no object that it, more than any other phenomenon, resists objectification in language.'[52] Besides, proposed Scarry, although pain's interior abstraction can be linked to visible objects, like, for instance, a scalpel to a scar, it owns no substantive faculties *in and of itself* by which it can be identified or described.[53] Contrast pain with imagination, she suggested, framing consciousness within these polarities: 'While pain is a state remarkable for being wholly without objects [...] the only evidence that one is imagining is that imaginary objects appear in the mind.'

Not all informed commentators agree with Scarry's central premise. As Louise Hide, Joanna Burke and Carmen Mangion (the guest editors of *19: Interdisciplinary Studies in the Long Nineteenth Century*, 2012) have noted, Scarry's claim that 'the experience of pain is unshareable because it is a private, subjective event that "[...] has no referential content" has been vigorously refuted by a growing number of historians and literary scholars'.[54] While they acknowledged that Scarry's theory 'opened a rich new vein of scholarship, which has turned the focus away from pain as an entity in and of itself towards the narratives of "people in pain"', they were also of the view that '[s]uffering bodily pain [...] *can* generate language and creative expression'.

Vincent Crapanzano thus asked in *Imaginative Horizons: An Essay in Literary-Philosophical Anthropology* (2010), 'Are there not in fact other "states" that are as "objectless" as physical pain? Does it follow that the "objectlessness" of a state prevents it, nearly prevents it, from being rendered in language? Were this so, we would have to deny the power of figuration. Our whole poetic tradition.'[55] Interestingly, Hilary Mantel has taken issue with Woolf's statements about 'poverty of language'.[56] In her personal narrative 'Diary', written following abdominal surgery for intestinal obstruction (the likely legacy of seven years' endometriosis), Mantel explored a recovery marked by drug-induced hallucinations, exhaustion, the 'shaking progress to the bathroom', post-operative complications, including apparent wound dehiscence, and days when 'the difference between a neutral experience and an experience of slowly building misery' was as little as a nurse taking 'a single extra minute to settle a patient comfortably'.

Mantel wrote, of Woolf:

> For the sufferer she says, there is 'nothing ready-made'. Then what of the whole vocabulary of singing aches, of spasm, of strictures and cramps; the gouging pain, the drilling pain, the pricking and pinching, the throbbing, burning, stinging, smarting, flaying? All good words. All old words. No one's pain is so special that the devil's dictionary of anguish has not anticipated it. There is even a scale you can use to refine it. [...] Pain may pass beyond language, but it doesn't start beyond it. The torture chamber is where people 'speak'.

And she questioned Woolf's credentials for commenting on the language of physical pain, suggesting that, in the 'shuttered room called melancholia', 'Virginia only has decorous illnesses'; that 'she is seemly; she does not seep, or require a dressing trolley'. (Since the context of Mantel's essay is the temporary 'itching, burning of the process of repair', was she saying that the ready-made words for pain – the words that do not start beyond language, including the sounds of excruciation extracted in the torture chamber – relate to communication of acute pain? And was she implying, in the light of her own history of persistent pelvic pain, that the pain that 'may pass beyond language' is more complex chronic pain?[57])

Ten years earlier, Lucy Bending, too, denied Scarry's referential assertions. In *The Representation of Bodily Pain in Late Nineteenth-Century English Culture* (2000), Bending was less concerned with ideas of pain, as she put it, 'as an ultimate sensation, than with arguments over the meaning and interpretation of pain'.[58] She posited that although language may 'disintegrate' in the presence of extreme sensations (say, of torture and war), ordinarily, the reference of pain to, or the association of pain with, other experiences in order to give it meaning, 'draws suffering into association with something else'.[59] Pain, as a 'shared cultural phenomenon [...] can be incorporated into structures of language and expression'.[60] Bending examined this argument against the ways in which pain was expressed in Victorian literature – when 'fiction was awash with physical suffering', and many authors wrote in the belief that enduring physical suffering underpinned human existence.[61] This shared understanding was found in the linking of metaphors and similes with physical sensations and suffering. As an example, Bending cited Dickens's *A Tale of Two Cities*, in which the character Jarvis Lorry finds that 'the coach (in a confused way, like the presence of pain under an opiate) was always with him'. (In Book 1, Jarvis Lorry – travelling on the mail coach along a robbery-prone route towards a mysterious mission, distrustful of his three physically anonymous and vaguely disquieting travelling companions – drifts in and out of a restless sleep.) Addressing the capacity of Victorian writers for describing the reality and alien nature of significant physical suffering, Bending did, however, agree that the language of pain may, in Woolf's words, 'run dry'. But she noted also the strong belief that to maintain silence was to conform to the conventions of creation and demonstrate 'allegiance [...] to the suffering Christ'.[62] Further, she observed a tendency, on the part of writers of personal narrative, to withhold frank communication of pain in deference to reader sensibility. She was convinced, in other words, that physical pain can be shared, and that metaphor is a means of referring pain, or the meaning of pain, to external structures in ways that take account of this shared basis of pain. Scarry's claim that there is no language for pain, Bending concluded, is likely to cause sufferers to feel helpless in the face of their own suffering.

The debate has continued

Arne Johan Vetlesen, Oslo philosophy professor and author of *A Philosophy of Pain* (2009), considered Scarry to be turning our thinking towards the 'prejudice of our age' that has seen the subjectivity or introspection of mental suffering overshadow the objective actuality or fact of physical pain 'psychologically as well as morally'.[63] Have we forgotten, he asked, that, as Scarry pointed out, 'Physical pain is able to obliterate psychological pain because it obliterates all psychological content, painful, pleasurable, and neutral?'

David Biro, a New York dermatologist and literary scholar who found himself powerless to express his own physical suffering, is another who supports Scarry's concept of pain as objectless and therefore unshareable. In *The Language of Pain* (2010),[64] Biro – whose reflections integrate narratives from real life, and from literary non-fiction and fiction – considered pain's linguistic elusiveness in terms of its 'lack of intentionality' and its 'inaccessibility as a bodily event'.[65] Pain, he wrote, belongs to that inner part of our existence which consists of such states as thinking, perception, dreaming and feeling 'connected or directed to objects in a manner essential to our comprehension of them'. However, pain's absence of connection or linkage to concrete or tangible objects results in a want of the verification they bring to 'inner experience'. In effect, said Biro, 'the only thing pain is about is itself'.

Significantly, Biro acknowledged visible physical harm as a potential exception to the concept of pain as objectless, because the wounds or implements of harm '*are accessible* to others'.[66] In this respect, he said, the resultant pain, which is likely to arouse recognition in, or be more difficult to dismiss by onlookers, will be easier for the sufferer to describe. Nonetheless, the pain of an obvious injury, or of a weapon (say, a gun) or visible source, appears to remain 'more inside us than outside us'; besides, later, when the gun has gone and the tissue damage has healed, the pain may persist – a 'disconnection' not found in any other inner experience (a statement which raises questions regarding the comparability of the invisible lingering of pleasure and grief). Biro also found that injuries that can be seen by others function not only in terms of connecting pain to language, but also as precipitating pain language, as in the case of medical consultations and pain scales (such as the Visual Analogue Scale where 1= very mild pain, and 10 = agonising pain).

Biro wrote *The Language of Pain* in order to promote the development of a 'rhetoric of pain' – an objective, he believes, that would be assisted by strengthening the links between medicine and literature and encouraging the use of metaphor. Words, if and when they come, 'almost exclusively take the form of something or someone acting on our body, forming our core metaphor for the experience'.[67,68] The goal, he admitted, is 'idealistic': for while the initiatives he proposed may encourage linguistic communication of pain for some, expression will not always be possible.[69] Biro's belief that filling pain's hazy perceptual and conceptual boundaries with the metaphorical language of visible or describable objects is challenged by Susan Sontag, who rejected metaphoric concentration on the negative aspects of physical illness. 'My point,' Sontag wrote in *Illness as Metaphor* (1978) in the wake of the cancer that instigated her 'enquiry', 'that the most truthful way of regarding illness – and the healthiest way of being ill – is the one most purified of, most resistant to, metaphoric thinking.'[70] (Sontag's concerns were the epitomes of past and present chronic illness at the time of writing: tuberculosis and cancer – the latter now arguably overtaken by chronic pain.) However, as Anne Hunsaker Hawkins pointed out in *Reconstructing Illness: Studies in Pathography* (1999),[71] we live amidst images – and '[e]ven Sontag realises this, observing in *AIDS and Its Metaphors*, "Of course, one cannot think without metaphors."' More recently, Martha Stoddard Holmes, in her essay 'After Sontag: Reclaiming Metaphor', found the use of metaphors to describe illness to be 'transformative magic' in terms of their potential to support diagnosis and treatment and alter the attitudes of medical professionals 'toward embodiments and illness'.[72] After she was diagnosed with cancer, Stoddard Holmes discovered that, influenced by Sontag, she was unable to 'make metaphors or spin out narratives'[73] – a deficiency, she believes, that may have slowed the medical response. Her 'metaphor-making' capacity returned only when, undergoing chemotherapy, she felt a need to speak of the strangeness of her experience.

The isolation and reduced communication that chronic patients experience, and their need for a narrative, have been analysed by a number of medical and academic authors writing for a 'broad audience'. Among those who have written most perceptively and eloquently here are Arthur Kleinman[74] and David B. Morris.[75] 'Chronicity,' explained Kleinman in *The Illness Narratives: Suffering, Healing and the Human Condition* (1988), 'for many is the dangerous crossing of borders, the interminable waiting to exit and re-enter normal everyday life, the perpetual uncertainty of whether one can return at all.'[76] Kleinman (who, a small note advises, suffers from chronic asthma) found that this state of affairs, so taxing for the patient, is also difficult for the practitioner, as it is for the relatives and friends who share the land of 'limbo', who also experience hurt, bewilderment, anxiety and loss. In this respect, he stressed the need for clinicians to engage in 'empathetic witnessing' – to encourage patients to talk about their illnesses, because there is alleviation in witnessing and assisting them to make sense of their experience.[77]

David B. Morris, writing in what is possibly his most influential work, *The Culture of Pain* (1991), advanced the desirability of a biocultural, rather than a biomedical, approach to communicating pain.[78] Like Biro, he saw the need to develop a dialogue between medicine and literature, which will spill over into the general population. And, like Kleinman, he has sought to give voice to the neglected testimony of patients. But Morris has gone further, saying that it is also necessary 'to recover the voices that speak most effectively for patients in the essays, poems, novels, plays, and other genres we call literature'.[79,80]

Lines of vision

The challenges for a writer bringing pain, particularly chronic pain, to the page are manifold. While words may be summoned for the 'raw sensation' of acute or temporary pain – whether in plain speech, instinctive or constructed metaphor, or the more extended imaginings of metonymy – conveying personal physical distress that is severe, constant and chronic or terminal, means negotiating the dark 'heart and soul' of the pain experience. It also involves making an individually complex pain universally acceptable – a task marked by Virginia Woolf's observation that '[w]e do not know our own souls, let alone the souls of others. Human beings do not go hand in hand the whole stretch of the way.'[81]

The unburdening of cause, ordeal and effect that embodies a writer's impetus to move beyond straight description of personal suffering in search of rationalisation or meaning was examined by sociologist Arthur W. Frank in *The Wounded Storyteller: Body, Illness and Ethics* (1997). Frank, for whom *Storyteller* became a 'survival kit' as he attempted to make sense of his own experience of a heart attack followed by testicular cancer, wrote of shifting the negativity inherent in such narratives, including notions of passivity and the 'ill person as a "victim of" disease and then recipient of care, toward activity'.[82] Frank's view was that just as the wounded may be taken care of, as narrators empowered by their injuries and through the force of their stories, they may, in turn, take care of others. In doing so, they both awaken the will to be heard and restore the facility for expression that trauma and treatment have lessened.[83] Storytelling of this sort, according to Frank, broadly encompasses (and, arguably, interweaves) three categories of illness narrative: the 'restitution' narrative, with its emphasis on cure and the means by which recovery will be achieved; the 'chaos' narrative, which is concerned with long or chronic suffering, and an absence of relief and mitigating insights; and the 'quest' narrative, in which the transforming power of an illness enables the patient to become someone different'.[84]

But it is not easy to relate and to listen to such stories, no matter how therapeutic watching oneself write and hearing oneself speak. And physical pain, as a 'tightly interconnected and constantly shifting mesh of the physical, the psychological, and cultural – continually reforming and redefining the person-in-pain', is, by this definition, likely to be especially resistant to achieving all-important narrative and emotional proximity.[85] This problem of proximity is most readily directed to chronic pain, in which the contradictions between cause and cure and the components of 'the constantly shifting mesh' are least understood, and the need to explain is greatest. Theorists may shower pain with meaning, rationalists apply principles of reason and knowledge, behaviourists examine patterns of activity and thinking and writers of literary fiction pursue the readily dramatised interventions of acute pain. But in the first instance, chronic pain memoirists (writing against constant pain, mental fatigue and 'heavy-duty' medications)[86] must confront matters of veracity and 'subjective speculation' (can non-cancer pain *really* be that bad?). Such issues touch on the 'feat of manipulation' by which, wrote William Zinsser in *Inventing the Truth: The Art and Craft of Memoir* (1998), a memoirist 'arrive[s] at a truth that is theirs alone', and is, in the end, 'the only truth a writer can work with'.[87] They must also allow for the likelihood that unless the pain is physically overcome, spiritually transcended or released in death, the story will struggle to achieve shape, narrative drive, a definitive end. And they will be aware that unlike acute pain, which, 'familiar' and finite, readily evokes a reader's concern, chronic pain's faltering reference points and less audible 'keening and howling', may elicit a less sympathetic response.

After more than a decade of intense intractable pain, Lous Heshusius, in *Inside Chronic Pain*, indicated that narrating pain is as much a matter of others' receptivity to the message as to the form the message takes. She asked: how can one put such pain 'on paper?'

> Love would be easier. Or joy, or pleasure. Things people desire. Then you can evoke that which cannot be said. The reader will gladly fill in the meanings left unsaid by the words. Trying to speak of chronic pain, on the other hand, the unsaid meanings are not easily imagined. For who wants to know what constant pain is like? How to tell of this dark, dark place?[88]

As I have discovered during the writing of this book, chronic pain does not always yield to objective analysis, especially not by a sufferer.[89] My attention, therefore, in what follows, to memoir, personal essay, poetry (to the various forms of what has been described as 'pathography'[90]), has endorsed my decision to allow the poetic to give to reason 'its most famous license'[91] and interpret what has been observed. Because pain has many lines of vision, it may preclude narration in a language that writer and reader can share. With this possibility in mind, I accept that pain can be effectively communicated only between sufferers. I also deduce, given the inability of medical science to determine where the connections between pain and suffering lie, that it is the apprehension of suffering – of the elusive constituents connecting the melody and mood of pain's 'silent concert' – that, for me (as for many), is the greater challenge of narrating physical pain.

2 Going nursing

An autobiographical prelude

I quite agree with you that how to be ill is a necessary complement of how to nurse. One is not complete without the other. – But, on the whole, I think the first duty better performed, generally, than the second.

Florence Nightingale to Harriet Martineau, 1860[1]

Behind half-open doors

In one of my earliest memories, I visit a hospital. I am outside a building up high, as if being held, or on a hill. The sky is blue, the wind blows and I have a hazy impression that I'm dressed 'for best' in organza. I am three years old. My older brother Bruce died soon after birth. My younger brother, David, is one and a half. Our sister Pamela has been born with spina bifida and hydrocephalus and will pass away in the hospital, aged three months. I only recently discovered that the hospital at Te Kuiti was indeed on a hill.

On another occasion, I brush my mother's hair as she lies in a shaded room. There's a photograph in which she wears a nurse's veil and crossover cape. In a second photo she, and my father, a soldier, stand on the steps of a church surrounded by nurses – they have just been married. My profoundly deaf grandmother comes to stay. David and I develop measles. I ride down a lane between trees, balanced on the crossbar of my father's bike. A large black bird, covered with soot, falls down the chimney and flaps around the lounge. I have many memories of brushing my mother's hair in dark rooms.

My medical associations continued. When I was five we moved north from Te Kuiti to Kaikohe, and a year later my twin brothers, Philip and Brian, were born. Philip had a hernia and couldn't have surgery until he was three months old. I was responsible for watching him in case he coughed or vomited, and distracting him so he wouldn't cry. Words like 'truss', 'abdomen' and 'strangulate' stayed with me. I heard, for the first time, that I had been born by Caesarean section when my mother developed septicaemia after an obstetrical examination, and was rushed by ambulance from Te Kuiti to Hamilton, where she saw my father in the doorway looking tiny, only a few inches high. I felt sorry for my mother, who was busy with the twins and often unwell; and for my father, although I didn't know why: like other fathers he smoked and whistled, liked to swim and play cricket and had left with the First Echelon to fight in Greece and the desert. I recall stroking his fair rippled hair one afternoon as he knelt at the fireplace in his army jacket, wet after coming in with wood from the rain. It seems I saw, behind the summer of childhood, that my parents carried wounds of illness and war.

We stayed in the Far North until I was eleven. I accompanied my mother when she went to church or called on the sick, to whom she carried baking, flowers from her garden, an embroidered hanky, a small bottle of Potter & Moore's Mitcham lavender; if we were visiting a hospital, I waited outside the ward absorbing the smell and shine of the corridor, the lines of mysterious patients in cream iron beds, the sterilisers and trolleys gleaming behind half-open doors. Once, at the age of nine or ten, I was sent, on my own, to help a new mother with her baby. 'Stephanie's very capable,' I heard my mother tell the woman over the phone. I began to see that my mother, often shy and uncertain in company, was quietly assured and respected in the role of helper and nurse. Influenced by her example, lured by the uniform, tantalised by the stories of illness and injury and the camaraderie of the student, senior, staff and neighbour-hood nurses in Helen Dore Boylston's 'Sue Barton' series of junior novels, and fascinated by medical terms, I knew I would follow suit.

We shifted to Wellington, where I started secondary school and my parents hoped I would go on to university. Meanwhile, at the public library, I sought biographies of nurses, surgeons, missionaries, and, from the bookcase at home, the novels of doctor-turned-writer A.J. Cronin: *The Keys of the Kingdom*'s trials of a priest in China; *The Citadel*, held to have influenced the introduction of pub-licly funded healthcare in Britain; the semi-autobiographical *The Green Years* in which Cronin traces his own vocational origins. But, unlike my father who once hoped to study medicine, I had no wish to become a doctor – to treat people, as I perceived it, briefly and intermittently. In class, I marked time in chemistry and was easily distracted in mathematics, preferring, to borrow from Shelley, 'the consummate surface and bloom'[2] of the sports field, the choir, the house plays, subjects like English, Latin and French where 'the owl-winged faculty of calcu-lation'[3] cannot fly. After I passed School Certificate my father, unable to dis-suade me from nursing, and reasoning that skills in shorthand and touch typing would stand me in better stead than University Entrance, enrolled me at a busi-ness college for a year. I left school, aged fifteen, frustrated but about to find speed typing and Pitman's symbolic language of shorthand surprisingly satisfy-ing. By the middle of the year, I would also be proficient in the vocabularies of surgery and bedside nursing.

As the first term at the business college started, I developed what the doctor called a 'grumbling appendix'. The condition duly became acute and I was admitted to Wellington Hospital, where – freshly aware of terms like 'referred pain', 'rebound tenderness', 'McBurney's Point' and 'localisation in the right iliac fossa' – I was taken to theatre and had an abscessed appendix removed. But some days post-op, I began to feel sick and to experience cramping abdominal pains – symptoms I kept to myself, reluctant to make a fuss, believing them to be normal and minor in comparison with the ulcerative colitis suffered by Barbara in the next bed. In fact, the cramps signalled the onset of acute intestinal obstruction, a complication of abdominal surgery requiring urgent intervention.

The pains intensified. I started vomiting, unobtrusively in the toilet block. The next afternoon at visiting time, I told my mother, who had not seen me during the week (daily visiting was not introduced at Wellington Hospital until June 1961). She realised what was wrong and, with the ward sister off duty, rang the Deputy Matron-in-Chief, who contacted the specialist surgeon. By now the vomiting was so violent that it was drawing up black matter from my intestines, and my abdomen, still tender after the appendicectomy, was noticeably distended. My cubicle was curtained off. A Nil by Mouth notice was attached to the top of the bed and the tumbler and jug of cordial were removed from the locker. The house surgeon arrived and fed what he introduced as 'a Ryle's tube' through my nose and, as I gagged and retched, down the back of my throat to my stomach. A nurse attached a large-barrelled syringe to the tube and suctioned off a copious quantity of black liquid. The doctor attempted to locate a site for the drip, only to find the onset of dehydration had caused the superficial veins to collapse. A registrar took over and prepared for 'a venous cut-down'. I watched him expose the deep, white vessel, insert a cannula and suture the skin. A bottle of replacement fluid and electrolytes was hoisted, and a trolley-bed, waiting outside the cubicle, rushed me along the corridor to the X-ray department. Back in the ward, school friends peered nervously between the curtains and then disappeared, and the consultant surgeon on call, wearing a suit, decided I was too ill for surgery and should first be stabilised. 'The general condition remains more or less stationary for a time,' I later learned in *Surgery for Students of Nursing* (1961),[4] 'but eventually sudden collapse is liable to occur and to produce a fatal result within a few hours.'

Throughout the night, injections of pethidine took the edge off the pain, and suctioning via the naso-gastric tube stopped the vomiting. But there was no relief from the raging thirst of electrolyte imbalance and severe dehydration. The night nurse, who was patient and kind, set up a mouth tray on the locker alongside Doris Leslie's *House in the Dust*, and swabbed my gums, tongue and teeth with moistened cotton wool swabs. I pleaded for a drink. 'You'll start vomiting again,' she said, explaining the need to relieve pressure on the stomach and small intestine, as she suctioned through the tube and checked the drip was running to time.

But I was in survival mode. When she wasn't looking I drank the sour glycerine and thymol mouthwash on the tray – only to see it return during the next aspiration, frothy pink in the syringe. The intravenous infusion gleamed in the night light. Drips of fluid bounced like crystals into the reservoir between the bottle and tube. If I'd had a pair of scissors I would have snipped and sipped from that plastic tube. I was desperate with thirst. I knew how people who died in the desert felt. I remembered the two girls in *The Back of Beyond*, the documentary about Australia's Birdsville Track I had seen in my first year of high school.[5] When their mother became ill, the sisters had left their outback home and gone in search of their father, and vanished, presumed to have perished wandering in a circle. Stunted bushes, trackless sand, the dust of dried wells and creeks. I shook my mother's bottle of lavender, but the liquid only dripped from its narrow neck.

The next day, in the operating theatre, the gangrenous intestinal loop was resected and anastomosed end to end. I returned to a bed by the window. My abdomen, with its large wound, felt abraded, raw. The slightest movement jarred. From time to time I was roused to move my legs and injected with pethidine, but not all the shots delivered suffusing relief. (Later, when as a nurse I had access to the hospital's medical records and inspected my file, I found that on occasion sterile water had been administered lest, still a juvenile, I become addicted to the drug.)

Outside the window, student nurses in the junior pink and senior mauve striped dresses they wore beneath their white on-duty smocks, staff nurses in tailored green and sisters in blue, passed by on their way to lunch, clutching their caps and veils in the wind and hugging their red capes. Between cubicles, the students, pushing trolleys stacked with washbowls and linen, sang 'Calendar Girl' and 'Where the Boys Are'. They wore up to three stars on their pockets, according to their year of training. I looked for nurses who were practised and gentle when the crinkled draw-sheet needed smoothing and tightening and I had to be rolled; or my heels, elbows and back, red with the pressure of lying in bed, were rubbed with spirit; or, with early ambulation newly in vogue, I was helped out of bed to take a few steps. And I learned from the few who, regardless of stars, were careless and heavy handed – the ones who bumped the bed or, worse, sat on it with a thump, whose injections didn't find their mark, whose lifting was ineffectual, sponge water lukewarm and pillow arrangements hasty and 'any old how', as my mother said.

In stages, the sutures were removed and the drip and uncomfortable Ryle's tube were discontinued and I started to recover. The day before I went home, the Deputy Matron-in-Chief, stately and smiling, came to see me. She asked if I was pleased to be leaving, a gentleness and studied awareness in her large blue eyes. I told her I would soon be returning to start nursing. She was accompanied by the slim efficient sister who had removed her starched cuffs, rolled up her sleeves and expertly sponged, lifted and made me comfortable when I was most vulnerable – and would also be a model to follow.

Six weeks later in the Outpatients Department, the surgeon remarked when he saw my abdomen, zippered with scars, 'She's had a rough passage.'

'Yes,' said my mother, 'she's been through the mill.'

'Slept well. Slept well. Pethidine for pain'

I entered the Wellington Hospital School of Nursing in the winter of 1962, a month to the day after turning seventeen. I was to undertake the recently instituted three-and-a-half-year New Zealand Registered Nurses' programme leading to registration as both a general and an obstetric nurse. Of the intake of forty, only nineteen would graduate – an attrition rate commensurate with the combined pressures of shift work, study and high levels of responsibility placed upon students, many of whom had joined with scant understanding of the profession or its demanding training. (Most of the class considered leaving, at some stage, for less stressful and better-paid employment.)

I trained on the cusp of the transition in nursing from the 'strong service ethos' of the 1950s to the 'medical ideologies of cure rather than nursing ideologies of care'[6] that developed in the 1970s, and continue today: from the Florence Nightingale 'patient-centred' tradition, to the 'nurse-centred' model;[7] from hospital-based training to campus education, degree status and the opportunity of a more flexible career path.

The 1960s heralded the rapid diagnostic and medical advances that would lead to the financial shortfalls, health reforms, increased patient turnover and bureaucratic proliferation of the next four decades. These progressions, together with the 'conflict of interest between the educational needs of the student'[8] and the obligations of nursing administrations to adequately staff hospitals, began to raise doubts about the British apprenticeship exemplar of care. From 1973, training in New Zealand was gradually replaced by American-influenced polytechnic and university education, supplemented by part-time practicum. The Nightingale-inspired 'synthesis of both art and science'[9] was redefined as 'a multidimensional profession [that] reflects the needs and values of society, implements the standards of professional performance and care, meets the needs of each client, and integrates current research and evidence-based findings to provide the highest level of care'.[10]

By and large, nursing education worldwide moved in this direction. The changes proved controversial, particularly among hospital graduates, some of whom contended that 'increasing the professional status of the nurse meant decreasing the vocational ethic and attracting a differently motivated recruit'.[11] I met registered nurses who, although academically proficient and technically adept, were unversed in the arts of patient comfort – who, in an absence of practical experience in the full spectrum of nursing settings, were unlikely to have had first-hand experience of an emergency department, an operating theatre, a birth, a seriously sick child, the wider processes of pain, the sudden and the lingering conditions of death. I spoke to new graduates who felt out of their depth but were suddenly 'expected to know it all' because 'you're a nurse'.[12] I heard experienced nurses complain about being 'dragged down by bureaucracy and documentation', the 'pressure to work faster and smarter and be more flexible', the expectation that they would 'acquire many skills' which was causing them to become 'masters of none'.

As a student, my view of nursing was largely unambiguous, despite the stirrings of the Nurses' Union and the 1960s climate of protest and personal freedom. While I supported pay claims, complicated by my moral obligation as a nurse not to strike, my immediate concern was obtaining registration. I was still learning: a status, I could argue, that was commensurate with an apprenticeship salary. I considered the role of the nurse trained to give close care, and that of the doctor to treat more distantly, to be professionally equal. I believed nursing education, at both student and postgraduate levels, would keep pace with medical developments, at least in the larger hospitals, and that nurses would pursue postgraduate qualifications and wider research and employment opportunities, just as they had always done. Although, at times, I resisted the disciplined hierarchical system, I also saw its sense, given the stringent checks and balances essential to safely supervising a large student workforce. And, as challenging as the training was, I acknowledged the value of experiential learning. In this respect, many of us as students in the 1960s, although capable, were not necessarily natural nurses. However, immersed daily in the hospital culture of caring and coping, we pressed on – acquiring the combination of concern and resilience that leads to good practice, developing 'the compassionate character [that was] the impetus for the practice of care [...] until its rejection in the 1970s'.[13] The tertiary sector educates, but the ability to respond to real life, which often comes out of 'left field', is learned only through experience.

My own first experience from left field occurred early, while I was in 'Prelim', confined for three months to the classroom and to carrying out minor tasks once a week on a ward. (Such was the general level of apprehension about approaching patients and godlike sisters that a girl in our class fainted en route to her first duty.)

I was in the Ear, Nose and Throat Ward (ENT), on loan from the Eye Ward, which was quiet. I'd been sent from feeding patients with bandaged eyes and wiping empty beds with Dettol to assist with the ENT ward tidy before the doors were opened for afternoon visiting. As I cleared locker tops, replenished water jugs, smoothed counterpanes and straightened bed castors – routines I would later interpret as training in attention to detail and maintaining a calming sense of order – I was stopped by a staff nurse and asked to 'find a commode chair and wheel Mr Finch to the toilet, and hurry, because *he's* in a hurry'. Mr Finch, heavy and elderly, had been transferred to ENT from a men's medical ward, where there was a shortage of beds, and was due for discharge the next day. I parked my trolley, located a chair and sped Mr Finch to the ablution block at the end of the ward where, because he declined the convenience of the commode, I assisted him onto the toilet – a time-consuming manoeuvre on account of his ill-fitting hospital pyjamas and sagging weight.

As I settled him and stepped away, he made a strange grunting sound and flopped forward. His face was grey and wet.

Cyanosis – was he about to faint? Had I done something wrong? Could he be having a heart attack? I pushed against his shoulders, struggling to hold him up. He didn't speak. I hung on. His breathing was stertorous, as if he was snoring. What should I do? There was no call light and no one in the vicinity. Should I rush for help and let him crash to the floor? He was too heavy to lower on my own. I shook him and repeated his name. He emitted a strange sigh, and his false teeth dropped and protruded, wedged between his lips. I had to let him go. I ran to the ward and grabbed the first nurse I saw – a one-star junior. 'Go and hold onto him,' she said, 'and I'll get help.' I raced back to find Mr Finch propped between the toilet and wall, his face mottled, his leaning weight barely supportable. I held onto him. He didn't seem to be breathing.

Without checking his pulse, I, even at seventeen, knew he was dead – puff, just like that, without forethought or pain, on an ordinary day, one minute ready for his afternoon tea, expecting visitors and due to go home, and the next purple, squeezed out of his skin.

The staff nurse rushed in and listened to his chest with a stethoscope. She sent the junior to delay visiting and return with a blanket. 'He's had a massive pulmonary embolism,' she explained as we waited. 'He's a classic case – a patient who recovers well, then suddenly calls for a bedpan and collapses. I had a feeling about him, which was why I asked you to get the commode.'

The junior returned and the three of us inched and swivelled Mr Finch, his eyes wide open, back onto the chair, swaddled him in the blanket as if he'd been out for a walk, and supported and pushed him back to his curtained bed.

The house surgeon was paged. The sister intercepted his wife. Negotiations were carried out between the outgoing morning and oncoming afternoon staff regarding his laying out. And I was sent, legs suddenly shaky, my pristine uniform rumpled, to boil the Zip and set a trolley for the patients' afternoon teas.

Two years later, aged nineteen, again in the ENT ward but this time on night duty, I underwent the defining experience of my nursing career. The patient involved, Mr Whyte, was a middle-aged man with advanced cancer of the larynx and the sole occupant of a cubicle outside the main ward, opposite the kitchen and sterilising room. He had been in hospital for some time. His larynx – his voice box and the passage from his lungs to his mouth and nose – had been removed and a stoma, or opening, created in the base of his neck. A curved stainless steel laryngectomy tube, with an inner cannula through which he breathed and coughed and I suctioned the secretions that built up, was in place. As he was unable to speak, he communicated by pencil and pad, and when he was distressed he gestured, his arms throwing angular shadows in the night light against the wall. Sometimes, in frustration, he undid the ties knotted behind his neck that kept the outer tube in position and threw it on the floor. A sterile replacement tube was kept at the ready for the house surgeon or supervising night sister to carefully reinsert, but as there was a shortage of registered staff at night, and the ward was some distance from the supervisors' office, I was given permission to replace it myself. Mercifully he appeared to suffer little, if any, pain.

After a couple of weeks I was asked to report by day to the ward sister who warned me that Mr Whyte's cancer was advancing on his carotid artery. 'There will be a sudden, fatal haemorrhage,' she said. 'If it starts during the night, ring the supervisor's office. The switchboard will give priority to your calls. All you can do is maintain his airway and assist him to stay calm.' A supervising sister would arrive as soon as possible and check a phial of morphine so that I could sedate him, and a 'night extra' would be sent to keep an eye on the ward. He would not die immediately. His wife had been told, but he himself did not know – it was kinder that way. Mr Whyte had shown me photos of his wife, whom he had only recently married, in the scrapbook she'd entitled 'Happy Days' – a dark-haired woman wearing sunglasses at the beach, a floral dress at a picnic, a headscarf blurred by wind. He kept the soft-covered book within sight, in his half-open locker drawer.

The ENT ward, with its tracheostomies, tonsillectomies, nose bleeds and delicate work within ears, could be busy. Night duty following an operation day was a continuous round of timing drips, manually recording pulses and blood pressures, administering pain relief, monitoring blood loss, reassuring patients whose noses were packed with gauze. A transfusion was often in progress, and the tonsillectomy patients who spat and vomited blood, sucked ice and were in a lot of pain needed constant attention, especially the children on the glassed-in veranda who cried. Familiar routines. But what about Mr Whyte in the side room, suddenly streaming arterial blood?

Each morning, as I went to bed, I allowed myself to imagine that while I slept he would die. If I heard a bird when I woke, I was hopeful. There were other signs I could favour – a pink evening, a dog in the car park. At dinner in the nurses' home I questioned the day staff. At supper I contemplated calling in ill. At 10.45 p.m. as I fastened my collar with a stud, tightened my belt, put on my cape and walked to the ward in the echo and yellow shine of the corridor, I willed the haemorrhage to start before the afternoon shift went off duty and I was on my own.

Each night I counted down the hours. Coaxed dawn over the rim of the moon. Wished I were Carole, who was a teacher, Alison, who was a secretary, Helen, who worked in the safety of a bank.

During ward rounds when I stopped at his door – saw his outline high and taut in his bed, heard the rasp of air mixed with mucus in his tube, smelt the sweetness of the carbol in the suction jar, the freshness of the antiseptic lotion on his dressing tray and the sickly stale flowers in the vase on the stand in the corner of the room – I held my breath. And as I suctioned him – fed the thin catheter into the cannula in his throat – I hesitated, even though his breathing depended on it, fearful a cough would provoke the calamitous moment. Afterwards, misting the dry air, adjusting his position and whispering, 'Dig your heels in and I'll hoist you,' I told myself, 'Stay in check, it won't happen tonight.' His arm was only the weight of its sleeve as I lifted him, his back a ridge against my shoulder as I bent across the bed supporting him and arranging his pillows. 'Take your time,' I would say as he choked with the effort, his head jerking. 'I'll wait.'

At the end of the week, I had a leave day, a sleep day. I went to the beach. 'Sail him away,' I said to the sea, darting between marks left by the tide.

That night, at a party, I danced, drank vodka from a large glass and dozed on a bed covered with coats.

A day later, between four and five in the morning, in the two-hour time zone when the body temperature is at its lowest, his bulb on the office call panel reddened. Had he removed his tube? Did he need suctioning? He had been edgy earlier. I had made him milky tea. Held the feeding cup as he sipped from the spout. Lingered in the warm kitchen with the comforting hum of the refrigerator and vibration of pipes, as I rinsed the cup. Returned to reposition his pillows and found him asleep.

I took my torch, paused to check a transfusion and saw, in the distance, that the light in his room was on. Something was amiss. I ran. As I reached his doorway, I could see blood, alarm, his hands at his throat. I slowed, trained to reassure. I folded a towel across his chest, conditioned to comfort. I said, 'A small bleed – this can happen.' His throat gurgled. I unhooked the suction hose from the wall and attached a catheter. The apparatus hissed. His eyes were on my face. 'That's fine,' I said, as the blood snaked through the plastic and into the jar beneath his bed. 'Your airway's clear. Take it easy. I'll leave now and make a call. Don't worry, I'll be back in a second.'

The phone in the supervisor's office was answered immediately. But in the minute I was away, the bleeding had not lessened. 'Hold tight,' I said, wiping a clot from his lips, 'you're doing well, just lie back and let me look after you.' The catheter struggled with the flow. I unblocked it. It re-blocked. His bed filled with blood. The morphine marked time, locked in a cupboard. The running footsteps of the supervising sister were a long time coming.

After I had given him the injection, I stroked his hand. Reminded him I was there. Waited for his eyes to close, for the opiate to overtake him, for the flow to diminish so I could change his bed, sponge him, pat him dry, dust him with talcum powder, clothe him in clean pyjamas: create a consolation of care. Did he know he was dying?

His wife arrived and sat with him. I returned to the office and wrote the patients' reports – 'Slept well. Slept well. Pethidine for pain. Transfusion through on time.' Then I drew up the six o'clock intramuscular penicillins from phials in the kitchen fridge, took the morning recordings, drained the sterilisers and counted the Dangerous Drugs with the oncoming senior. The ward curtains were opened and the clink of thermometers and rattle of trolleys carrying jugs of hot water and bowls for hands and face washes before breakfast could be heard.

I looked in on him as I left at seven: my mind turning – from the fearful waiting, the well-meant deceptions, the sudden horror of his death and the knowledge that when the time came I could do what was needed – to his own weeks of waiting (for what?) in a windowless side room, and his unimaginable minutes of haemorrhage with only a student nurse to assist him. His wife was still there. She sat, without moving, her back to the door, while I floated, with each step, into deeper levels of relief. His light had been switched off, the suction was silent, and despite his body in the bed, the room already felt empty.

Towards the end of our training, as we approached registration, we applied for positions as staff nurses. I was working in Women's Orthopaedics, a ward I had not enjoyed as a junior. The patients tended to be immobile and long term. Some lay flat in pelvic and cervical tractions; others were nursed upright in a variety of splints; a number suffered from severe arthritis and experienced much pain; and there was a small but constant population of elderly women who had fractured the necks of their femurs, required basic nursing, and could be heavy.

Having dismissed the sameness of medicine, the quick turnover of casualty, the technical emphasis of intensive care and the impersonality of the operating theatre, I'd imagined myself requesting a surgical or paediatric ward. However, there was a new sister in Women's Orthopaedics – a former nun in, maybe, her late thirties – and she was opening my eyes to the art and rewards of long-term and sometimes unglamorous nursing. I saw her, leading quietly by example, institute routines of consideration and comfort – compassion by another name – and reveal the chronically incapacitated, often of limited interest to young doctors and nurses, to be much more than they seemed. I observed the way in which she took 'the tiny tasks of daily life and [made] something rich out of them':[14] tasks not normally undertaken by ward sisters, tasks as small and large as brushing away crumbs, turning a hot pillow, tightening a wrinkled undersheet, or arranging flowers to their best advantage. I was drawn to the care she took when making beds, as if she deemed it 'a privilege to prepare the place where someone else will sleep';[15] to her gentle, methodical manner when washing, shaving and applying the adhesive strapping and bandages of skin traction to fractured legs; her measured mixing of tincture of Merthiolate with zinc and castor oil cream (her personal 'recipe' for preventing and treating bedsores) in the utility room (not normally the preserve of ward sisters); her early arrival in the ward each morning to ensure anyone in pain received medication before breakfast was served. I especially noticed her talent for enabling each patient to feel tended and special, and the absence of anxiety among her patients. I decided she had a lot to teach me.

Although this sounds earnest and sober, my time in Women's Orthopaedics was anything but. Here, I realised the enrichment of patients who needed to share their lives, and were keen to be part of mine: who, looking to balance indefinite confinement with joking, laughter and small excitements, illuminated Nightingale's precept that nurses care 'for bodies and no less living minds'.[16]

In time I moved on to a paediatric ward, a coronary care unit, night supervising. I travelled and nursed abroad. Embarked on unrelated studies, entered dissimilar careers. Continued to monitor the profession as a mother, a patient, a wider family member.

These days I examine nursing through the magnifying lens of chronic pain. Individual exceptions and hospice ministration aside, I note the shift from caring for patients to 'managing clients'. I encounter healthcare technicians, less reliant on nuance and applied knowledge than on theoretical conjecture and machines; perfunctory attention given to 'comfort and reassurance' – nursing's guiding principle when I was a student; medical environments cluttered with the paperwork of policy and administration.

I feel privileged to have trained in less ambiguous times, in the tradition of nurturing that first drew me to nursing and shaped me in my formative years.

And I remember Boris Pasternak's words in the last month of his life to Marfa Kuzminichna, his nurse, 'who had been at the front during the war and had a high sense of her own worth', who would hold his head in her practised hands at the end: 'When I get better, I won't write about politics or art. I'll write about the work of nurses. Oh yes, you are real workers. The world is in such a muddle, everything people do has become so difficult and involved, but what you do is so straightforward, so genuine and selfless. That's what I want to write about.'[17]

3 At the end of the mind, the body[1]
A memoir, 2003–2004

*

The pine tree leaning over the Kumutoto Stream rocked. Its crown, the highest in a stand of three, moved from west to east, brushing the clouds, gathering light from behind. Its foliage, high and low, rippled equally. I watched it sway through binoculars from my bedroom window. Framed the stumps on the mid-section of its trunk. Searched unsuccessfully for nests. Elongated the waving branches until there was stillness between them, and the city hill on which the pine stood became a mountain. Taoist Masters believed in the efficacy of trees, in their ability to absorb energy out of the earth and the 'universal force' from the sky. The more strongly rooted the plant, they claimed, the higher it extended to heaven. Plum trees were said to calm the mind, maples to disperse ill winds and lessen pain, and the tallest trees, notably pines, to be best for healing, especially when growing near running water.

*

A coal smouldering

December 2003. I had a pain deep in the pelvis. It had started slowly, six weeks earlier, after a fall in Poland where I was researching a novel, *The Fountain of Tears*, and promoting the Polish translation of my memoir-biography, *Unquiet World: The Life of Count Geoffrey Potocki de Montalk*. I slipped on the marble floor of our bathroom in Warsaw's Bristol Hotel and bounced off the sharp edge of the bath, breaking three ribs on the lower left side. I thought myself fortunate at the time. I could have hit my head, fractured my spine, or punctured a lung. Or ruptured a kidney, the possibility of which caused concern at the Szpital Kliniczny Dzieciątka Jezus (Clinical Hospital of the Infant Jesus) to which I was whisked by ambulance.

'It's Potocki, from beyond the grave,' exclaimed my biography's translator, Maria, when I returned to the hotel; she was phoning from Kraków where I was due to be filmed for a television arts programme, and had remembered my poet cousin's capacity for denunciation when displeased, and the infections that I contracted while working with his archive: infections referred to as the 'Curse of the Count'.

'Not at all,' I reassured, as room service delivered a tea trolley laden with complimentary savouries and cakes, and an *allegro agitato* ushered in Chopin's *Fantaisie-Impromptu* on the in-house sound system. 'I'm his executor and trustee launching his story in his spiritual homeland. I'm paying my respects to our trusty and beloved cousins. Besides, the infections were only to be expected – the archive was rat-bitten and mouldy.'

I delayed the trip by train to Kraków for a few days, and settled awkwardly to resting my ribs and staying warm in the calm but bitingly cold northern autumn.

The pain was intermittent at first. It was also familiar. I had experienced the intense dragging discomfort sporadically for twenty years. Difficult to locate and explain, it was typically absent overnight and on rising, but gathered pace during the day. In 1985 a specialist detecting tenderness at the sites of the left and right ischial spines (the bony extensions at the base of the pelvis) had diagnosed an ischial tendonitis or bursitis, explained as a complaint common in the shoulder, similar to tennis elbow, soldier's heel, housemaid's knee. 'It's usually caused by a minor but repetitive irritation,' he said. 'Weavers get it, writers, maybe, and others who sit for long periods. There's no treatment necessary. Exercise and rest as pain dictates. It could take months to come right.' I had checked the diagnosis in the library, in a medical textbook. It confirmed a widespread condition, and mentioned a chronic form contracted by animals, especially horses, which lay on hard floors. In 1985 I was not a writer, but I had been sitting for extended periods on a wooden chair researching and scripting a film documentary. The symptoms made sense.

On my return to New Zealand the condition intensified. My doctor diagnosed a recurrence of the inflamed bursa and was sure the discomfort would settle. I continued to sit long hours at the computer drafting *The Fountain of Tears* – my retelling of 'The Fountain at Bakhchisaray', Alexander Pushkin's *poema* of the impossible love of a Tatar khan for a Polish countess held captive in his Crimean harem.

During February 2004, I waited for the inflammation to recede, as it had in the past. I gritted my teeth in cafés and restaurants, shifted from hip to hip during movies, excused myself early from social occasions, alluding to my ribs, or saying 'I've injured my back', aware that pelvic pain was a vague term and 'ischial spines' meaningless to most. By March the pain had escalated beyond any level at which I had known it before. It dragged: a cat at the curtains. It burned: a smokeless flame, a coal smouldering. It drilled. It needled like crushed glass. It radiated out and pressed down, a non-existent weight from the vicinities of the left and the right ischial spines. On glorious Indian summer afternoons I lay on a sofa oblivious to the buzz of sun and cicadas, wondering why mainstream analgesics were having no effect, how pain of this degree and debilitation could be caused by a bursitis or tendonitis. Repeated consultations uncovered nothing. An MRI scan of the pelvis and lumbar spine was normal. A bone scan picked up the three fractured ribs but found no sign of ischial enthesitis, or inflammation. The blood tests were clear.

Wearily, I decided that if I was to live with this unanswerable condition I should try to follow the example of Robert Louis Stevenson, who wrote of his recurrent respiratory illness, 'I begin to hope I may, if not outlive this wolverine upon my shoulders, at least carry him bravely like Symonds and Alexander Pope. I begin to take a pride in that hope.'[2] John Symonds had lived his life around tubercular symptoms. Pope, with a curvature of the spine, had failed to grow and suffered lifelong headaches and a heightened sensitivity to pain. Had these men sought refuge in writing? Was I being directed to do so? To what end? To interpret the message of a mysterious wind? To write *about* pain, like Alphonse Daudet (*In the Land of Pain*), who daily battled 'the fear that pain inspires';[3] Aleksander Wat ('Diary Without Vowels', an essay), who observed the 'nervous pained quality of [his] writing';[4] Harriet Martineau (*Life in the Sick-Room*), who sent words of understanding and sympathy to fellow invalids from her 'shadowy recess'?[5] Was chronic pain to be the effect of the fall, with the ribs merely collateral damage?

But the pain was too consuming. Unlike these writers, I could expect that in the medically advanced twenty-first century, the pain, although inexplicably insistent, would eventually be treated.

Moreover, Stevenson's burden had revived memories of John Bunyan's *The Pilgrim's Progress* – a Christmas present when I was nine, and still on a bookshelf. The pilgrim, vividly illustrated in a dusty blue tunic with a water flask, staff, and a creeping shape on his shoulders, had wept, trembled, cried, 'What shall I do?' Then he had set forth on his hazardous journey, achieving hard-won arrival at the Celestial City, more concerned with the shedding of his oppression than its management.

I would extricate myself from the swamp, head for the Wicket Gate, dodge the proximal arrows, pay the keeper and enter the King's Highway. Aristotle had said, 'not pleasure, but freedom from pain, is what the wise man will aim at'.[6]

I needed to regain my bearings, keep making decisions. Why sit blindly, albeit bravely, trying to write and hoping to get better?

The sunlit uplands would not easily be found. The medical literature on pain was blocked by theory and assumption, peppered with words like 'think', 'believe' and 'suppose', bewildered by individual responses, hedged like an inaccessible poem with hidden internal workings.

René Descartes' seventeenth-century model of pain, which first recognised the role of the brain in sensory perception, held sway with few modifications until the mid-1960s; it likened the nervous system to a grid of electrical wires carrying pain signals directly from sites of injury to the brain where sensations appropriate to the degree of tissue damage were recorded as pain. Pain is produced, states Descartes in *Treatise of Man* (1662),[7] 'just as pulling on one end of a cord, one simultaneously rings a bell which hangs at the opposite end'. In 1965, Ronald Melzack's and Patrick Walls's Gate Control Theory (GCT)[8] of pain replaced Descartes' hypothesis, and despite ongoing modifications and expansions essentially remains in place; according to Melzack and Walls, certain nerve cells in the spinal cord admit and intensify or reduce pain impulses before either transmitting them to pain centres in the brain or impeding transmission altogether. In 2002, Clifford Woolf and Michael Salter, noting physiological changes in the pain conduction pathways of chronic pain patients, raised the possibility that long-term neurological alterations function as a 'pain memory' akin to that of brain-maintained memory.

Beyond these neurobiological frontiers, all that could be said with certainty was that while significant progress had been made in subduing the symptoms of physical distress, the mechanisms that produced pain were not fully understood.

I was well aware of the consequences of this incomplete understanding of pain.

In 1977, in Hong Kong, while undergoing a Caesarean section, I was given a general anaesthetic that appropriately paralysed me, rendering me unable to move a finger or open an eye, but which also left me able to hear, feel and remember.

Already in labour, I'd greeted with relief the decision to proceed to surgery and left the threshing woman in the next bed (epidurals were not then widely available). On arrival in the operating theatre I was lifted, between contractions, onto the table, catheterised and painted with iodine. My arms were positioned on either side of my body and matter-of-factly strapped down. An intravenous needle was inserted. A mask was placed over my face. I was invited to count backwards from ten.

As I knew from previous surgeries, the routine was not in question. I closed my eyes and anticipated a quick delivery (to limit foetal anaesthesia); a sub 'bikini line' incision (with fewer complications, less bleeding and a more comfortable recovery than the classical vertical midline approach); surgical oblivion, the reversible coma, the most welcome of sleeps.

However, seemingly within seconds, I heard an overloud rush of Cantonese punctuated by English. I wondered, was I waking – was the surgery over? The voices settled and became clear. I tried to open my eyes but my lids were too heavy. I waited to be shaken and roused. Braced myself for the lift back to the trolley.

'P.O.P.,' said the familiar voice of the surgeon.

Persistent occipito-posterior,[9] I thought. Neither transverse lie nor breech presentation (as ventured in the absence of prenatal sonography). No need for the Caesar, but good to be spared the long labour.

The surgeon paused and continued in Cantonese. Was he speaking to me? I tried to reply. I couldn't speak. I felt oddly submerged, mentally alert but physically sluggish, as if the post-op anaesthetic reversal had been halted. Instruments clinked. Was the scrub nurse checking the retractors, clamps, forceps; the circulating nurse counting the sponges; my baby lying nearby in a linen crib with a plastic tag on its wrist blinking at the whiteness of the room?

Then, without warning, something hard and wedge-like was being forced into my throat. I choked. The choke echoed silently – a gulping cough, in my head. My chest was immobile. In a second, in rising panic, I realised that the endotracheal tube was going in, my gagging was not visible, the operation was just beginning and I wasn't properly under.

I strained to raise my head. Turn. Move a leg. Lift myself off the table. Nothing. I was immobile, pinned, flattened as I pictured myself at the time, as if beneath concrete.

The scalpel perforated my abdomen just below my umbilicus. I screamed. The scream passed through the roof of my mouth into my head. I couldn't recoil. The blade ripped relentlessly downwards, magnified, jerky, unexpectedly clumsy, jagged, like the neck of a broken bottle (a beer bottle, a wine bottle), shredding skin, fat, fascia (less incision than crude wound), on and on through the abdominal wall to the uterus. In the background, the surgeon's requests, followed by the scrub nurse's muffled replies. In my head (with no sense of a face, with no mouth, open or closed), reverberating screams, images of sound – of waves exploding against a curved wall of grey bone.

'A boy.' The voice of the surgeon.

'Two-twenty-seven.' A nurse for the medical record.

Proof, with the classical midline incision, this was no ether dream.

A pause.

A scorching plunge either side. In my mind's eye, hot iron, branding, numbers, the sizzling hides of cattle in close-up. I registered scar tissue, sterilisation, the pre-arranged ligation of my fallopian tubes.

Silence.

A sentence in Cantonese.

A reply. The tones of the language.

Another sentence, interrupted by English with 'suture' and 'closing' and in English again, 'She seems to be light, better put her under a bit deeper.'

The direction was no sooner given than an unfamiliar voice close to my ear said, 'Wake up.'

I sensed a shift in surroundings. The room felt nearer, smaller. Was I in recovery or back in the ward? Or was I still in theatre?

'Is it over? Is it over?'

'It's all over,' said a nurse.

'Are you sure?'

'It's all over, you're fine.'

'I felt the whole thing. I wasn't properly under.' My eyes opened. Where was I exactly? I felt slow, as if still submerged. The walls were hazy. Was I off the table? Was the conversation real?

'What's wrong?' The surgeon and anaesthetist appeared alongside.

'I wasn't under.'

'What do you mean?'

'I felt everything – it's a midline incision.'

'Yes – in keeping with your previous scars.'

'It's a boy, born at 2.27 – P.O.P.'

The surgeon confirmed all I told them. I was starting to surface, becoming restless. 'Twitching was apparent throughout,' he said, horrified he'd mistaken my attempts to move for involuntary responses to stimuli. He conferred in Cantonese with the anaesthetist.

John, sitting on a bench in the corridor, was called in. 'You were distressed and frightened,' he recalls. 'I was shocked. I'd never seen you like that.'

I was lost between anaesthesia and reality and couldn't be placated or convinced he was John. As the trolley swung into the corridor, and all the way to the ward, I rambled. 'Are you real, John? Am I dreaming? Am I still on the table? How can I be sure that it's over?'

The house surgeon ordered an injection of strong sedative.

'She thinks she felt it all,' whispered one of the nurses at the foot of the bed.

The next day, the chief anaesthetist came to see me. We discussed the transient and painless consciousness with incomplete recall occasionally reported by patients, especially after the light anaesthesia of Caesarean sections. He stressed that my state of sustained awareness and pain was so rare as to be almost unknown. A technical malfunction was mentioned, my slightness, the low dosage of anaesthesia administered to similarly sized Chinese women, a referral for psychological assistance.

I declined the therapy. I was a nurse – medical misadventures occurred. I was thirty-two – youthful, resilient. I had four healthy children, a happy family; I had a live-in amah who lit incense and left fruit on the altar in her bedroom to appease restless spirits, and swept the graves of her ancestors during Ching Ming in the Third and Ninth Moons. At sunset, junks sailed past our balcony overlooking the South China Sea. On Saturdays and Sundays we played tennis, shopped at Wah Fu, swam at Deep Wave Bay. As a member of the Red Cross mobile blood collection unit (moving from the colony's boardrooms and shopping malls to housing estates, colleges and prisons – yes, even secondary school students and prisoners were encouraged to donate), I observed the workings of a pragmatic society. I preferred to detail the event on paper – a firm narrative I could repeat, if necessary, without thinking – and tuck it away in a file, where it couldn't haunt me.

Had my personal circumstances been less positive, or the procedure more prolonged, the mental consequences of the trauma might have been significant. As it happened, the immediate effects seemed surprisingly few. For some months I felt threatened when I lay on my back, and would cover my abdomen with my hands. And if I was tired, a pulsating rhythm would begin in my head, as if waves were pounding a sea wall, and I would hear, *one, two, three: try now, try now* – the repetitions with which I'd urged myself to move, to break through the weight of the anaesthesia. A flashback also occurred, one hot humid afternoon during Tropical Storm Harriet a few weeks after the operation, as I sat in a minibus in traffic on Pokfulam Road below the hospital – reminding me, as I focused on the rain, that beyond common knowledge the connections between the body, the brain and medical science are frail and erasable.

However, the moment of intubation and realisation that I was suspended without communication between consciousness and insensibility continues to hover. It is reminiscent, if I allow myself to think about it, of Edvard Munch's work of anguish and alienation, *The Scream*. The only other emotional repercussions have been a stirring of inward panic, as a patient, at the immediate prospect of approaching the doors of an operating theatre – overcome by taking a sedative in advance and closing my eyes on the trolley; and a reluctance to speak of the experience – not wanting my children to fear hospitals, wary, as some wonder in disbelief why I had not lost consciousness, of dissecting the horror.[10]

The most enduring effects (still present) proved to be physical. Within six weeks of the surgery I had developed problems with balance. I became dizzy in fast lifts, lost my sixth sense (that is, the physiological sense which prevents falling when one is walking or standing motionless) and tripped if unable to see my feet: symptoms confirmed by a nystagmus – a jerking movement of the eyes (related to the fibres between the brain and the eye that control eye movement), when I was directed to look to the side. Investigations, including a brain scan and a lumbar puncture, produced no conclusive pathology. A neurologist thought I might be developing multiple sclerosis. I put the symptoms down to 'the fuse I blew on the table'.

Recollection of the surgical pain's intensity faded with time, and I remembered the sensations as less agonising than my notes suggested. I imagined that, over the years, my memory had telescoped those sensations into rational fact and lodged them deep within the cerebral cortex's convolutions and fissures – confirmation that acute physical pain, once past, is all but forgotten.

In the years since, other patients who have been 'awake' and 'feeling' throughout surgery under general anaesthesia have come forward. Lawsuits for emotional trauma have been taken and compensations awarded. More importantly, monitors that record levels of consciousness by detecting and measuring changes in brain waves during sedation are now available to assist anaesthetists to mix hypnotic and analgesic agents with greater accuracy. Yet despite such advances, the parameters of consciousness remain indistinct and the precise functioning of general anaesthesia is not fully understood. Patients continue to experience minor episodes of anaesthesia awareness, even when their index readings are within anaesthetic limits. And the exact cause of 'anaesthetic aware-ness with explicit recall' – or *Silenced Screams* (2002)[11] as psychologist Dr Jean-ette Liska entitled the book she wrote after her ordeal during a hernia operation – is a mystery. Liska's account of that surgery – of 'searing agony' and 'screams that reverberated again and again off the cold walls of [her] skull' – is eerily similar to my own.

*

The pine lurched in an unseasonal gust. A pair of magpies playing chase-and-fly in single file along an upper limb disappeared into foliage. They were back. Last year, a group of four had threatened my morning walks in the park. In August, they had swooped over the rugby and soccer fields. In September, they invaded the croquet lawn, establishing a ritual of surveillance: on my first circuit, they stayed out of sight; on the second circuit one magpie appeared as if to test my territorial response; by the time I completed a third round, all four were there on the smooth grass, strutting like storm troopers. 'One for sorrow, two for mirth, three for a funeral, four for a birth.' Concerned for the small birds they frightened away, I considered reporting them to the regional council. I'd seen a single magpie flying across the field cause a dozen sparrows on a fence to rise as one into a cabbage tree, from which there was an invisible outbreak of tweeting, followed by a cowed silence. There were local body protocols for dispensing with magpies. In rural areas, shooting with a .22 calibre, or a high-powered air rifle, was permitted. In urban locations, the use of a cage trap, humanely covered with a tarpaulin, was encouraged, since without such protection a magpie, whose plumage is not waterproof, could become cold and stressed while awaiting collection. Either way, a bait of fatty meat, or a mirror and magpie distress tape, could be useful. The caretaker knew all about magpies. He told me he had watched one appear out of nowhere, intercept a pigeon in midair and sever its neck at speed. The gusts intensified. The pine responded in time, building momentum, drawing metronomic force from its movements and from those of the shorter, bushier trees alongside.

*

A violin string on its bridge

April 2004. The difficulties of diagnosis and treatment posed by the hidden processes of pain seemed to be especially prevalent in the assessment and relief of chronic pain – a term applied to pain of known or unknown origin that has been present for six months, or continues beyond a course of normal healing. All too frequently, that uncertain landscape beyond the known impact of acute tissue damage languished within a confusion of disorders, syndromes and cycles; the impact of unique personality, past experience and interplay of family, social and employment environments; referrals for psychological and psychiatric attention.

I turned to an online Pelvic Pain Society brochure;[12] in trying to name, and contain, the pain in an absence of diagnosis, I'd been reversing the rule of cause and effect. Discouragingly, the finely balanced basin below the umbilicus, bounded by the hips, spine and abdominal muscles, brimming with musculo-skeletal structures, organs, canals, passages, glands, ducts, nerves, blood vessels, and associated soft tissues, was home to the symptoms of sixty or so separate and overlapping medical conditions. Unsurprisingly, it was described as a diagnostic and management challenge, as a result of which much pain, unnamed and undertreated, became chronic.

'As this long-term, unrelenting pain process continues,' the brochure advised, 'as conventional treatments yield little relief, even the strongest person's defences can break down.' The outlook was grim: limited physical and social activity, depression, displacement in the family and society. I 'ticked' the section on diagnostic testing and moved on to discussion of individual perception of pain in body and mind, the rise of related problems, the importance of patience, the assistance of mental and physical therapies, medication as a temporary measure until a therapy proved effective.

But I was beyond patience and nebulous therapies, beyond breathing and relaxation. I needed conclusive solutions and unequivocal medications. The biofeedback, distraction, imagery, mindfulness and other 'transmission modulating cognitive activities' could come later. The pain was intractable, intense – surely this signalled significant physical injury?

One bleak morning, under the power of Bunyan's Giant Despair, I typed 'ischial spine', the location of my supposed tendonitis, into Google. The Internet was not yet the repository of medical advice it would become, and my action was tentative. I hoped, at most, for an overlooked diagnostic clue. The words took me to a pelvic pain forum, and from there, via a process of medical logic and guesswork on my part, to the site devoted to a rare and obscure disorder known as pudendal nerve entrapment (PNE).[13] I stared at the screen in disbelief. The pain described matched my own. It was nerve-related. No wonder it flared and played games. Of course it would not respond to the usual medications.

The lists of fruitless visits to physiotherapists, chiropractors, osteopaths, acupuncturists, orthopaedists, gynaecologists, urologists, proctologists, neurologists, psychiatrists, even dermatologists, together with the litany of misfortunate investigations and treatments, made unsettling reading. Especially perturbing were the unnecessary, often major surgeries, and the diagnoses of somatoform pain dis-orders. A young man in Tucson spoke of consulting twenty specialists in five months. A woman in London wrote, 'I want my life back, I can't go on.' I closed the computer down.

The next morning I returned. For the rest of the week, at once relieved and apprehensive – the pain at last had a name, but there was no certain cure – I roamed the Internet, downloading information and excluding conditions, among them ischial bursitis, with which the condition was sometimes confused.

I learned that the pudendal nerve arises from both sides of the spine's sacral plexus (a network of intersecting nerves in the lower back, which provides motor and sensory capabilities to parts of the pelvis, most of the thigh, the lower leg and the entire foot). Entrapment of this nerve – a circumstance unknown in med-icine before 1988 and little recognised since – causes, often for no apparent reason, a 'chronic, disabling and often intractable' pain unresponsive to physical and drug therapies. The pain was described as characteristically heightened by the mechanics of sitting, bending and lifting – activities that increase pressure on the pelvis, further constricting the compromised nerve. Occasionally (and thank-fully not in my case) incontinence resulted. Determinants were said to include accident trauma, such as a heavy fall onto the buttocks or hips; adhesions from previous pelvic or abdominal surgeries; protracted childbirth; long-standing irri-tation and scarring of the nerve, resulting from prolonged sitting and sports-related activities like high mileage cycling, weight-lifting and rowing; and inflammatory pelvic conditions, notably endometriosis. Variations in tissue mass, nerve positioning and even tightness of the nerve – in theory, a con-sequence of a hereditary musculoskeletal irregularity – were thought to explain why (when most people can endlessly sit, ride or row) the nerves of some become irritated and inflamed and, in the case of an unfortunate few, confined by scar tissue and adhesions.

The pain of this entrapment, I read online, could be so intense as to prompt thoughts of suicide. But since limiting or even desisting from sitting and other nerve-irritating activities might lessen the pain, it was possible to make those changes and manage the pain that remained. While varying degrees of neuralgia might have been present for as long as twenty years, the majority of cases docu-mented online recounted a five- to ten-year history, presumably because that was the length of time taken to find a doctor who could diagnose the condition.

I was alarmed to discover that only a handful of specialists worldwide – in Cairo, Houston, Nantes and Aix-en-Provence – offered conclusive testing for, and decompression of, the entrapment.

The world expert on PNE, anatomist and neurosurgeon Professor Roger Robert, was in Nantes, France. He had pioneered the transgluteal surgical approach to freeing the nerve. In 1987, Robert, together with neurologist Jean-Jacques Labat and radiologist and pain specialist Maurice Bensignor, concerned about 'the consistency of complaints of severe pain with sitting'[14] expressed by sufferers of deep, chronic, pelvic pain, began to investigate the possibility of entrapment of the pudendal nerve.

A hundred or so years ago surgeons used to sever the pudendal nerves of patients suffering this intolerable pain without knowledge of the underlying condition. But the catastrophic effects of incontinence and sexual dysfunction, and the risk of the pain continuing (in the manner of phantom limb pain), had quickly caused withdrawal of the procedure, and left the pathology of the pain undiagnosed.

Initially, working with cadavers – six men and six women – Robert and his colleagues identified the area known as Alcock's Canal, and sites between the two ligaments of the right and left ischial spines, as points on the route of the nerve and its three branches where entrapment could develop. They discovered, by simulating sitting in the cadavers, that the nerve does not lie flat but 'describes a curve which drags it around the regions of the ischial spine which it straddles like a violin string on its bridge', hence the pressure applied and the pain caused by sitting and bending. (As a child violinist, nervous when tuning my instrument should a tightening string snap, I winced at this description.)

The team members had confirmed their findings in 1988, in *Surgical and Radiologic Anatomy*. They found that the character of the pain – which they described as 'piercing and very comparable to acute toothache' – additionally comprised 'sensations of burning, torsion or heaviness' and 'foreign bodies'. They also ascertained that the symptoms, including those precipitated by a fall, could develop slowly; and stated, crucially, that 'activities requiring the seated position [...] are no longer available to these patients, whose mental attitude is one of chronic pain sufferers so obsessed with their miserable state as to be rapidly regarded by their doctors as psychiatric cases'.

The Nantes specialists reported that the non-surgical approach to settling and freeing the nerve – a series of precise, CT-scan-guided injections of steroid into the likely areas of entrapment – worked for some. Of surgical patients – whose 'progressive and relentless' symptoms rendered steroid infusions impractical – 33 per cent were said to achieve a cure or significant relief and 33 per cent a degree of improvement; for another 33 per cent, however, there was no change following surgery, and for 1 per cent a worsening of pain, usually because the nerve had been irreversibly damaged. As well, the handling of an already traumatised nerve could increase the pain for an extended period.

There was no pain scale in consistent use. Of the commonly used assessments, the McGill Pain Questionnaire (MPQ) offered seventy-eight 'sensory, affective and evaluative' words to consider in order to calibrate a numerical score; the Visual Analogue Scale (VAS) intensity indicator was based on ratings from 0–10; and the Wong-Baker Faces Scale (WBFS) for children illustrated degrees of distress.

I passed over the MPQ in favour of the more straightforward VAS, on which I placed my own pain at its worst between the Horrible Eight and Unbearable Nine. I scrutinised the WBFS, where I hovered between the Eight upside-down-mouth of 'Hurts A Whole Lot' and the Nine of the tear-dropping 'Hurts Worst'. I had noted that the pain of this entrapment was frequently described by sufferers as a Ten – Agonising in VAS terms – and wondered if the pain I experienced was genuinely less severe. On my individual scale, a Ten meant total incapacity, near collapse. Was my rating lower because I was more familiar, than some, with physical pain? Would it rise as time went on?

In his essay 'The Language of Pain' (1994),[15] Richard Selzer, Professor of Surgery at Yale, wondered 'whether man has not lost the ability to withstand pain, what with the proliferation of pain-killing drugs and anaesthetic agents. Physical pain,' he suggested, 'has become a once-in-a-while opportunity for most of the industrialised world. Resistance to pain, like any other unused talent, atrophies, leaving one all the more vulnerable. What to a woman of the late 19th century might have been bearable is insupportable to her great-great-granddaughter.'[16]

I queried the extent to which the sliding scale of subjectivity skewed the diagnosis and treatment of pain generally. Interpretations of pain could alter according to just about anything – age, ethnicity and gender; genetic tolerance (the ability to tolerate and manage pain), genetic threshold (the level at which pain is registered by the brain) and past experience of pain; duration of current pain, physical exhaustion, mental fatigue, the time of day.

I also checked the Comparative Pain Scale (CPS),[17] formulated in 2002 by a US systems engineer who had developed PNE. The colour-coded register provided for comparison of the varying levels of persistent pain with clinically established levels of pain and behavioural change. This scale divided Minor Green, Moderate Yellow and Severe Pink pain sections into subgroups of three or four options per section. The descriptions ranged from the Green One of 'very light barely noticeable pain' akin to 'a mosquito bite or a poison ivy itch' – during which, for the most part, 'you never think about the pain' – to the Pink Ten of the 'unimaginable', 'unspeakable' consciousness-losing pain of, say, a crushed hand.

I decided that I swung between Yellow and Pink. This meant I was experiencing unstable pain, typical of nerve involvement, which rose in minutes, as if a gremlin were twiddling a dial, from a 'distressing' mid-level Yellow Four to an 'utterly horrible' mid-level Pink Eight. The former was listed as comparable to toothache – 'so strong you notice the pain all the time and cannot completely adapt', and the latter was placed on a level with childbirth – pain 'so intense you can no longer think clearly at all, and have often undergone severe personality change if the pain has been present for a long time': pain so insistent that 'suicide is frequently contemplated and sometimes tried'. I wondered – never having known, and unable to conceive of the Pink Ten's consciousness-losing agony of a crushed hand – if my 'intense' was another's 'unimaginable'.

The value of this scale appeared to lie in its reference to behavioural response to chronic pain. I could relate, say, to the comparison of a 'very distressing' Yellow Five which supposes that 'not only do you notice the pain all the time, you are now so preoccupied with managing it that your normal lifestyle is curtailed', with an 'intense' Yellow Six, which suggests that 'you begin to have trouble holding a job or maintaining normal social relationships'. Yet, as someone inclined to push on during illness and pain, I queried whether my behavioural Yellow Five equated with another's Yellow Six.

Moreover, I was of the view that equating the known, relievable pain of toothache, and the self-limiting pain of childbirth, with that of a singular, unappeased entrapment was too approximate to be useful, even though the comparative terms 'distressing' and 'utterly horrible' were close to the mark.

Nonetheless, my options were clear. Either I was to consult an overseas specialist, verify the entrapment and work towards a form of recovery; or I was to hope for a remission, as had apparently happened in the past. The PNE surgeons abroad urged early diagnosis and treatment before the nerve damage became irreversible. But I chose the latter option. France was hardly around the corner. The outcome of surgery was uncertain and my twenty-year history of pain rendered the odds doubly unfavourable. The nerve might not be entrapped. I might have a temporary neuralgia caused by muscular compression. I might have a psychogenic disorder – a haywire connection between body and brain, remedied by psychological intervention. The pain might even be due to a repressed event – why not: all states of being, including thinking, are chemical and, in the end, physical. It was easier to stop sitting.

*

The autumn sky detailed and diminished the pine. In early morning the tree, which faced east, glowed. Backlit in the late afternoon, only its spiky outline was visible. The danger of a wildfire in the green belt close to the house had passed. Although summer had produced a flash flood and morning mist over the airport, it was only with the arrival of a bank-slipping storm that the spectre of winds, fuelled by dry grasses, dead branches, wooden houses and the leaves of ghost gums filled with flammable oil, had faded. My prevailing concern was the pine's ability to remain upright, its crown intact, until its height, or an intense blaze at the base of its trunk, directed a safe fall forward. Not, I reasoned, that conflagration would be necessarily catastrophic. The pine could use heat to its advantage. While its structure might fail, its seeds, secure in their cones, would scatter when the hot scales sprang open, planting themselves in needle-free ground. I protected the pine with a thousand inaccessible valleys and peaks. At night I meditated on its pale trunk, lit by the city below. And because I detected memory of movement in the tree's autumn stillness, I opened a window to share its tension – even though it remained mute, as if storing vigour for winter.

*

Milky juice into powder

May 2004. I strove to bring the pain under control. All the while the 'pessimism of the intelligence' strained against the 'optimism of the will' – to appropriate Antonio Gramsci's activist motto.[18] As I persuaded myself that rest and hyper-avoidance of sitting would allow the inflammation and swelling to ease and the nerve to glide freely, I also agitated. For how long was I to stop driving, dining out, going to the cinema; to eat and drink standing at the kitchen bench or the sideboard, on the fringe of conversation? How could I be expected to write standing all day, keyboard wobbling on a cardboard box on top of an ironing board? Was I being discouraged from writing? Who or what had taken hold of my life, and to what end?

In searching for a sense of direction, was I to consider supernatural forces – in which case was the pain good ghost, goblin or ambivalent djinn? Should I set conventional medicine against amulets and small synchronicities; explore metaphor, myth and random events; embrace the dictum of sixteenth-century German-Swiss physician, alchemist and astrologer Paracelsus, that 'The magical is a great hidden wisdom, and reason is a great open folly?'

Or was I to pursue the fruits of philosophy? I flicked restlessly between the thinkers. Marcus Aurelius reasoned that 'What we cannot bear removes us from life; what lasts can be borne.'[19] Michel de Montaigne advised that we should 'learn to suffer whatever we cannot avoid', adding that the key to living a complete life is the ability to make positive use of adversity.[20] Friedrich Nietzsche believed that just as 'a tree that is supposed to grow to a proud height [cannot] dispense with bad weather and storms', a fulfilled life is not possible without pain.[21] Schopenhauer proposed that 'At all times everyone indeed needs a certain amount of care, anxiety, pain or trouble, just as a ship requires ballast, in order to proceed on a straight and steady course.'[22] Little of what was said appeared profound; much seemed obvious: 'Many are the sayings of the wise/In ancient and modern books enrolled,' sang the chorus in John Milton's *Samson Agonistes*, '[…] Little prevails, or rather seems a tune,/Harsh, and of dissonant mood, from his complaint.'[23]

I liked the sound of Paracelsus, who rode home to Austria from Arabia with the wads of opium compound, known as the Stones of Immortality, in the hollow hilt of his sword, so that the poppy of sleep and relief, prohibited following the Inquisition when all things middle-Eastern provoked suspicion, could be reintroduced to Europe.[24]

The isolation from informed medical expertise was magnifying my credulity, the doubt of self-diagnosis my uncertainty.

I delivered PNE printouts to my GP and specialists. The condition was not known to them, but unlike some of the medical professionals condemned on the Internet they were keen to be informed.

In accordance with my diagnosis of nerve entrapment, amitriptyline[25] – a tricyclic anti-depressant with analgesic benefits in doses at a fraction of those specified for depression – was prescribed. The amitriptyline, taken at night, was befuddling and dried my mouth, but enabled sleep; it would only take the edge off baseline pain and prove powerless during flares. I was also prescribed codeine. A natural derivative of opium at the low end of the opioid scale, today codeine is either manufactured from morphine to which it reverts in the body, or produced in the laboratory by synthesis alone. Opioids,[26] I read, besides being habit-forming and quick to build tolerance, provide incomplete relief for nerve pain. I brushed aside questions of dependence, determined an opium-related drug would work for me. I responded to the idea of using a derivative of the Aspirin of the East, valued since antiquity, extolled in Arabia as a Gift of God, in Greece as The Juice, and on the battlefields and in the hospitals of the American Civil War as God's Own Medicine. Above all I craved soothing, luminescent laudanum (from the Latin, *laudare*, to praise) as Paracelsus first mixed it: scoring the unripe seeds of poppies with a knife in the morning, drying their milky juice into powder, then combining the fine dust with amber, musk, the whisper-thin softness of gold and the delicate rose of crushed Indian pearls. Thomas de Quincey had taken tincture of opium to relieve facial neuralgia and succumbed to a misty mind and dreamy visions. Addiction had also been the lot of Samuel Taylor Coleridge. Perhaps an enhanced literary output would compensate for the inevitable withdrawal and harsh descent to reality.

'Nerve pain is unlike that of trauma or surgery,' a pain specialist concurred, 'and when severe it's difficult to control. Amitriptyline will be a question of trial and error, codeine at best an ancillary tool.'

I asked him about a TENS (Transcutaneous Electrical Nerve Stimulation) machine, the leads of which, worn on the skin, instigate a distracting tingling and confuse pain impulses, thereby closing a gate of transmission. 'The nerve's too deep,' he said, setting the suggestion aside.

*

I lay awake, curtains open, eyes fixed on the pine. Earlier in the week an arborist, preparing an estimate for reducing the overgrowth dampening our lawn's northern border, expressed surprise the tree had lasted so long in an exposed position. 'It's dangerous,' he said, recognising a beacon for lightning and gales, squinting as he reckoned the distance from its crown to our roof. I was hesitant about his plans for the garden, even though it was clear that culling was necessary. He insisted the shrubs were constricted and struggling for light. The camellia would flourish released from the lemonwoods, and the sago palm from the density of the holly. The laurel bay had lost shape and in its present condition served no useful purpose. He crouched down and plucked at the lawn. Opened a pocket-knife, scraped the soil, said of the turf, 'It has shallow roots and will dry out with the increased exposure to sun. Cut it less often with a good sharp blade and water it in the early morning when there's less evaporation. Summers end, like everything else, and grass is a great survivor.' I remembered seeing a documentary about an arboretum, in which instructions were given for communicating with trees. 'Find a small one,' the guide suggested. 'Don't start with a very old or a very tall one – you will look so small, so like a child, that the tree which has been growing and a part of the world for a long time may not accept you. Stand on the outside of its leaf fall. Hold your hand on your heart. Smile to your heart. Your heart will radiate your smile out to the tree.'

*

Far point to near point

June 2004. The pain was indeed difficult to control.

When there seemed no way forward, John drove me to a recommended chiropractor, some hours away. I lay flat on the back seat feeling diminished, dizzy, car sick, watching an overcast sky flick by. The practitioner took X-rays and pointed to an 'asymmetrical pelvis'. I handed him the medical literature on PNE, including Professor Robert's groundbreaking paper. He consulted his wall charts, advocated two weeks' pelvic adjustments and promised a positive outcome; my recently broken ribs, he reassured, would not be affected. John returned to Wellington, while I stayed uneasily in a motel to undergo treatments at a clinic in a room overlooking a twisted oak tree. I was treated kindly with heat packs and reassurances even though my pelvis was said to be the most 'locked' the chiropractor had seen. The day my ribs became painful, I discontinued the corrections with relief.

I carried a handkerchief embroidered with yellow and white flowers which had been offered by a friend for prayer at her church, together with a slip of paper on which I had written 'The nerve is smooth and free in a cool breeze' in my left pocket.

I composed paragraphs of happy, healing words: words like *optimism* and *good health*; *better*, and *best*, and *best step forward*; *violet* and *yellow*, the colour of pansies and crocuses; *orange*, the colour of poppies; *pink*, the tinged peace of roses.

I turned my small herd of elephants and occasional ornaments on the bookshelves, so they wouldn't feel trapped, their trunks and noses facing the door.

I investigated Buddhism and pondered my accumulation of negative karma, and Zen Buddhism, which suggested that as long as I continued to be a slave to 'words and logic' I would experience measureless suffering.

I sought the teachings of Confucius who advised against speaking when eating and conversing when in bed, believed that in language 'perspicacity was everything' and hated the way in which purple was robbed of its lustre by red.[27] The theological intelligence of C.S. Lewis, who admitted that his thesis *The Problem of Pain* (1966) was written without personal experience of pain, from which I most usefully deduced that animals suffer less because they have no capacity to imagine the future. The Celtic wisdom of John's grandmother, parent of eleven children, who used to say, 'You'll always be where you're meant to be' and 'If you're meant to be punished you will be.' The spinning thoughts of the Persian mystic Jalal al-Din Rumi, who wrote in 'Enough Words':

> You must have shadow and light source both.
> Listen, and lay your head under the tree of awe.[28]

I considered growing hashish, or rascals' grass, as Arabs once called it, and mixing it in biscuits; trialling methadone; falling into the strong arms of Morpheus, god of dreams, son of Hypnos, spirit of sleep.

In the lowest moments, when the pain escaped the pelvis and developed a pallid, external life of its own, when it became a cloud filling the room, closing me down, and it seemed neither words nor 'the world of men' could help me, I fantasised about oblivion. I eyed the squat, brown bottle of codeine, carried it in my pocket, counted and recounted the tiny white pills; contemplated the weightlessness of stepping late at night from a high window or bridge into the wind; curling beneath a fern into oneness with nature; sleeping at the foot of the pine, on the bank of the stream, in the transforming softness of moss and of gathering leaves. And I thought about the power of suggestion, and finding online that suicide was an option.

Later, when the pain was less relentless, I did not find this wish to surrender unreal. The memory of severe chronic pain is not diluted by time. It waits in the mind as if haunting the wood of an instrument long played, storing and orchestrating sounds for the future.

As my novel *The Fountain of Tears* languished, its khan unrequited in love and the captive countess in his harem beset by the heaviness which, 'like the night before and the day ahead, never leaves her';[29] as the days shortened; as each evening I drew the curtains and lit and heated the house; as I repeated my encouraging mantras and paragraphs of positive words; as I read Henri Charrière's *Papillon* and Jean-Dominique Bauby's *The Diving Bell and the Butterfly* – I felt locked, without recollection of summer and little prospect of lifting spring, between Warsaw's autumn and the Wellington winter.

John came home for lunch. The children called in with gifts: a burner and a selection of bergamot, lavender tree and orange sweet oils, a lambskin rug for the sofa, a pair of opossum fur boots, a wheat pack, a hand-stitched hot water bottle cover, a bright pot plant, a regular supply of dark chocolate.

I absorbed the support. I achieved a measure of acceptance. The world became simpler, gifted with time and the fascination of small things. The clutter of life – deadlines, appointments, extraneous obligations – fell away. Energy and optimism slowly returned. I began to focus for short periods on writing – on placating the 'animal in perpetual unrest' with the controlled stories of less immediate worlds: *Cover Stories*, a collection of poetry; 'The Fountain at Bakhchisaray', a free translation of Pushkin's *poema*.

The pain held on, a cohesive influence, a necessary edge to my thinking. I am reminded that Wordsworth compared the spontaneity of childhood expression with the measured 'philosophic mind' of later years;[30] and that Louis Simpson spoke of the 'natural force' of ideas arising of their 'own accord' in 'things'.[31] Pain was those later years, that force of things.

What of the neurosurgeon, Professor Robert in France, I started to wonder, as poetry – the relief of rhythm, the grace of words, the strength of thinking in lines – cleared my mind, and the medications and hyper-avoidance of sitting, lifting and bending moderated the pain? What of Nantes at the Atlantic mouth of the Loire, childhood home of Jules Verne; three hours by fast train, or an hour by plane, south-west of Paris?

Appointments in Nantes proved difficult to arrange. Emails and faxes, *Urgent et Confidentiel*, went unanswered. Key people were not available to take phone calls, their secretaries all-shielding. My GP, fluent in French, spent half an hour on the phone one evening speaking to doctors in hospital corridors, and gave up.

The uncertainty caused the pain to rise.

I emailed Houston instead. Over the phone at four in the morning, I finally spoke to a knowledgeable medic: a sports medicine specialist, who had trapped his nerve in an accident and undergone surgery in France. Two years later, when he had his 'life back', he'd returned to Nantes with a neurosurgical team to work with Professor Robert and Drs Labat and Bensignor. As a result, in 2002 Houston offered the first PNE diagnosis and treatment facility in the United States.

'Don't do anything that brings on the pain,' he advised.

'The pain is constant. I've scarcely left the house in three months. Should I be out walking?'

'Not if it brings on the pain.'

'I've stopped sitting. I lie down all day. I stand only to eat. Could the nerve settle, as it seems to have done in the past? Could it spontaneously disengage?'

'No,' said the specialist who was happy for me to come to Houston but agreed that, financially speaking, I would be better to go to France. 'The nerve's had enough. You're at the top of the curve.'

Like Sir Richard Burton, whose biography I was reading – weak and depressed having barely started the march that would lead to the discovery of Lake Tanganyika – I fretted about 'the sorry labour of waiting and reloading asses' and 'the wear and tear of mind at the prospect of imminent failure'.[32]

Like Burton's wife Isobel, who permanently injured her back and ankle after slipping in a Paris hotel, I might have written, 'Strong health and nerves I had hitherto looked upon as a sort of right of nature, and supposed everybody had them, and had never felt grateful for them as a blessing.'[33]

A day later there was a message to contact Professor Robert. He spoke English, and was receptive to the symptoms I listed by phone. In due course, an email questionnaire arrived; then, after intercessions from friends fluent in French, dates for testing and surgery, if necessary, in August.

I had my hair cut, standing. On better days I met friends for coffee in cafés with counters and bars.

I made progress with *Cover Stories*. The act of writing was stabilising, the concentrated and absolute order of the language of poetry supported the shapelessness in which I was suspended and steadied the diary entry of despair at the end of the day.

I composed not, as I preferred, while walking or pacing, but lying flat on a sofa obstinately turning words in my mind and drafting them in pencil onto a lined A4 page, asking them, 'where will you take me today?' I prised journeys of projection and memory from the ceiling and walls, the lamp on the sideboard, the vase of cut flowers, the flicker of birds entering and leaving the kowhai tree close to the window. Ideas were lured from far point to near point, details from blurred to sharp focus, images as if from three-dimensional shadow boxes of the sort that once attracted motionless travellers to distant places with mirrors and prisms.

The stories accumulated with little revision or recourse to the neural reconcil-iations of sleep (amitriptyline's dense dreams delivered few waking insights). Unlike Marina Tsvetayeva's 'celestial, four-petalled guest'[34] growing slowly through flagstones, or the dreamlike dissociations of Lukeria, Ivan Turgenev's ailing serf[35] lying alone as if the only person on earth, open to thoughts pouring through her like rain, they took shape deliberately, as ice, crystal on crystal, each shard a cover[36] for 'a story within a story, perhaps a story within that',[37] in which I cast myself as an outsider, or spy – a tourist in Warsaw, in the company of poets:

> swirling vowels around
> on their tongues,
>
> singing songs best sung
> in the rain,
>
> saying 'Good evening,'
> and 'Thank you,'
> and 'Madame, as you can see,
> I have a fever, please
> may I use the telephone?'[38]

a strolling player:

> posting myself
> wherever I please
>
> in headgear not necessarily
> of my choosing:
> panamas, bowlers,
> a fez, a crash helmet ...[39]

a monumental trumpet-necked vase:

> from an Ottoman palace
> in the hands
> of a master restorer [...][40]

the composer of a slim volume of obscure verse asked:

> for the straightforward
> expression of torment
> and other tragic
> manifestations of the heart,

[…] a story
with blockbuster potential
about battles, wounds,
wolves trying to raise
viable cubs …[41]

a shape shifter, seeking an agency for physical pain:

tackling terrain
as difficult now
as it has always been –

peaks almost too perfect
to abandon,
hairpin descents,
nameless lakes
shining below –

with no mules,
no markers,
no pale orange poppies

only a local brochure
and a tight lipped guide
to hotels in my pocket,

information
my commanding nirvana,

transformation
my stock in trade,[42]

a camper beside the Axeinous (Black) Sea, calling:

'Unaccountable daughters of Gaea,
ease your retribution,

detach yourselves
from the mountain,

light our paraffin lamp:

the moon has almost
no colour in its face,
the shoreline no reflection.'[43]

The poems rested on a ridge of unease, yet expressions of personal pain were concealed in the narrative associations of metonymy. Why was I unwilling to employ the direct comparisons of metaphor, to name and engage with the hard edges of pain? Was this because I was reluctant to imply vulnerability, a want of stoicism, an obsession with self? Or was I becoming aware that, while literature readily conveyed mental or emotional pain, the expression of physical pain, particularly multidimensional chronic pain, necessitated the wider negotiation of bodily *and* mental distress?

But this was no time to linger in a haze of conceptual and linguistic entanglements.

I was wanted in Nantes, where, as I imagined in my poem 'Talking Pictures', *le docteur, le professeur*,[44] would promise to consider the case after lunch. He wore chino trousers and a watch with Roman numerals; when he said *de la consultation et du traitement*, syllables would slide from his balconied tower like silver.

I was finalising consultations and buying plane tickets, eyes fixed on the light between hilltop and sky.

For the moment, for all I cared – as relayed in 'Waxing and Salting' – pain was halfway to India in search of a forest of exotic monkeys, preparing to chatter, swing by its tail, adopt a more flexible vocabulary; or rolled in the luggage of a language peddler, original, with maybe a dozen translations stapled together.[45]

Shortly before leaving, the pain's base level dropped from a CPS Yellow Four to a Green 'blow to the nose' Three. Was this self-resolution, at last? Should I cancel my arrangements?

I rang Atlanta, Georgia, and spoke to the author of the Comparative Pain Scale, devised in response to the pain of his own entrapment. He too had stopped sitting early on and reduced his symptoms. On arrival in France almost pain-free, he had been sent home, only to return the following year.

'It's playing hide and seek,' I said. 'It's capricious and devious. Soon I'll need it for testing and it might not be there.'

'Start sitting,' he advised. 'You should aim for at least a Three for the tests to show cause and effect.'

*

The tree feller awaited a decision. I was comfortable about culling the holly and lemonwoods but debated the laurel bay's removal. It was Apollo's sacred tree, deemed forever youthful, forever green – a metamorphosis of Daphne whose skin became its bark, hair its glossy leaves, arms and feet its branches and roots. The ancients believed the plant breathed poetry and radiated the light of prophecy; that an aromatic leaf placed beneath a pillow at night beckoned the muse. Pliny held that a bay planted close to a house guards the doorway and garden and is never struck by lightning. 'Taking it away could cause the bank behind it to slip,' I dithered. 'Its shallow roots will die back,' admitted the tree surgeon. 'But its taproot structure will remain intact for ten years. The bank will be safe.' 'The stump could look ugly.' 'The stump will re-sprout, even if the tree is taken at ground level – a bay can revive, even after dying all the way back to its roots.' 'Should we prune it? Clip it into a hedge or some other practical shape?' Recent research in Iran had determined the leaf oil of *lauris nobilis Linn* contained anti-inflammatory properties that produced analgesic effects comparable to morphine – in mice. The tree surgeon shook his head, explaining that the under-wood was too spindly for pruning, and the leaves had been reaching for sunlight too long for the core to re-form. I should ease my conscience by thinking coppicing rather than cutting: in Europe, trees regularly felled for firewood have been kept alive for centuries in this way. He waved at the pine. 'Pines are also good for harvesting – their wood's lightly structured and burns quickly, and the aerated cones make good kindling.' I picked a bay leaf. Apollo had a reputation as a healer, but his arrows had brought death and disease. 'I could fill the space with a low-growing daphne,' I reasoned. 'Let the laurel bay go,' the surgeon agreed, 'and then watch it return. The tree is still there in the stump.'

*

Sleeping on saffron

July 2004. Nantes straddles the Loire River – the last untamed, unlocked waterway in Europe – 50 kilometres from the Atlantic Coast. The sixth largest metropolis in France, and main city in the West, it has a population of 250,000 and a wider reach of 800,000.

'Born unto the river,' said a travel guide. 'A child of the water.'

'Once a centre of European surrealism,' said another.

The city's history is marked principally by Henri IV's Edict of Nantes, 1598, evoked during the Catholic–Protestant Wars of Religion. The Edict granted the persecuted Huguenots freedom of worship and civil rights; it was revoked after religious hostilities resumed following Henri IV's assassination. Also of note, Nantes' eighteenth-century status as France's foremost and wealthiest port: a consequence of slave trading during which some 450,000 Africans were shipped to America.

In 2003, the weekly *L'Express* had appointed Nantes as France's greenest city. During my visit, *TIME* magazine (August 2004) would vote the cultured, relaxed centre 'the most liveable city in Europe'.

Of interest to a New Zealander, there was the 1986 Rugby Battle of Nantes, when the All Blacks were beaten 16–3 by *Les Bleus* and Wayne (Buck) Shelford, in one of the toughest test matches of his career, tore his scrotum while at the bottom of a ruck. Myth had it that Shelford insisted the physiotherapist stitch it up at the side of the field, from where the act was broadcast live to the nation, so he could return to the game.

Jules Verne recalled his home town with affection, and based much of his maritime writing on his early adventures there. André Breton, the 'Pope of Surrealism', remarked that 'Nantes, alongside Paris, is perhaps the only town in France where I got the feeling that something worthwhile might happen to me.'[46]

I travelled with John, precariously, protecting the nerve, sitting for take-offs and landings, lying flat during international flights, standing in galleys on domestic flights, attempting to maintain the pain at a tolerable level until I reached Nantes. I carried a medical letter of explanation for the airlines, and another for Customs as I was well stocked with codeine.

Between sleeping and standing to eat, I studied my entrapment file, pausing to picture the cadavers' quiet contribution. To be reassured by the photographs and explanatory diagrams of ligaments, muscles, fascia and vascular patterns they had made possible; the absence of supposition; the irrefutable language of anatomy. John, ensconced in an English/French version of *Jeeves Takes Charge*, with *Stiff Upper Lip, Jeeves* to follow, or sitting comfortably with a glass of wine and cheese board on his tray anticipating an agreeable French vacation, shuddered when he looked over at the images and said, 'What the eye doesn't see,' but as a former nurse these were details I needed to know.

I wanted, moreover, to be sure of my quarry. 'If you know the fighting capability of your opponents,' the fourteenth Dalai Lama said of suffering, '...then you're in a much better position when you engage in the war.'[47] War was an apt metaphor.

We arrived at Charles de Gaulle airport at six in the morning. The reception clerk at the Sheraton, close by, astride a train station, could not check us in until noon. He gave us a key to the Club Lounge, empty, surreal, in which a buffet spread with cheeses, grapes, crackers and dried apricots, and small tables set with glasses and complimentary drinks, waited for guests who might not arrive. We opened a bottle of Badoit mineral water and watched planes take off only metres away.

There was an adjoining bathroom – an uncanny replica of the Warsaw scene of my fall: the same grey, mottled marble; the vertical tube lights either side of a bevel-edged mirror; the same shower over the same deep bath. I spread a towel on the floor for protection. Here, too, the hovering of unseen guests: a used ashtray and empty bottles of red raisin and grapefruit juice grouped to one side of the basin.

The suite was very quiet, with barely a hum from the air conditioner and no hint of the workings of the airport, or of the large train station below. I lay on a narrow magazine stool with a velvet nap, my head in a soft chair. John tinkered with a samovar and tried to make tea. A lanky porter in a white jacket silently entered, and left with the empty bottles.

At twelve we took a corner table in the dining room. I stood discreetly against a wall. The pain, ever the genie, was rising, as if it knew Nantes was near, overtaking the codeine; the Australian wine; the sole, potatoes and broccoli, steamed to perfection; three Englishmen at an adjacent table discussing pasta and olive oil with a hint of tarragon, and a married woman they all knew, who was having an affair.

Finally, entering our room, we found a voucher inviting us to redeem a supposed 4,000 star points for a bathrobe or a bottle of Laurent-Perrier-Brut Champagne. Then, the telephone rang and a strange voice said, 'Oh darling, I've been trying to find you, where have you been?'

'France,' I said to John, 'is beginning to feel superstitiously appropriate and coincidental.'

That night we both dreamed of pigs: John's pig had a velvet shawl over its shoulders; mine was poet Dinah Hawken's favourite pet. John decided we had seen an animal resembling a pig in a TV report on flooding in Bangladesh the previous evening, and the magazine stool in the Club Lounge accounted for the velvet napery. I thought my connection could be a couple of lines from 'Where We Say We Are', Dinah's poem of travel to the islands:

> [...] I've come
> for the drums, and the drumming, and the drumming of the
> drums. I've come for the pig asleep in a ditch.[48]

The following afternoon we took a fast train to Nantes. We waited on the platform with backpackers, excursionists shouldering camera bags, families manoeuvring pushchairs and suitcases: holiday-makers tanned, agile and speaking a dozen languages. The nerve burned. I felt adrift and afraid. I took my notebook from my pocket and fiddled with the line breaks of an unfinished poem, 'Soliloquy for Sir Richard Francis Burton', en route to Mecca:

> where the sun
> rose and set with
> the same intensity
> and you could only
> mimic the fervour
> of fellow travellers
> because apart from
> surreptitious observation,
> documentation and sketch
> you had no prophets
> or gods in your heart,
> no angels or flying
> white horses
> to assist you to heaven.[49]

On the train, I loomed intrusively from the aisle over the surrounding passengers; pitched and rolled in the baggage compartment; lay curled across my seat, head in John's lap. Finally, with the express established at full speed, I wedged myself between the carriage wall and the last seat, across the corridor from a woman in a wheelchair, secure in a space reserved for the purpose.

Nantes was the remembered France: melt-in-the-mouth fish, crusty breads and crisp vegetables; sweet tomatoes and impeccable peaches; the courteous French, their mellifluous language: it was impossible not to speak French, no matter how flawed, in the slipstream of the language.

I browsed in perfumeries, stood in the shop of *le chocolatier* where the aroma alone was sufficient, laundered our clothes using fine soaps, bought slim-fitting sandals, forgot about sunblock, was stopped twice in one day for directions and three times for market research.

The temperature averaged thirty degrees, but the sun had a bathing quality and the light was redemptive, golden. Our room, with its small balcony overlooking the tops of the tilleul (linden, or lime) trees in the rue du Couedic and the potted daisies and sun-yellow awnings of the Entrecôte café, was golden. The old stone was golden. The doctors, nurses and the general population and its many dogs tucked into baskets on buses and trams and in banks, were golden. Shops closed for lunch, as expected, and didn't open on Sundays. Nobody dined before seven. The shade and early morning air were dry and pleasantly cool.

I pushed pain, as if at will, to one side. This strange time of malaise was the summer I had missed.

In the hotel lobby and lifts I scrutinised guests for signs of nerve entrapment. A woman with an American accent stumbled over *Bonjour* at the desk and alighted on the second floor when she meant to go to the third. She looked tired, unlike a tourist. Breakfast was delivered on a tray to her door. Was she a contender? Would we share a hospital room?

Masha, a Russian friend from New Zealand holidaying in Pornic on the coast, drove through. We spent the afternoon at an outdoor café beside a fountain sipping martinis and toasting the synchronicity of our visit. The 'dusty aromatic smell of old lime trees coming into blossom drifted in a wave as tall as a house and lingered in the air', straight from the pages of *Doctor Zhivago*.[50]

'I'm sleeping on saffron,' I said.

'France is the land of indulgence,' Masha agreed, smoking her cigarettes and tossing her newly blond hair.

I sat, calling in *la douleur* for the diagnostic nerve blocks and motor latency test the following day (*douleur*, from the Latin *dolor*: both words mean physical pain, grief and suffering). I was aiming for the upper limits of the Comparative Pain Scale, for an Unbearable Nine if necessary – 'Pain so intense you cannot tolerate it and demand pain killers or surgery, no matter what the side effects or risk' – and asked a man at the next table to take a photograph to prove it.

The four CT-guided nerve blocks were no problem: an average visit to the dentist. A long needle carrying local anaesthetic reached through first the left, then the right gluteal (buttock) muscles into the depth of the pelvis to infiltrate, twice each side, tissues adjacent to the nerve's likely areas of entrapment; if relief resulted, compression was suggested. Precision was essential: an inaccurately placed needle tip might damage the nerve; if not sited within one millimetre of the target, the numbing liquid could be delivered to a point too distant to have the required effect. I lay prone, scarcely daring to breathe. The pasta-like nerve, just the width of a coffee straw, was surely among the body's most inaccessible structures. After each set of infiltrations I climbed out of the scanner, sat on a chair and, closely watched by a doctor and radiographer, assessed the diminution of pain. I'd read of patients who wept when they found themselves free of their symptoms for an hour, two hours, even longer. I also knew, the inaccuracy of needle positioning aside, that a very short period of amelioration could mean either the entrapment damage was severe, or the nerve was compromised beyond the 'point of the block'. I experienced a cessation of less than a minute one side and seconds on the other.

The thirty motor function shocks to the deep nerve were worthy of the Inquisition. But the pain caused was productive. It put forward a three-page graph indicating abnormally slow nerve response times and the conclusion: *Il existe donc des arguments en faveur d'un syndrome canalaire du nerf pudendal bilatéral.* 'Testing suggests bilateral pudendal nerve entrapment.' But it was short-term pain: *un mauvais quart d'heure*. It confirmed my diagnosis. It wasn't running my life.

*

What was this – a conifer growing sideways on a public lawn beside a thorough-fare in the middle of the city? I crossed the road to take a closer look at the stunted trunk supported by iron trestles, forking without side branches like pincers into the two limbs of its crown. Its posture and grooved bark bespoke old age, its stunted growth a once-crowded forest or low light source. Had a branch assumed control when the central trunk faltered? Sprouted from a decomposing plant? Grown over a boulder retaining its bowed form when the obstruction was removed? I smoothed the furrowed bark, ruffled the waist-high brush and gath-ered a handful of needles for good luck. Traffic passed at a steady pace. A white tram with green markings glided to its stop. Damp air from the direction of the river fanned a woman shouldering a canvas bag, and a young man in blue jeans and a T-shirt lying on the grass in the sporadic shade of a neighbouring tree.

*

In adequate dosage

Early August 2004. There was a gap of ten days before surgery.

John left to visit his mother in Scotland. I was tired, and elected to stay in Nantes. The holiday season was underway. The sun was out, the streets were crowded and the canopied restaurants and brasseries beckoned. I wanted to linger over a sidewalk pain au raisin and coffee, the mild breeze tousling my hair and swirling aromatic steam from my cup, but I didn't feel brave enough to stand alone at a table. I walked to the fortress Castle of the Dukes of Brittany – site of the signing of the Edict of Nantes – only to find the bridge across the moat blocked because restoration was in progress. On the way back to the hotel, I lit a candle in the cool, neo-Gothic Basilica of Saint Nicholas. A pile of prayers had been placed nearby. I selected Cardinal Newman's *Ce que tu voudras*, an extract from Pierre Teilhard de Chardin's *La Messe Sur le Monde* and Mother Teresa's *La vie est une chance, saisis-la* from the stack of coincidentally coloured Comparative Pain Scale Minor Green, Medium Yellow and Severe Pink leaflets.

A cousin phoned from Toulouse. 'When John returns, come down,' Peter said. 'We'll take you to the country and escape the heat.'

I lay on the bed reading Stephen Mitchell's translation of *The Selected Poetry of Rainer Maria Rilke* (1987).[51] In 'O Lacrimosa', Rilke had written:

> Ah, but the winters! The earth's mysterious
> turning-within …
>
> …
>
> Where imagination occurs
> beneath what is rigid; where all the green
> worn thin by the vast summers
>
> again turns into a new
> insight and the mirror of intuition

From time to time I stood in my new sandals confiding expressions of pain to my diary on the laptop, which I'd positioned on the dressing table on top of the shoebox; where I also ate takeaway pastries and *tartines* – watching myself in the mirror.

The only television channel in English repeated news stories about the armed theft, from an Oslo museum, of Munch's *The Scream*; and about the tallest living man, who plucked the sweetest apples from the highest trees, struggled to live life at ground level and said from Ukraine, 'I must adapt to the world rather than the world to me.'

On the weather front, the east coast of Scotland was covered by a haar, and southwest Europe was having a heatwave.

The French channels carried footage of the Pope's visit to Lourdes. Jean Paul II was shown nearing the ivy-covered Grotto of Apparitions on his mobile throne. Pilgrims applauded and reached forward to absorb divine radiance. A nun spoke directly to camera about his courageous example, and a former nurse with a back injury said with conviction that she had 'a lot of faith in a cure'. A rhythm from an imagined journey to Lourdes, completed for *Cover Stories*, underpinned the commentary.

> She waits to be taken
> beyond dawn
> to the foot of the Pyrenees,
>
> to the bank of the stream
> where the fortress and medieval
> spires of the basilica
> pierce the blue morning ... [52]

'If the Pope remains afflicted,' I said to the screen, 'how can I expect any improvement?'

I watched Lourdes's long lines of pain. It was more than three decades since I had trained as a nurse. Although steroidal and non-steroidal anti-inflammatory drugs were making inroads into the treatment of acute and chronic inflammatory conditions, derivatives and permutations of the ancient poppy had not been superseded in the management of terminal and other great physical pain. Advances had, however, been made in the *delivery* of relief. The convenience of intravenous lines and the constancy of Patient Controlled Analgesia units, for example, had replaced four-hourly injections for surgical and terminally ill patients and enabled a measure of patient control over pain. Epidural anaesthesia, which had revolutionised childbirth, could be substituted for general anaesthetics in abdominal and lower limb surgeries and continued in the ward. Opioids were commenced during general anaesthesia, even as the operation took place, so that the days of waking after surgery and registering each painful bump of the trolley were long gone.

I remembered Mrs Mathews whom I had nursed through the final stages of breast cancer: her darkened room; her fragility and bone-thin body as I sponged her, and held her against me when, unable to use a bed pan, she painfully made her way to the bathroom. During visiting hours her husband had sat beside her bed, his head bent, asking, 'Is it time for her next injection?' When he wasn't there she had called for it as I went to and fro past her room, also longing for the regulated moment when I could unlock the Dangerous Drugs cupboard, draw up the morphine, administer the harsh intramuscular needle.

I remembered Hurst, yellow with liver cancer, his abdomen tight with ascites, the first patient in terminal pain I cared for as a junior nurse. He'd sat in bed cradled by pillows, without books, radio silent, his head turned to the window, young enough to be called by his first name.

I remembered Mrs Saunders, with an open wound that discharged intestinal contents onto her abdomen after a surgery gone wrong; who cried while I cleaned and dressed her excoriated skin, day after day; of whose distress I wrote in detail in the end-of-duty report to alleviate my outrage that she should have to suffer so much. And Miss Stevenson, the French teacher, who'd had to give up her job, bed-bound with severe rheumatoid arthritis, regularly admitted for surgery or nursing care. She marked university exam papers sitting rigidly upright, and took an age to settle for the night: the contents of her locker top had to be arranged just so, within reach, each pressure area gently massaged at length, each limb precisely positioned and re-positioned between pillows. I have a photo of her in her dressing gown in a wheelchair outside the Wellington Hospital Nurses' Chapel at my wedding, a dark wisp of hair in the wind, smiling sideways at the camera, guarded, unable to swivel her neck.

I turned off the television.

I thought about my brother David, aged eighteen, dying of motorcycle injuries and rare, undiagnosed gas gangrene, asking me, a third-year student nurse aged nineteen, why the injections for the escalating pain in the stump of his amputated leg were not working. He had fallen when his motorbike skidded in gravel rounding a corner south of Whanganui. A horse float, close behind, unable to swerve, had crushed his pelvis and all but severed his right leg. He remained fully aware through nine pints of blood on admission to hospital and, after amputation, the agony that followed.

I travelled to Whanganui from Wellington a few days after the accident, where I found my brother in a side room outside a ward (there were few intensive care units in those days). He was lying flat, his lower body hidden beneath a bed cradle, his head rolling from side to side. A plastered arm was hoisted to a pole; the other arm received a transfusion. Tubes drained bloodstained fluid into bottles beneath the bed. As I entered the room, his eyes, deep in the pillow, followed me, as if from the back of his head. He questioned me restlessly. I was a nurse, his knowledgeable older sister. As a child, I had played pranks with him, raced him on my bike, watched my mother rub his chest with camphorated oil and wrap it in warm flannels when he had one cold after another. Despite his 'weak chest' he had been a live-wire, popular, with a cheeky sense of humour. At college, he had been a gymnastic champion, graceful on the beams, able to walk the length of any hall on his hands. In my album, there was a photo of the two of us at Paihia, in our togs, in front of our Zephyr Six. I checked the drip and the drainage bottles and charts, reassured him, told him that, slowly, the pain would lessen and pass. I lifted his head and turned his pillow, sponged his fingers, cooled a facecloth and wiped his damp white face. Stroked his brown hair. Felt, for the first time, fear's physical clutch. So distressing was his condition that my twin brothers, Philip and Brian, six years younger, were allowed to see him only briefly from the door. In the passageway, the ward sister whispered of his distress the night he touched his stump and realised he had indeed lost his leg, and of the raging pain in that stump. 'He's got a long way to go,' she said.

I returned to Wellington; despite his fractures, amputation and extensive internal injuries David was expected to live. By the end of the week he was dead. I was working a late afternoon shift in Casualty, monitoring the vital signs of the severely injured young man I had accompanied to the X-Ray Department, when the news came through; news that an anaerobic, spore-forming bacillus had infected David's unchecked, tightly bound stump and multiplied in an absence of air, releasing toxins into his circulation. His rising pain and agitation, apparent on the day of my visit and typical of gas gangrene, had failed to alert the nursing and medical staff to his condition. As his clinicians later explained, the disease was a feature of battlefields where the soil was infected by horses carrying the bacillus in their gut, and rarely seen in modern hospitals; by the time they had unbandaged his stump, sighted the purple gas bubbling on its demarcation line and rushed him to theatre for further amputation, David was in irreversible toxic shock. He died on the operating room table where my parents, who had been waiting in the corridor, saw him for the last time. The involvement of the horse float was seen as significant. His pelvic injuries, it was now claimed, may have been insurmountable.

I thought too about how, for many years, the memory of my brother in the side room and the circumstances of his death had caused an ache in my chest indistinguishable from physical pain. So acute was the ache, I rarely spoke of David. I rarely visited his plaque in the lawn at the Makara Cemetery and was unable to enter his room at home where his bottle of Mennen aftershave lotion stood on a tallboy. I had no words with which to allay my parents' distress, nor they mine. Death evoked awkwardness and avoidance, the expectation that one deal with distress and silently move on. As a nurse I was trained to do this. But I took a long time to move on. Alongside the separation and 'cold truth' of loss, there was an abiding grief caused by the suffering I had been powerless to share or relieve, and by the knowledge I had not recognised David's symptoms. I was about to sit my State Final exams. I knew all I should know. My copy of *Surgery for Students of Nursing* (1961)[53] had warned, 'The mortality of gas gangrene is high', and advised that its development should be suspected in accident cases experiencing a rise in wound pain, at which point intravenous anti-toxin was essential. 'In the last war,' the text said, 'the best results were obtained when both anti-toxin and penicillin were given in adequate dosage.'

C.S. Lewis, in *A Grief Observed* (1961), described grief's physicality as akin to 'fear', 'dread', 'suspense', as a 'sudden jab of red hot memory'. 'The same leg is cut off time after time,' he said of the recurring emptiness, following his wife's death from cancer. 'The first plunge of the knife into the flesh is felt again and again.'[54] And he contrasted the temporal nature of his emotional distress with the constancy of his wife's suffering, likening emotional pain to the discontinuous dropping of bombs, and severe prolonged physical pain to the relentless onslaught in the trenches. 'What is grief compared with physical pain?' he asked. 'Whatever fools may say, the body can suffer twenty times more than the mind. The mind has always some power of evasion.' Lewis also wrote of the impossibility of sharing another's pain, observing that while the mind may condole, the body cannot – a concept which had prompted me to reflect on the bodily pain endured by my mother one night in a Whanganui motel room the week she waited for David's condition to stabilise. So intense and prolonged was the occurrence that my mother, convinced of the powers of prayer and mental telepathy, believed she had taken her son's pain on herself; the next day in the ward she learned that David had slept, without the need for medication, during the very hours of her torment.

I have wondered since if this apparent sharing, or even complete transfer of pain, could be attributed to coincidence: if a physical manifestation of stress, or of intense imaginative empathy engendered by the bond between mother and son, my mother's loss of two children in infancy, her personal knowledge of pain, Christian convictions and restlessly dreaming mind (she insisted she had been wide awake), had coincided with David's sleep of exhaustion.

I've hesitated, reluctant to assign the possibility of an act as profound as pain transfer, or sacrificial suffering, to chance. Had a supernatural event taken place, as my mother maintained? Did elucidation lie with Carl Jung's notion of synchronicity: in which the emotional mobilisation of psychic patterns, precipitated by an overwhelming circumstance, attracted affiliated happenings? Jung's theory was reflected in Arthur Koestler's view of the psyche as a 'psychic resonator', and in Koestler's description of the 'universal hanging-together of things, their embeddedness in a universal matrix'.[55] This belief was shared by Schopenhauer, for whom the finite status of causality was questionable since all was 'interrelated and mutually attuned'. 'When once compassion is stirred within me by another's pain,' Schopenhauer explains, 'then his weal and woe go straight to my heart, exactly in the same way, if not always to the same degree, as otherwise I feel my own. Consequently the difference between myself and him is no longer an absolute one.'[56]

In 2007, I would find a tentative neurological explanation for pain by proxy, although not for pain transfer, when cells in pain processing areas of the brain known as mirror neurons were shown to fire simultaneously, albeit nonsymptomatically, in both a person experiencing pain and a loved one observing infliction of the pain. Subsequent research would establish empathetic brain registration of pain in an observer when a loved one was subjected to pain out of sight (it was sufficient for the observer to simply know that pain was in place), suggesting that over-sensitive mirror neurons might, in part, hold the answer to my mother's shared experience. Empathy and compassion, researchers postulated, were likely to be strongest in those who have known extreme emotional or physical pain.

'From now onwards,' wrote Maxim Gorky, recalling a vicious beating as a young boy by his grandfather, 'my concern for others never let me rest for a moment, and, just as if my heart had been laid bare, I became almost intolerably sensitive to any insult or physical pain, whether I, or someone else, was the victim.'[57]

'The self and the other are just two sides of the coin,' elucidated neuroscientist and psychiatrist Marco Iacoboni.[58]

My mother passed away nearly thirty years after David's death, in a hospice, in the twilight sleep of a continuous morphine pump. But, as is the way with pain, all may not have been as it seemed. As the cancer progressed, an idiosyncratic response to morphine had caused her to hallucinate for weeks, believing she was in a concentration camp. When the medication was stopped and the world returned to normal, she preferred pain to the side effects of relief. She asked me to watch her closely for signs that she would need morphine again at the end. She had seemed peaceful, but what, I had agonised, of her state of mind and hidden dreams?

The sun had left the side of the building. I turned off the air conditioner and stood on the balcony. Below, a queue was forming outside l'Entrecôte – awaiting salad starters, sirloin steaks with garlic butter, fries and well-chosen house wines. Patrons dining alone read at their tables. John had quickly become a regular.

Later that evening I couldn't find the peaches I'd bought at the supermarket. The next morning, when I opened a bottle of Badoit, the two glass tumblers were missing. In the wake of the testing and alone in the hotel pain, the opportunist was trying to run away with me.

*

Standing on the balcony of our hotel room in Nantes, eating toast spread with honey and thinking about an article I'd read on wild hives in Poland, I saw, in the corner of my eye, a man at home in Kelburn, with a wire-netting trellis tied to his back and a lidded can, hammer and small hatchet to his belt. I watched him negotiate the steep rise to the pine. His progress was slow – a step forward, half a step backwards – but remarkable given the slope's absence of traction. Upon reaching the tree, he strapped himself to its trunk, which he gripped with his knees, and began hauling himself aloft cutting footholds ahead in the bark. A third of the way up he stopped, chopped an oblong hole in the bole and placed a syrupy comb from the billycan in the recess. Then he licked his fingers, nailed the trellis across the opening and descended, hand beneath hand, feet notch to notch. The entire operation, including his slippery moves on the hill, took less than an hour. 'Imagine that,' I said to John who was sitting at a patio table, his head in a newspaper. 'Soon there'll be a wild hive in the pine.'

*

Beam and throb

Late August 2004. We flew to Toulouse then drove to Languedoc, and La Balbaugette, my cousin's *maison de campagne* three kilometres from the village of Sorèze on the edge of the St James pilgrimage way to Santiago de Compostela.

This is sunflower country; on either side of the road, crops bow east and west, acknowledging the changing light, waiting for rain.

It is a region of spirited winds, the wild dreaming and interpretation of winds, the chronic bending of trees.

It is home to the *autan*, which makes autumn seem like spring and brings malice and happiness in the same breath.

From the eleventh to the thirteenth centuries it was a stronghold of the Cathars – converts to the greater religious purity of early Christianity's gentleness and poverty, before their denunciation as heretics, hunting down by crusaders, suffering at the hands of the Inquisition and the eradication of their faith. The Cathars believed the world was created, not by an omnipotent eternal God, but by a malevolent begetter, who had fallen from Heaven's perfection. Adherence to the strict creeds of Catharism (fasting, vegetarianism, pacifism, acceptance of reincarnation) were the means by which, over many lifetimes, earthly souls – held within the prison of the body – could be perfected and released to Heaven.

We spent an afternoon with Peter and his wife, Geneviève, at Carcassonne, a working walled city, once a Cathar fortress, in the hot dust of a tilting ground watching mounted knights recreate jousting and hand to hand combat between the Crusaders and the Trencavel nobles, protectors of the Cathars; and exploring the restored ramparts and towers from which sieges were repelled and lost while the population within perished in epidemics and died of thirst in the summer's intense heat. As we were leaving, storm clouds gathered overhead funnelling thunder, rain and a midnight wind through the streets. Lanterns swayed. Tourists converged in a narrow dash to the barbican and car park. The heatwave had broken.

At La Balbaugette, after the wind had died down, the shutters had stopped banging and the loggia and pool had been cleared of branches and leaves, time was given to the leisurely preparation and serving of food.

I lay as if in a field, beneath Indian lilacs, flowering laurels and the sky of the sieges, balanced between the Crusades and Inquisitions of Languedoc and the short-lived relief of the Edict of Nantes; themes of pain and transcendence.

Here, pain, skilled in the art of intrigue, spoke with a medieval tongue, posing questions about the blending of the pain of body, mind and soul with salvation; the dependence of ecstasy upon agony; the influence of the Middle Ages when the owners of hospices – centres of enlightenment as well as curing – sought portraits of suffering for their chapels so that, in the contemplation of intensely visualised distress, the sick, wounded and possessed might be persuaded to confront and come to terms with pain, to pray and, through prayer, achieve healing belief.

I pictured the life-sized figure of Christ on the Isenheim Altarpiece by sixteenth-century Bavarian painter Matthias Grünewald, commissioned for the hospital of the Antonite monastery in southern Alsace, where the triptych remained until the French Revolution and the secularisation of art and healing. And the centre panel of Grünewald's masterpiece, the crucifixion, which embodied not only unimaginable suffering – graphic wounds; the grey distortion of shock, exhaustion and the body's dislocating weight; the hidden suffocation caused by the pull of the stretched arms and sockets constricting the rib cage and lungs; the added torment of poor quality nails, inexpertly made, according to some medieval accounts, by women, used during crucifixions to intensify the pain – but also, through the symbolism of the lamb at Christ's feet, patient and sacrificial suffering as a means of redemption. On the panels either side of the pictorial disquisition, wings, supportive saints and images of the Annunciation and Resurrection were depicted, like Nantes, in the bathing, golden light of salvation.

I conjectured that the quiddity of serious chronic pain is uncertainty. This is pain, I thought, which even as it eases, seeks to return; escapes shape yet becomes a shaping force; raises walls but during phases of relentless attack breaks walls down; causes life to lose its leniency and also its steadfast form. Was there any coming back to the self I once was?

I closed my eyes and saw swinging doors: doors behind which I had found neither rampart nor crenellation, 'mirror of intuition' or rite of enlightenment and, while it would have been reassuring to believe otherwise, no new tolerance, patience or proof of learning. Only a heightened sense of Time, sometimes stoic, sometimes teasing, which replied when I said, 'I am sadder and more aware, but can I really say I am wiser?' 'You take what comes your way. You are what you are, as you were born, as you were raised, as you will always be.'

Today, I reflect on this view and find it still stands.

I consider, too, the example of Pope John Paul II, for whom the meaning of suffering was said to be found in reminding the rest of us that we cannot control our lives, and in eliciting from those who observe pain and its process an ennobling compassion. The view of the fourteenth Dalai Lama that suffering is unremarkable, and occurs because it is a 'part of nature and a fact of life', simply because the body exists. Thomas De Quincey, continually battling opium withdrawal, whose writings suggest a conviction that without pain the creative spirit and intellect will not fully develop. Voltaire's practical Pangloss, in *Candide*, who said of adversity: 'Private misfortunes contribute to the general good, so that the more private misfortunes there are, the more we find that all is well.'[59]

An aircraft hummed out of sight.

The pool robot wandered lazily around its tiled floor, tail sweeping, eating water.

John, Peter and Geneviève slept.

The house, once a byre and hayloft, its timber living-room pillars worn with the rubbing of cattle, absorbed the ancient silence of nearby Mt Berniquaut, dark with forest conifers and oppidum remains.

At twilight, a five-kilometre circuit of the nearby reservoir lake was scheduled. Afterwards, we would watch a firework display in honour of the Assumption, and return home to dine in the leisure room, previously a barn, open to the surrounding meadow.

Tomorrow we'd breakfast alfresco in the former hutcheries and sties adjacent to the well, visit a craft market, and lunch at a café famous for its strength-giving cassoulet before returning to Nantes.

'Say no to as much as possible,' a sufferer had advised online. 'Prune your life, forgo social occasions, don't plan ahead. You can only manage this condition day to day.'

The sun dipped and the sky lost its brilliance, but the air remained warm. Geneviève wandered out carrying chocolate biscuits and tea. Trying not to bend, I got to my feet.

A couple of days later, in Hôtel Dieu at the Centre Hospitalier Universitaire de Nantes, a 915-bed teaching hospital, the pain-producing nerve was released from sites of 'severe' entrapment on the right and left sides of the pelvis in separate surgeries, and transposed forward of the right and left ischial spines, in order to lessen tension.

'It's free in fatty tissue, in a more protected position,' said Professor Robert, crisp in a white coat on his ward round the next morning. He had treated over 3,000 patients with the same nerve pain from France and abroad since identifying the condition in 1987. Of this number, around 1,000 had required surgical decompression to free the nerve from mechanical entrapment. The operation was hardly routine. Nevertheless, Robert had reassuringly quipped, he could carry out the procedure blindfolded.

Less reassuring was the state of the nerve. Long compromised – the result, maybe, of adhesions following abdominal surgeries and stretching during difficult childbirths, further impaired by the Warsaw fall – Robert had found it to be 'folded', 'flattened', 'laminated and adhering to everything around it, including inside the [Alcock's] Canal' and 'along its whole length' – a situation he described as 'extreme' on the left side. I had read that the older the patient and the longer the entrapment (with seven years the critical indicator), the less likely surgical relief.

'I consider the nerve to be young until it's aged seventy,' said Robert.

The nerve, at fifty-nine, was young enough to recover. The accident in Poland was assuming new meaning. Without the exacerbating fall, I might unwittingly have pressed on, sitting, believing the pain to be a bursitis, until the nerve was no longer viable. Was the injury a rare *miraculum secundum naturam*? Had an event of wind and sun brought me to Nantes where poet René Guy Cadou observed he had encountered enough 'subjective coincidences' to suggest he lived in the city of Orpheus, tamer of wild animals and writer of mystical books?[60]

My experience of Hôtel Dieu was positive. The methodical, unhurried, mimed consultation with the non-English-speaking anaesthetist, the stringent antibacterial Betadine shower and the thoughtful drop of pre-operation sedation on my tongue encouraged confidence. I came to in the Awakening Room, with a cool rush of oxygen across my face. In the ward the nurses, immaculate in white fitted tops and tapered trousers, hair discreet, were attentive despite my halting French and the pressure of the *neurotraumatologie* environment. Alluringly scented lotion was rubbed on my back. There was a glass carafe of water on the locker. White rolls and butter were served on the breakfast tray. In the hospital's shiny yet solid common-sense order I felt secure, supported by a traditional European model of medicine.

Only the post-operative morphine was problematic. Delivered intravenously, its relief was unequivocal. But so was the glistening Māori warrior with the painted red face it sent in close-up on the first night, on the edge of sleep, to menace the room between three and six in the morning. The cubicle begged for a breeze in the heatwave, between bouts of thunder and lightning. The emergency helicopter took off and landed at intervals outside the window with a disruptive beam and throb. Intravenous drips running low beeped, call buttons buzzed, feet pattered, uniforms rustled, self-closing doors creaked. I lay on my sutures (necessary to keep pressure on the operation sites and prevent bleeding), stared at the small red glow of the ON light on the wall-mounted television set, and tried to stay awake. Where was the tattooed visitor from? The haka performed on the field where the Rugby Battle of Nantes had been lost? Convinced of the warrior's opioid origin, remembering my mother's response to morphine, I had the drug dispenser attached to the drip removed. '*Morphine, ce n'est pas accept-able!*' I said in phrasebook French to the questioning nurse, and to my aston-ished French roommate, a nurse, her nerve also decompressed the previous day and keen to keep her intravenous relief.

'I need to think of the pain as constructive,' I said to John ten days into recovery, as we leaned on a table, at bar height, sharing a sesame-coated panino and raspberry tart in the Nantes Monoprix café.

In his 'Second Manifesto of Surrealism' (1929),[61] Breton declared: 'Every-thing leads us to believe that there is a certain state of mind from which life and death, the real and the imaginary, past and future, the communicable and the incommunicable, height and depth, are no longer perceived as contradictory.'

The nerve, without the restriction of scar tissue, irritated by handling, was registering base level pain at an intense Yellow Six, described on the Com-parative Pain Scale as 'comparable to a bad non-migraine headache combined with several bee stings, or a bad back'.

I was reminded of my poet cousin, Potocki de Montalk, and his belief in the mystical power of words. And Paracelsus who had urged doctors to take lessons from 'old wives, gypsies, sorcerers, wandering tribes', writing, 'Resolute Imagi-nation can accomplish most things.'[62]

'I need to believe that pain is a welcome or appropriate presence,' I con-tinued. 'A brisk wind after monotonous calm. A burden with a purpose.' The scrutiny of rationalisation and curing magic was turning full circle.

'You could convert to Catholicism,' suggested John, remembering the prayer sheets in CPS green, yellow and pink from the Basilica of Saint Nicholas. 'Follow the example of the Pope.'

'Create my own miracle, you mean, by achieving acceptance and patience?'

'Or you could become a Buddhist?'

'Recognise that this is a physical pain, and know it is no more than a physical pain,' I said without assurance.

I walked cautiously from the café to the hospital for my final post-operative follow-up. My buttock muscles were in spasm. I felt as if I were walking through sand.

In the Service de Neurotraumatologie, a nurse showed me to a treatment couch. I lay face down as she swabbed the incisions, snipped the stitches at either end and noted a surface haematoma.

Professor Robert was called. He pressed either side of the wounds and helped me to my feet. 'Good,' he said. 'Remember that the original pain could be worse for six months, perhaps more. This is normal: the nerve has been assaulted. You may increase your medications. Don't return to work for eight weeks. Don't ride a horse or a bike.'

'The muscle spasms?'

'During surgery the gluteal muscles were forced apart with retractors [in order to uncover the nerve]. The spasms will lessen. Nature provides.'

'The flattened nerve – will it recover?'

'It's not possible to assess the success, or otherwise, of this operation until a year after surgery, or even longer.'

We passed from the cubicle, to the corridor where his students clustered respectfully at a distance, to the office. His secretary collated a travel authorisation and *Compte Rendu Opératoire* in French and, because of the entrapment's rarity and obscurity, a letter of explanation in English. The letter advised that the branches of the nerve on both sides were also affected and concluded that only time would determine the surgical outcome and ability to fully resume the activities of daily living and employment.

In a few days I would be on the other side of the world. I was seeking a lyrical moment, a prevailing wisdom, a conclusion worthy of the journey.

Professor Robert said, demonstrating, 'Bend and lift your knees so the nerve slides back and forth.' He held out his hand for the letter.

'The Edict of Nantes,' I murmured, the pain limited by the effect of his presence.

He clicked his pen.

I asked, 'Can I sit?'

He nodded. 'You can sit – according to pain.'

'How should I exercise – should I walk, can I swim?'

He spread the letter on the desk. 'Yes, but again, according to pain.'

A bed was wheeled past the office, sides raised, drip stand attached, the tube running between the drip and a mechanised syringe barrel timing and dispensing relief from inside a plastic orange case.

Professor Robert paused as if in thought, or perhaps for dramatic effect. 'Pain is the leader,' he said, signing the page.

4 But at the end of the body, the mind[1]

A memoir, 2004–2009

*

Warm air from the north pushed against the uninterrupted air of Antarctica, troubling the Great Southern Ocean. The wind lifted, releasing pine cones out of season, shaking the laurel bay's elliptical screen, tossing the kowhai's gold. The holly, shiny with rain, clung to the last of its small red fruit. In the town belt, the Kumutoto Stream rose without reserve and the hillside beneath the pine thickened with weeds, sooner than collapse and slide into the valley.

*

A shimmer of thistle

I returned from Nantes in September 2004, convinced of the power of positivity, confident of recovery, ready to regard the pain as finite and take up life where I had left off. The surgery had brought clarity and a way forward. The nerve had been sighted, the damage defined: pain, the mysterious puppet master, now existed in its own unemotional medical right. I signed on as Victoria University writer-in-residence for the following year, completed *Cover Stories*, commenced a second draft of *The Fountain of Tears* and, applying Professor Robert's instruction regarding the use of pain as a guide, occasionally sat for short periods.

The pain simmered and flared. This was to be expected.

At times it was surprisingly low. Early amelioration was not normally part of the plan. Had the nerve been moderated by its release and transposition, or by optimism and a placebo effect of surgery (*placebo*, in Latin, 'I shall please')? The placebo effect, whether a result of inert medicines used in drug trials or tonics and herbs in everyday use was well established; and the studies of pain-relief medications, in which more than 50 per cent of placebo subjects reported short-term relief, were especially persuasive.

I was aware of a study that had suggested a mind-body connection in the apprehension of pain. During World War II, US military physician and anaesthetist Colonel Henry Beecher observed that only a third of the wounded soldiers he interviewed in Europe had requested morphine post-operatively. Yet, in his pre-war study of injured civilians, he'd found that, despite less serious tissue damage, four out of five patients had called for relief. Free of the threat of battle and positive in outlook because they'd survived, the soldiers' pain tolerance thresholds were raised; anxious about not surviving surgery, the civilians' thresholds were lowered. Expectation, surmised Beecher, could impact on how one feels and heals.

What then of a sugar-pill influence of surgery, or even of place? Recent research suggested that 'just being in the healing situation accomplishes something'.[2]

The idea of a placebo effect, with its blurring of medicine's limitations, was appealing. Had I subconsciously designated Nantes and its golden light a 'portal of healing'? Was the Hôtel Dieu's expert, empathetic team part of the prescription? Perhaps the strong expectation of a return to normality, together with the reassurance of finally putting myself in somebody's hands, was also contributing to an unexpectedly rapid recovery?

'The individual on whom we operate,' wrote French physiologist and surgeon René Lerich in *La Philosophie de la Chirurgie* (1951), 'is more than a physiological mechanism':

> He thinks, he fears, his body trembles if he lacks the comfort of a sympathetic face. For him nothing will replace the salutary contact with his surgeon, the exchange of looks, the feeling that the doctor has taken charge, with the certainty, at least apparent, of winning.[3]

What of the television images in the hotel of Pope Jean Paul II amidst the *malades* at Lourdes – maybe they had imbued both location and process with a spiritual dimension akin to that of the surreal and symbolic thinking I'd adopted as I awaited relief? Certainly, the rituals of the religious excursion – the trains, the wheelchairs and stretchers, the Grotto – had invaded my imagination even before I left for France. 'In accordance with the Almanac,' I wrote in *Cover Stories*,

> she will travel in April
> when the blackthorn hedge
> is in blossom,
>
> before its prune-like
> fruit is taken for jam,
>
> before the shimmer of thistle
> and wild grass,
>
> to connect with the third
> daily train from Paris
> which arrives in time
> for cassis and white wine
> in the late afternoon,
>
> when the sun is still strong,
> the shadows truly restful.[4]

Were there also parallels between the pilgrims' search for the conventions of acceptance and caring at Lourdes, that released them from medical misunderstanding and 'linguistic abstraction', and my own awareness that pain's physical and emotional processes struggle for expression?

As to my original proposition of a placebo effect of surgery and place, it seemed possible that if sleights of hand and illusive manipulations were capable of bringing if not a cure, then relief, the backdrops and protocols of mainstream surgery, introduced at an appropriate psychological moment, could be similarly efficacious. 'The bigger and more dramatic the patient perceives the intervention to be, the bigger the placebo effect,' commented a placebo researcher on the results of a study that had found fake and regular arthroscopies had returned persuasive power-of-suggestion results.[5] 'Big pills have more than small pills, injections have more than pills and surgery has the most of all.'

But my partial reprieves, for whatever reason, were short-lived. Pain levels rose and fell. Battering flares arrived with no way of anticipating their onset or knowing for how long they would last. Fatigue was ever present. When the nerve eventually settles, I read, the pain mechanisms may need to be recalibrated – although some researchers question whether, in the case of long-standing pain, the wedged key can ever be completely freed.

*

From the second-floor bedroom, the pine dominated the sky. From the adjacent balcony, its clearly visible rough bark and soft brush breached the sough of city and wind. When I stood on the front path, the tree, dwarfed by the house, and the laurel, lemonwoods and holly not yet coppiced, was neither magnet nor distraction, even though its roots bordered the lawn.

*

Gathering mushrooms after a strident sky has run to black

I had stepped from eight purposeful months of diagnosis, travel and surgery, into a time of hoping, coping, trying to hold back the tightening circle of pain.

That first summer I wrote in my diary: 'Hot. Exhausted. Flares intensifying. Last night a moth, like a fan, at the window.'

A day later, head heavy with medication, walking into the city determined to live normally, I met a friend, a poet, who asked, 'How have you been?' Affected by her gentle concern, I told her, in tears. 'You caught me at a low moment,' I said.

In truth, the moments were days – 'viaduct days', when the pain was so relentless the bridge twenty minutes' walk from our front door was ever seductive. Like the woman in Aleš Šteger's 'Grater', I was being whittled away.

> Inside the madness of pain a window opened
> She stepped out and stepped out of her body.[6]

'You don't know what's on the other side,' John would say, recalling Hamlet.

'Pain can kill,' warned pain specialist Jennifer Schneider in *Living with Chronic Pain* (2004),[7] making clear that chronic non-cancer pain, which is notoriously undertreated, can cause patients to 'attempt to suicide more often than people without pain', and two to three times more successfully. Schneider observed that while depression is often a precipitant, sufferers who were not clinically depressed wanted to die because they were 'simply no longer able to tolerate their undertreated pain'.

'Chronic pain is a thief,' concluded Claudia Wallis, *TIME* editor (of a special report on pain, 2005).[8] 'It breaks into your body and robs you blind. With lightning fingers it can take away your livelihood, your marriage, your friends, your favourite pastimes and big chunks of your personality. Left unapprehended, it will steal your days and nights until the world has collapsed into a cramped cell of suffering.'

On the darkest days, I hid my head beneath a sheet and retreated to a cave in the Carpathian Mountains, in the high Tatras south-west of Kraków. It seemed right that I return to Poland. I liked to think that as the place of the pain's onset it held the power of reversal.

I approached the cave through cooling, knee-high wet grass and a small forest lodged in a cloud (visualising their dampening effects on the nerve).[9] Stopped to pick raspberries (my favourite fruit) from a bush as tall as a man (so there was no need to bend). Entered the cave's generous mouth (wide, so I could see the sky) and lay down on green felt at the base of its spine. I lay very still (the nerve was aggravated by movement), projecting my mind into the blue or night space beyond. The strain of the pain's physical and mental totality was assuaged by solitude – not by aloneness conducive to meditation or deep thought, for my brain under siege shut down, but by weightless, enveloping blankness.

During 'reprieves', apart from not sitting or bending, I forced myself to continue as usual. Fear of disconnection and fundamental alteration, jostled with

denial and the possibility that recovery was hiding nearby and opportunities need not be wasted. When I could have paced my activities to coincide with medication peaks and lulls in the physical bedlam brought on by moving around, I remained stubbornly mobile.

Continuing as usual meant reporting each day to Room 101 as writer-in-residence at Victoria University's International Institute of Modern Letters. (In George Orwell's *1984*, Room 101 was a 'torture chamber' in The Ministry of Love, in which one confronted one's own worst nightmare of fear.) Here, at a standing desk overlooking the city and the morning sun on the harbour, energised by the hum of conversation and bursts of laughter from the creative writing students in the workshop room next door, I pressed on with *The Fountain of Tears*.

The eighteenth-century legend of Maria Potocka – said to have been abducted by Tatars during a slave raid into eastern Poland and held in the harem of the palace of the Tatar khans at Bakhchisaray on the Crimean Peninsula, where she died – had haunted me for years. I'd first encountered Maria in Lesley Blanch's *The Sabres of Paradise* (1978). Blanch, researching her story of the 1834–1859 Caucasus Wars, had visited Bakhchisaray and seen the Fountain of Tears. The sculpture, she wrote, was thought by some to honour the memory of an 'adored Christian woman, Marie Potocka'.[10]

My family and middle name had leapt from the page. When a quick check in the *Encyclopaedia Britannica* confirmed Maria as the captive in question, and noted her immortalisation in 'The Fountain at Bakhchisaray', Alexander Pushkin's long poem of the khan's impossible love, I went in search of her. The story behind Pushkin's *poema* proved confusing, inconclusive. Nonetheless, by late 2003, prior to leaving for Warsaw (and falling), a first draft of the interwoven narratives of Maria Potocka and Alexander Pushkin was complete.

However the work felt source-laden and leaden, and Maria in particular seemed shadowy, removed from her psychological base. Although I had filed my research, she continued to hover, turning my ear, producing new snippets and insights. I'd departed for Poland in 2003, assuming the influence of place would subdue her and fill the story's emotional gaps.

Meanwhile, a friend, the literary editor Andrew Mason, was reading the work. On my return from Warsaw he'd called in to comment. I made notes as we sat at our dining-room table. But with the pain undiagnosed and rising, the challenge of bringing the khan's melancholy, Maria's alleged murder and the harem's indelible mood of romantic sorrow to life had seemed insurmountable.

In 2005, at the standing desk, fortified by distraction, outpacing the burning nerve and fog of medication with a sense of urgency and minimal revision, I deleted the research-driven detail and reframed Pushkin's poem of the faces of love with those of pain. The Warsaw fall had opened Maria's mind to me in ways I could not have imagined.

I transferred all that tormented me – confinement, displacement, vulnerability, uncertainty – to Maria's story of abduction, incarceration and exile. The khan's helplessness and grieving, the dislocation of Zarema the demoted first wife, the

faded dreams of Molesmes mistress of the harem, also played out as if from memory. So too the actuality of physical pain: in the castration room; the harem's birthing room; and in Maria's secretly embroidered tale of 'Tereus, Procne and Philomela' from Ovid's *Metamorphoses.*[11] (Tereus the Thracian king, husband of Procne, visits Athens, where he persuades Philomela – sister of Procne and aunt to his son Itys – to sail home with him. Upon reaching land, the king defiles Philomela in a cabin, severs her tongue and imprisons her with but a loom for company. Speechless, Philomela weaves a fabric on which she tells of her captor's savagery. The needlework is smuggled by a maid to Procne, who rescues Philomela. The sisters, wild with revenge, kill Itys, joint him, cook him, and serve him as a feast to his father.)

Links between detachment, memory and the transforming power of the imagination emerged as principal themes. Maria looked to her former life only to admit that although scenes were sufficiently close in her memory to touch, they were lost to distance 'unaccompanied by the imperceptible breath of the moment'. 'The most familiar,' she wrote,

> are as individual snowflakes,
> only visible
> before they reach the ground.[12]

Using as a canvas the strips of Crimean sky visible from her window, she repainted familiar artworks, knowing that 'while contentment is softly hued, there is little detail without brush strokes'.[13]

On pages supplied by a biddable eunuch, and under the pretence of drafting tapestry patterns, one thin grey sheet at a time, she compressed the fears and frustrations of everyday life into verse, asking

> Why keep this record –
> these questions,
> this conversation in pages,
> this rise and fall of reply –
> when no one will read it?[14]

She assumed the khan, who otherwise forbade the use of pen and ink in the harem, would dismiss the irregular spaces and lines as 'an odd infidel or European design'.[15]

Like Philomela, sewing in the close lights of window and candle, she secretly embroidered Ovid's balancing of the acts of mortals against the mythical acts of gods, as her own tale of change and transformation. 'Admire the swiftness of message, the immediacy of description, the way cadence directs connotation,' she recalled her father saying of the *Metamorphoses*. 'This is the wonder of words. They are painting and music. They alone carry sound and image together.'[16]

Alongside *The Fountain of Tears*, I wrote a personal essay titled 'Pain'. Maria's story was a layered affair. The essay, which documented the pain of the

previous year, was more direct. In Room 101, detached from domestic distractions, writing within a community of writers, impelled to place 'the best words in the best order' (as Coleridge defined poetry), I believed that whatever I wrote at the standing desk would be valid.

Later in the year, a colleague handed me an English translation of Alphonse Daudet's memoir *In the Land of Pain* (2002). 'This book has your name on it.'

I took a break from writing to lie on the foam rubber squab I used instead of a chair and read Daudet's brief but explicit account of the nerve pain and disability of *tabes dorsalis*. I was consoled by his honesty, grateful for the shared experience, thankful for his sanctioning of my own pain. One *could* complain about intractable non-cancer pain, and do so in graphic terms.

'How much I suffered last night,' he says. 'Sheer torture ... there are no words to express it, only howls of pain could do so.'[17] On another occasion he writes, 'Crucifixion. That's what it was like the other night. The torment of the Cross: violent wrenching of the hands, feet, knees; nerves stretched and pulled to breaking-point. The coarse rope bound right around the torso, the spear prodding at the ribs.'[18]

He spared nothing: his moments of terror, hopelessness and self-pity were as evident as his struggle for mental resilience.

I bought my own copy of Daudet's book and read it repeatedly, admiring the strength of his writer's eye, and the conciseness of the style from which his depths of resolve and endurance emerged. I noted that the translation was made from the unedited jottings he had kept for a final, semi-fictional work to be entitled 'My Suffering' (the jottings were found among his papers thirty years after his death), and wondered how frankly Daudet, a self-titled Vendor of Happiness, would have written his definitive work? Whether, in the manner of Auguste Renoir – crippled with arthritis, confined to a wheelchair for the last fourteen years of his life, painting with his brush wedged between his fingers or tied to his wrist – he might have erred, from time to time, on the light side?

I also questioned how many of those who had hailed Daudet's unflinching reflections truly comprehended what he had been through. Had they visited the land of physical pain other than occasionally or briefly? Had they engaged with a language beyond the capability of occasional guests?

'Are words actually any use to describe what pain (or passion, for that matter) really feels like?' Daudet muses. 'Words only come when everything is over, when things have calmed down. They refer only to memory, and are either powerless or untruthful.'[19]

On a sunny Saturday afternoon

I was in the garden. The family cats, Bozhbie and Bizhbie, sat on the slatted seat. They were sturdy British Short-hairs, one a feisty bi-colour, the other a gentle blue. I knelt on the lawn to stroke their dense velvet coats, hear them purr, watch their amber eyes squint with pleasure.

Nearby, an infant cedar. I rubbed its fragrant needles between my fingers. The conifer was a gift from an immigrant, a friend who had since returned to Russia, where he lived on a small plot in the countryside from which he called on Angels from the North, South, East and West to heal me. He also sent bottles of blessed oil and framed icons of Saint Matrona from the Pokrov Convent in Moscow – Matrona Dimitrievna Nikonova (1881–1952) who, blind and gifted with inner vision and the ability to heal since age seven, had calmed and stroked the heads of the sick. 'Stay away from hospitals and doctors, until it arrives,' he directed by phone when a parcel was delayed.

'He will plant another,' I wrote of his small tree in *Cover Stories*:

> He will light his fire
> with its cones.
> He will bottle
> its aromatic oil
> and send it by fast post
> to protect us
> very soon.[20]

The cats curled into sleep on the wooden slats, rough with dried lichen. At dusk they would slowly stand, stretch, and after a cursory check for prey would station themselves on the path declaring their territory. That evening they would wait without stressful expectation or neediness to be fed. Tomorrow morning they'd inspect the garden and neighbouring properties and return brushed with cobwebs and pollen, carrying the scent of viburnum on their paws from the damp lower lawn.

They were said to live within the repetitions of heredity, domestic conditioning and the largely colourless moment, with no accumulation of memory, no sense of progression from an understood past to an unfamiliar or imagined hereafter – for which reasons their capacity for suffering had been dismissed as minimal, rendering them suitable for pain research. Cats were reputed to be stoic, and less demonstrative of physical and emotional distress than dogs (which, as pack animals, were inclined to call for sympathy from humans and support from the pack). This stoicism had reinforced the belief that cats register little pain.

A few weeks earlier, Bozhbie's bile duct had become obstructed and her pancreas acutely inflamed. She'd crouched on the floor, unwilling to move. Approached, she flicked her tail. Picked up, she stiffened. Palpated by the veterinarian she bared her teeth and screamed, her eyes locked on John's. In keeping with contemporary human protocol that aggressive pain be treated aggressively, intravenous fluids containing an immediate release opioid were administered, and a pad containing a slow release narcotic was taped to her paw until antibiotics tamed the infection. She lay in a veterinary cage for three days, sedated, silently healing, soothed by puffs of feline pheromones from wall-mounted spray dispensers, rousing herself only to shake her bandaged paw and try to rid herself

of the drip. She was discharged with the opioid paw patch in place until recovery was complete. The vet said that if Bozhbie were afflicted with chronic pain she'd require pain management like my own, including daily scheduled medication for both relief and to prevent 'neural wind-up'.[21] Despite her higher threshold for extremes of temperature, and a superior production of natural endorphins, the physiology of our respective nervous systems was very similar.

Bozhbie's display had indicated excruciating symptoms. In the past, she had masked fever and pain, presumably so as not to alert adversaries to her vulnerability, and she would have been similarly circumspect in the presence of the vet. Her reaction, when examined, had evinced not simply a reflex action, but a conscious perception of pain.

I had found myself reading about cats and developing a new appreciation of our own cats' radiating warmth and calming, self-healing purr (the low-frequency sound waves of which are thought to result in cats experiencing fewer bone, ligament and muscle traumas than dogs). Our common responses to pain extended further. Behavioural studies of felines indicate states of withdrawal typical of depression, and the vocalisations of grief and loss. Far from living in a beige and grey circle fixated on prey, they respond at close range to a spectrum of purple and blue, yellow and green.

I stood up, rubbed my knees, leaned against the warm stone of the wall. The nerve was timed to heal at the rate of one millimetre a day. If its damaged pain-carrying fibres didn't regenerate, it would continue to fire off pain signals. If scar tissue had reformed following surgery, the nerve would once more become entrapped and the cycle of injury repeat itself. Either way, under constant and chronic bombardment by pain messages, the central nervous system would also become dysfunctional, refusing relief, extinguishing hope, closing the circle.

'At the end of the mind, the body,' Paul Valéry's Monsieur Teste reminded me, as he attempted to understand the 'geometry' of his own pain. 'But at the end of the body, the mind.'

The rosemary growing along the top of the wall released its scent, said to improve memory. The plant was top heavy and its roots were losing their hold in the dry earth. I broke off a twig. The plant needed little more than a damp breeze to keep it alive. A sprig beneath the pillow warded off nightmares.

*

The pine thrummed with cicadas – for seventeen years wingless nymphs sipping root juices in the tree's subterranean tunnels. Gums split sickle-shaped leaves, releasing the scent of incendiary oil. Wild spraxia trumpets burst into bloom vibrating with orange and yellow. At the edge of the lawn, near the entrance to the green belt, the late-blooming magnolia shed a large white petal.

*

The same, but another

As the momentum of diagnosis and surgery had waned and recuperation been deemed complete, pain, the extraordinary, ingenious, physical mechanism, was generally seen as having fulfilled its mission.

Increasingly, I struggled with the tendency of the pain-free to turn away. I recalled Brueghel's ploughman in *The Fall of Icarus* (1555),[22] for whom a boy falling from the sky into the sea was of no great moment, and the unperturbed ship in that painting which, as Auden reflects in 'Musée des Beaux Arts', 'had somewhere to get to and sailed calmly on'.[23]

'Pain is always new to the sufferer,' Daudet testified in *The Land of Pain*, 'but loses its originality for those around him. Everyone will get used to it except me.'[24]

I struggled in particular with the codes of 'dignity in silence' and 'let's pretend and the less said the better'. I rehearsed nuanced replies: *Not too bad. Not so good. As good as. Waiting and hoping.* In response to casual enquiries about my back, I joked, 'It's not my back that's the problem – I've a rat trapped in my pelvis.' In company, I was the odd one out, the one with an invisible, dismissible ailment. In my heart, I was pre-pain – at Wellington airport, en route to Warsaw, with a white Nike tick on my jacket.

This was a difficult pain to explain. I could call up descriptors and metaphors, but they alluded to physical trauma and ignored the mental ordeal. Moreover, conditioning had taught me that they were not the sorts of words the world wanted to hear. And I worried about wearing out family and friends. As Arthur Kleinman made clear in *The Illness Narratives* (1988), relatives and friends 'sit in the same waiting rooms' and 'travel through the same land of limbo, experiencing similar worry, hurt, uncertainty and loss'.[25]

I became uncharacteristically hesitant.

On the one hand, I was warmed by the trustful understanding of those for whom the nature of the pain was not in doubt.

On the other hand, a distancing 'I hear you're still having issues with pain' likened me to an underperforming department. Advice to 'breathe through the pain' from the survivor of a sutured finger irritated. Recommendations regarding diet and exercise rankled. A reminder that 'we all have problems' caught me short. An airy 'think positively and look forward' made me fume for days. '[W]hat a convenience it would be,' says Florence Nightingale in *Notes on Nursing*'s 'Chattering Hopes and Advices', 'if there were any single person to whom he could speak simply and openly, without pulling the string upon himself of this shower-bath of silly hopes and encouragements.'[26] I was as alert to misconception, whispers of exaggeration and suggestions of self-pity – to 'the genius and awkwardness of consolation', as Harriet Martineau observed – as a weakened animal to the threat of predators.[27] 'We are not the same, but another [...] all the time we are out of our own country,' William Hazlitt wrote in his 1822 essay 'On Going a Journey'. 'We are lost to ourselves as well as our friends.'[28]

John saw both sides. 'What else can you expect?' he said. 'People see you out and about and hear you laugh on the phone. They think pain's treatable and temporary because it usually is. They don't get to see your trench warfare one-thousand-yard stare.'

He saw my 'equanimity' as part of the problem. 'You put on a face. You don't always give a straight reply.'

'The difference between stating a truth and complaining is one of tone, and not everyone recognises that difference.'

He wondered if this reticence was inherited from my pioneer ancestors, or if it was to some extent generational. 'You were born as World War II ended, when people just got on with things. You were raised not to make a fuss.'

'As a nurse, I learnt to stay steady.'

'Your father never spoke to you about what he'd been through in Greece and North Africa.'

'Why would he, when he knew I couldn't imagine what he had been through?'

After my father died I had read, in the thinnest of sketches, his accounts of the New Zealand Division's campaign in Greece, and of his eight-man scouting party caught behind enemy lines during the Division's evacuation, on the run until a cruiser could be sent to uplift them. He concluded that he could write 'reams and reams', but the details might be 'boring to others'. I also learned that, in the desert, he was standing beside his best friend in battle as his friend's head was blown off; and that his claustrophobia, of which I was unaware, was the result of having been dragged from his burning tank.

'There's a fine line,' said John, 'between protecting people and shutting them out of your life.'

With Aristotle

I took the opportunity to find out how John felt about our life's change of direction. We were having breakfast. John sat at the table. I stood at the bench, quickly dispensing with my toast and tea so that I could lie down. It was more than two years since we'd lingered, sharing the newspaper. Although I missed the activities that were no longer possible – restaurants, dinner parties, the movies, the theatre, driving and being driven in the car – with pain all encompassing I hadn't dwelt on them. But John was not in pain. How much did my constraints affect him?

I cleared my dishes. 'Can I ask you some pointed questions?'

'Interrogate me, you mean?' He refilled his cup and moved to an easy chair.

I found a pad and pencil (I'm a keeper of records).

'Fire away.'

'I've been wondering about the pain's impact on you – all those things we no longer do?'

'One adapts,' he said. He agreed that he missed our outings at the beginning, especially the relaxation of sinking into a seat at the cinema on a Friday night after work. 'I go with what's presented without wasting time thinking about what I can't do.' He poured more tea. 'There was a synchronicity about your fall and my leaving varsity and setting up in practice – I was busy and wouldn't have been able to be out and about much anyway. Your situation actually liberates me to concentrate on my work.' (John, formerly an academic, was now a lawyer specialising in Accident Compensation Corporation appeals.)

'What are your thoughts in general about pain?'

'Mainly that you need to avoid it. I'm with Aristotle on that. "The prudent man strives for freedom from pain, not pleasure." These days I tell people who ask me how I am, "I'm not in pain." I've only known pain of the moment, solved by the pill of the moment. I can't grasp the idea of being in constant pain, with the restrictions it imposes.'

'And if you can't avoid it?'

'I suspect I might withdraw into oblivion, and all the problems that would flow from it – which would be a worrying thing.'

'Are you frustrated that I'm not improving?'

'There *was* frustration early on, but I've moved beyond the male belief that I must fix things up. I'm aware that one doesn't suggest remedies – I know that if there's something to be done, you'll do it. In the meantime, my mind's eased knowing that you have an inner life researching, and writing poetry and the novel.'

'How do you feel about our diminished social life?'

'It doesn't bother me. I like meeting people on my terms and for short durations – which I still do. Large groups and small talk are an anathema to me, and there's never been a guest I've been sorry to see leave. I like solitude, and we're alike in this. I don't need any other person but you.'

'Has pain affected our relationship?'

'I don't think so. I read files where the partner gets fed up with the situation and leaves because they feel the one who's ill isn't pulling their weight. I can see how this might happen if there are other underlying problems. But the pain came at a late stage of our relationship. I knew you. I knew you didn't put things on.'

'What's it like, living with someone in pain?' (John has clients who suffer chronic pain. He sees the added burden caused by medical and social misunderstanding and is grateful for my perspective. Sometimes he tells his clients about me, and hears their voices lighten knowing they are understood.)

'The pain's a dampener,' he said, 'especially when I come into the house and there's no sound and I know that things have been bad. But it's uplifting coming home and seeing by your face, and the way you're lying on the couch, that there isn't that strain there.

'I love to see you smile, it lifts my heart, it has added meaning these days.'

*

Was the pine threatened by a contagious disease? After years of shiny leaves and perfectly proportioned fruit, the little lemon tree nearby was ailing. Leaf loss bared its branches. Lemons, although unblemished, dropped early. There was more dead wood than there needed to be. I checked it for aphids, blisters and cracked bark. Shook its trunk to release caterpillars and whiteflies. Blamed spraying of the kerbside thicket of blackberries by the City Council. Contemplated a virus or a canker bacteria – and spread of the weakening disease to the pine, inviting sapwood infestation by beetles, necessitating its immediate removal. Internet remedies abounded: a dose of Epsom salts; slow release blood, bone and potash; a scattering of grass clippings; a good pruning; insertion of a nail through the inner stem to counteract copper deficiency. I opted to water the small tree by hand, at its base, so that relief would go straight to its roots.

*

At the salon

I was in the cave. The pain was sickening, exhausting. It scorched. It radiated into the nerve's adjacent structures and organs. It invaded my bones, my core. An increased dose of codeine offered an hour's partial respite. Immediate release morphine might double that time, but with whispering hallucinations around the door. A slow release narcotic wouldn't rise to the occasion. Opiates, as I had known from the beginning, were of limited assistance for nerve pain.

Codeine, at the low end of the spectrum, was a thin slip of linen between mind and spirit – barely better than nothing. I doubled the dose. Put the tiny pills on my tongue and swallowed them slowly, tasting their bitterness. Added a couple of rapid-acting paracetamol and waited for the dissolving oesophageal fizz to hasten and boost the codeine's imagined effect. Lay perfectly still at the back of the cave, on the floor – from which I could fall no further. Pressed the pain into the earth. Daudet describes 'the *tin tin* of my spoon in the glass' before he took chloral.[29] Michael Ondaatje's English patient, Count László de Almásy, listened for the clink of a glass syringe in an enamel kidney dish and the crack as the tip of the ampoule of morphine was severed.[30]

Days later, I stood in a corner at the hairdresser's near the washbowls, reading *On the Suffering of the World*. Schopenhauer was discussing animals: 'With the animal, present suffering even if repeated countless times, remains what it was the first time: it cannot sum itself up. With man, on the other hand, there evolves [...] an intensification of his sensations of happiness and misery which can lead to momentary transports which may sometimes even prove fatal, or to suicidal despair.'[31]

The gremlin turned the dial. The nerve ground and burned by degrees. The once pleasurable salon visit was a race against pain. 'Ready in an hour,' said the stylist, positioning me beneath a hot lamp to speed the process, and sending a junior for a cup of tea.

The line of clients seated before mirrors waited for Red Revenges, Cheeky Blondes, Glamorous Brunettes and Irresistible Coppers to take hold. At the same time, I realised, animals locked in cosmetic laboratories suffered in the cause of safer and longer lasting colourants, shine-and-protect shampoos, extra-care conditioners. My mood was low. But I was not clinically depressed. A hamster on a runged wheel came to mind.

I sipped the tea and reopened Schopenhauer at 'On Suicide'.[32] He asserted that 'the destruction of the body [...] is a deterrent because the body is the phenomenal form of the will to live'. And yet, I thought, covering the chapter title with one hand as the stylist inspected a lock and reset the timer, a body in perpetual pain is also a phenomenal model of the desire to die. Its agony is a kind of light.

Nietzsche, who understood pain, and whose uncertain diagnosis swung from the torment of a slow growing tumour to that of tertiary syphilis, wrote (in the voice of a Persian sage) before his irreversible mental breakdown, in *Thus Spake Zarathustra* (1892):

But the awakened one and the knowing one says: Body am I completely, and nothing else; and soul is only a word for something in the body.

'I'he body is a great reason, a multiplicity with *one* meaning, a war and a peace, a herd and a shepherd.

Your little reason, my brother, which you call 'spirit', is also a tool of your body, a little tool and toy – a little instrument and toy of your big reason. [...]

There is more reason in your body than in your best wisdom. And who knows precisely what your body needs your best wisdom for?[33]

I shifted from foot to foot, walked in and out of the corner. 'Standing,' a physiotherapist had said, 'contracts the small muscles required to keep you upright, increases metabolism, burns calories, strengthens your back.'

Cole Porter and the Tatar Khan

Sun filled the turret. My year's residency at the university had ended and I was re-establishing a writing space at home. Frank Sinatra was singing Cole Porter. He moved into a slow version of 'What is This Thing Called Love?'[34] I hummed, paraphrasing Porter.

What is this thing – called pain?
This funny thing – called pain?

I had been a fan of Porter, Crosby and Sinatra since the age of eleven, when I was given an old wind-up gramophone and a pile of their 78rpm records for Christmas (that summer, David and I had played the records in our backyard tent).

Who can solve its mystery?
Why should it make a fool of me?

I was thinking about Porter's unpublicised life of pain: the riding accident at the height of his fame that had fractured his femurs; the latter half of his composing life – twenty-one years – blighted by his irreparably damaged thighs, chronic osteomyelitis, the pressure of scar tissue on nerves, more than thirty brutal surgeries, almost constant suffering. Incredibly, he'd continued to hide his physical and mental distress in stylish phrasings and rhymes, saying privately of the psychological solarium of composition, 'It's the only thing that gives me the courage to wake up again in the morning.'[35] His right leg was eventually amputated at mid-thigh. The loss of his limb, coming after the deaths of his mother and then his wife, was too much to bear. Porter, exhausted, declined into reclusion and the physical breakdowns that led to his death. After he died, his relatives, it was said, told of never seeing Porter in obvious pain, or dulling his suffering with alcohol and medications.

I hung a blue crystal ball in the window. Sinatra's pace quickened. Pain was pressing me to finish and lie down.

> I've got you under my skin.
> I've got you deep in the heart of me.[36]

I set a small brass gong on a sill. Transferred Sir Richard Burton's six-volume translation of *The Book of a Thousand Nights and a Night*, jammed with reference markers, to a shelf (Burton's comprehensive Notes detailing Eastern practices and customs had been invaluable while writing *The Fountain of Tears*). I had 200 nights until September 2006, until the incline reached a plateau – less than a year to relief.

> Night and day you are the one
> Only you beneath the moon or under the sun.[37]

I moved between the packing boxes and shelves in tight circles. Shifting a pile of files, I lost sight of my feet and tripped, thudding onto the wooden floor, jarring my pelvis and fracturing my left wrist.

'I'm jinxed,' I told the hospital registrar once the complicated break had been reduced. 'Cole Porter's involved.'

This wasn't the first time I'd entertained paranormal intervention. In Warsaw, in 2003, reading in the hotel lounge after my fall, I'd chanced on an article in the *Guardian Review* by a biographer who described herself as 'battered and scarred for life' while writing about Byron. Entitled 'The Curse of Byron',[38] the piece detailed a sobering catalogue of events – including a fall, three broken ribs and a two-year baffling and incapacitating pain syndrome. Were poets averse to posthumous attention, I'd mused, recalling the infections caused by Potocki's mouldy archive when I was researching his life, and the possibility, advanced by the Polish translator, that his influence had followed me to Poland? Did writers who delved into other people's lives become the unwitting recipients of their own psychic acts? Could a biographical variant of Carl Jung's collective unconscious be at work, instigated by one or more of *The Fountain*'s factual characters – Maria Potocka, Alexander Pushkin, the Tatar khan, Lord Byron in a minor role? Had the Curse of the Khan (or someone else) overtaken the reference to Potocki and 'The Curse of the Count'? Did William Carlos Williams not write in *The Doctor Stories* (1984), 'I defend the normality of every distortion, every disease, every amputation'?[39]

The wrist healed, accompanied by commiserations and attentive signings of the cast. A plastered limb is a minor rite of passage: a common, visible injury with no call for social awkwardness.

My pelvis raised its baseline pain from a CPS Three or Four, to a Yellow Five, before escalating into an intractable flare. Professor Robert wondered from France if a haematoma was disturbing the nerve. The ensuing investigations proved fruitless.

*

I awoke to loud squawking and wailing. 'Seagulls – a storm on the way.' The pine, framed by the window, rocked at the foot of the bed. The ghost gum, in keeping with the season, stripped its bark, exposing rain-rippled limbs. On the Chinese chest, within reach, a bee sleepy with sweet syrup gripped the bottle of chloral hydrate on the front cover of Daudet's *In the Land of Pain.* The door opened. John had returned from his morning walk. 'Is the park full of gulls?' 'Not quite, but a couple of "quardle oodle ardles"[40] flew low over the cricket nets and then perched on a wire staring at me.'

*

Free light chains[41]

My friend Andrew had cancer – multiple myeloma, a rare blood plasma cell disorder. He'd fallen while out tramping, injuring his spine, the trauma revealing the hitherto silent condition. He found sitting difficult and needed a stick to walk any distance. His work as a literary editor was on hold.

Soon after his diagnosis in March 2006, he had written from a 'bubble of pain, far from the productive world': 'Like you, I find myself now in a situation I had never prepared for, and it's hard work. [...] The real pain comes from an injury very similar to yours, but presumably due to bone weakening caused by the cancer. [...] In my case, because of a fall the bottom vertebra has collapsed and fractured. [...] I've read and reread your essay on pain in *Sport*[42] and taken a strange kind of comfort from it. That's also why I've gone into some detail above, which I normally never do.'

My email in reply concluded with: 'Last night I dreamt that I was SITTING in your lounge watching you DANCE A JIG!'

'I love your dream,' he responded at once, 'and will hold fast to it (even though I've never been able to dance!). You must hold fast too.'

I'd known Andrew since 2001 when, recently returned from living in Poland, he'd edited *Unquiet World*. We'd met to discuss his interventions for purposes of 'clarity and precision and simplicity only', as he defined editorship, at our house in Kelburn and, on occasion, in his hilltop home at Mahina Bay surrounded by bush, overlooking the sea. His generosity of spirit towards my eccentric cousin (including the glee with which he encountered the missive of outrage Potocki sent to the *NZ Listener* when Andrew, as literary editor, declined to publish his satire on Katherine Mansfield scholarship) had made the process unexpectedly pleasant. In 2004, soon after I arrived home from Warsaw, he'd called in to encourage me to move *The Fountain of Tears* forward. I made notes sitting at the dining-room table. I was in pain but trying not to show it. Andrew had put his hand on my arm and said, 'Are you all right, Steph?'

Following his injury in early 2006 he underwent repeated rounds of radiation and chemotherapy and a gruelling two-phase stem-cell transplant. I prepared *The Fountain* for publication and, for a year, lived amidst the chaos of remodelling our 100-year-old house into an upstairs and a downstairs apartment.

We corresponded frequently, at times daily. Like Zbigniew Herbert's soldier in his poem 'Report From a Besieged City',[43] appointed to 'the supporting role of chronicler', we each might have claimed: 'I write down – not knowing for whom – a siege's history.'

I kept much of our 'history', initially as a means of staying abreast of the twists and turns of Andrew's treatments and condition. As the weeks passed, I read it as a shared diary of listening and telling – an interchange of 'free light chains', measurement of which marked the progression and regression of his illness.

Hardly a message was sent without reference to the consolations of nature. 'You must come to visit,' he wrote, 'and you must choose a day like today, when the weather and view were absolutely perfect and the tui were cavorting in the kowhai and a kereru decided to stroll along the deck and then stop by the front door to admire itself in the glass. And we must do it soon, before the winds start and I go into the horrors of the transplant.' At the time, he was temporarily 'in quite good health', no longer needing morphine in the morning to alleviate 'the nerve pain' and the numbness that he had described as 'ferocious' and 'like a solid block of fire' in his ankle and foot.

Throughout, Andrew clung to 'the notion' that things would improve, recalling his old history teacher's conviction of 'the inevitability of gradualness',[44] proclaiming his 'faith in the future'. 'How do you learn to accept [pain] as a permanent thing?' he wondered. 'Or must there always be something in the future, like your writing and your newly transformed house with its light and views, that keeps you going forward? Or is it for you just a matter of endurance, knowing that the pain will ease at times, and that you may find relief either with time or with something unexpected? What is it that keeps any of us going in the end? Interesting that such issues inform *The Fountain*, if in very different ways.'

Nogs and dwangs

All the while, the renovations proceeded apace. Each time I turned around a builder waited behind me to cut a hole in a wall or ceiling. On-the-spot decisions were made about profiles, trims, heating vents and the positioning of the double-hung windows. Urgent trips were taken to showrooms to inspect baths, basins, showerheads and taps. Sparkies and plumbers tripped over each other on the stairs. An apprentice mixed thinners in the kitchen. Saws whined. Hammers banged. Dust collected.

I'd decamped to a downstairs bedroom where I flicked between the khan's attempted seduction of Maria, and the nailing of nogs (aka dwangs); the chants of Nirali the healer, and discussion of vermin guard (plumbing); the opium-prompted reminiscences of Molesmes, mistress of the harem, and measurements for rebated kitchen carcasses (cupboards). 'Just let me get my head out of an eighteenth-century harem,' I pleaded one morning, attempting to absorb an involved explanation as to why the beam that would support the turret had to change direction. That afternoon, the underside of the floor of the turret was stripped away, and thousands of maggot shells swooshed down into what would be a new lounge, showering a builder who later had an asthma attack. (The shells had accumulated in a space containing a petrified possum, directly beneath the chair at which I once sat at the computer.)

Upstairs, the house had been pared back to its bones to reveal structural inadequacies. Parts of the floor were missing and there were temporary supports in place pending the installation of permanent steel beams of significant weight and the engineer's report on the required bracing. At night, I padded cautiously around with a torch, followed by the cats, invading the house's last vestiges of dignity; imagining myself in the belly of a whale or the framework of an airship. I picked up pins and nails for Andrew, which, to the builders' amusement, I left on ledges for good luck.[45] One day I found a huge nail, the longest ever, and put it aside for his stem-cell transplant.

*

There were more storms on the way. A congregation of black-backed gulls huddled in the middle of the cricket pitch, as if sitting on a hollow mass nest, their backs to the harbour. I counted them as I circled the field: 'Ninety-nine gulls on the grass, and three on the rim of the fountain.' A couple of sparrows pecked beneath a clump of fennel. There wasn't a butterfly, bee or magpie in sight. The caretaker came out of his shed with a rake and a bucket of topsoil. During the night, students from the nearby university hall of residence had broken bottles and stomped on the croquet lawn. I stopped to express solidarity and lament the breakdown in hostel regulation. Groups of young people regularly ripped the side mirrors and windscreen wipers from cars parked on Salamanca Road, kicked in our fence palings and stumbled around our lawn. We'd upgraded our garage door and positioned a sculptured head near a window overlooking the street. Our neighbour had installed an iron mesh roller on his carport. A house a couple of doors down had been barricaded with a stout plank fence. The caretaker scattered and raked the topsoil and patted it with a light hand. His purple bucket was a nice sight on the grass. The next day, the croquet lawn was fenced off with blue twine, and a sign read PLEASE KEEP OFF RENOVATION IN PROGRESS. 'I don't know what's happening out at sea,' said John at the end of the week when the first storm hadn't arrived. 'The crows are not to be seen, and the gulls are still there, a hundred of them, on the field.'

*

Oh, for a gem necklace

Surgery's two-year touchstone passed without relief. My inclination, as a former nurse, was to let conventional medicine take its course.

'Adopt the pace of nature: her secret is patience,' advised Emerson[46] – who also claimed, 'He has seen but half the universe who never has been shown the House of Pain.'[47]

But there was no negotiating with the pain. It had developed a life of its own. The need for relief is primordial.

I underwent a course of Healing Touch, or energy healing. An article in *Kai Tiaki: Nursing New Zealand* (2003)[48] described a gentle hands-on or hands-off therapy, used in conjunction with traditional medicine, designed to reduce pain, relieve stress and facilitate healing by re-balancing one's energy fields. Encouraging results were reported from programmes implemented in Wellington Public Hospital's neonatal and obstetric and oncology units.

The practitioner I visited was a registered nurse of my generation, who saw patients free of charge in her own home. I climbed up onto a treatment couch in her sun-filled apartment overlooking the sea and lay, eyes closed. She swung a crystal and moved softly around the table, adjusting the energy fields in the surrounding air, occasionally and lightly placing her hands on my body. I left soothed, the pain lessened. The symptoms intensified as soon as I started moving around (as the nerve either failed to glide or was irritated by its adjacent muscles). But I believed the nurse's quiet, gentle attention had been beneficial: she was calming, and I liked to think that at some level a soothed mind assisted physical healing.

An Ayurvedic physician visiting from Kerala called at the house, his consultation facilitated by the owner of our local dairy whom he'd treated for a 'bad back'. I was keen to believe that his holistic science of healing and 'positive health', incorporating daily routines of diet, exercise and mental discipline, and living in harmony with the seasons, held an ancient secret to relief. The practitioner, reassuringly authentic in a Nehru jacket, listened carefully, asked medically appropriate questions, checked my tongue, took my pulse closely watching my face, and concluded that since the nerve had been damaged in an accident, relief was beyond his expertise. He offered to email herbal remedies tailored to offset the side effects of my medications and advised visualisation and meditative practices to distract the pain.

Neither transcendental meditation, which I had practised intermittently for years, nor mindfulness, which was on everyone's lips, was helpful, although I didn't doubt that recognition of thoughts, moment to moment, and adoption of an enquiring, open and accepting mind assisted the management of temporary and low level pain.

A visit to a highly regarded Chinese acupuncturist who'd relieved a friend of the pain of trigeminal neuralgia was unproductive. The acupuncturist listened intently and produced detailed anatomy books, which he laid out on a bench for perusal. He raised again the possibility of ischio-gluteal bursitis, and, refusing payment, concluded that apart from suggesting a heat lamp he could not help me.

A session with a cognitive behavioural psychologist, to whom I referred myself on the enthusiastic recommendation of a friend of a friend, was likewise disappointing. I stood against the pleasant young woman's consulting room wall on a grey afternoon, acid washing through my pelvic floor, muscles in spasm, listening to an explanation of 'healthy thinking' and cognitive modulation or reinterpretation of pain. I stared at the printout of a chart on which I was expected to record my pain management options and endorse my awareness of the potential outcomes of my choices. I might have responded like Richard Jefferies who wrote to a friend: 'If I wrote a volume I could not describe it to you, this terrible scorching pain, night and day. There is nothing in medical books like it, except the pain that follows corrosive sublimate which burns the tissues. […] I dread to go a few miles alone by rail lest I throw myself out of the window of the carriage.'[49]

A friend in Hong Kong had recently sent a book on 'gem therapy'. That afternoon, the prospect of a high-purity gemstone necklace dissolving blockages responsible for disharmony, pain and disease sparkled; and the wisdom of the Azerbaijani professor, about whom I'd read in Ryszard Kapuściński's *Imperium*, who healed using the scents of flowers and leaves, was also therapeutic, just to consider: 'Rx: Laurel leaves. Ten minutes a day. For three weeks.'[50]

I had held hypnotherapy, my strongest alternative, in reserve. Now, a *TIME* article reported the flourishing use of hypnosedation during surgery. 'The typical pain signal,' elucidated a University of Iowa study, 'follows a well-worn path from the brain stem through the mid-brain and into the cortex, where conscious feelings of pain arise'; however, in hypnotised subjects, the '"ouch" message doesn't make it past the mid-brain and into consciousness'.[51]

'I can see,' agreed Andrew, 'how, if pain has a physical cause which cannot be ameliorated, and so is constant and inescapable and varies only in degree, the only way to control it is by addressing it in the mind.' Andrew would seek relief from his own pain through complementary practices, including Healing Touch.

There was little doubt that I'd be a suitable subject. In 1968, I'd successfully undergone hypnotherapy with the eminent Welsh hypnotherapist Arnall Bloxham,[52] husband of Dulce de Montalk (Geoffrey Potocki's sister), during a visit to their Cardiff home. Earlier in the year, I'd experienced a protracted first delivery; since I was again pregnant, Dulce, a former nurse, suggested that Arnall, who'd practised obstetric hypnosis, predispose me to a less problematic second event.

In addition to conventional hypnotherapy,[53] Arnall was renowned for reportedly regressing, and recording the journeys of, hundreds of deeply hypnotised subjects into former lives. Some of the participants had been regressed in order to source an intractable mental or physical problem, others to prove or disprove notions of reincarnation.

John and I listened to a number of these tapes on the evening of our arrival. The incarnation that left the deepest impression was that of Graham Huxtable from Swansea, who was polite, mild and dismissive of reincarnation. In a trance on a couch in Arnall's office three years earlier, Huxtable had become an uncouth, illiterate eighteenth-century gunner's mate on a British naval frigate at the time of a blockade of the French off Calais. A battle was relived, during which Huxtable's leg was blown off. The raw force of the seaman's pain, and the urgency in Arnall's voice as he ordered him back from potentially fatal trauma and shock, were unforgettable.

As I recall, Huxtable awoke breathless and with pain in his leg but no memory of his regression. (Even so, Arnall declined to revisit that life despite a request from Lord Mountbatten, former First Lord of the Admiralty, who'd obtained a copy of the tape.) The blockade was subsequently dated, and Huxtable's incomprehensible naval slang translated by historians at the National Maritime Museum. Sceptics protested that the phenomenon of regression was attributable to 'cryptomnesia', or memory of facts one forgets one knew. 'Huxtable's either the greatest actor of all time, or there's truth in this,' John had decided.

I was not regressed. I did not even lie on a couch. The next morning I sat at Arnall's desk with my eyes shut and was talked into a relaxed state. The day was cold and misty, the office warm and cosy. Arnall, grandfatherly, pricked my hand with a pin and, as suggested, I felt only a blunt touch (after the session, the pinprick was still visible). During induction, the telephone rang in the next room and Arnall excused himself and left to answer it. I sat on, listening to the brief conversation feeling pleasantly present but uninvolved. Upon returning, Arnall (accurately) addressed the physiological processes of late pregnancy and labour and the roles each should play in facilitating a straightforward delivery; he instructed my pelvis that, should foetal malpositioning occur, it would enable negotiation without undue delay. I left Wales unconvinced. Later, in New Zealand, after a strong fifteen-hour labour, I sat up in a cubicle fresh with spring flowers, and said that I could repeat the experience next week.

Although Arnall's instructions had not held for subsequent deliveries, I retained a certain faith in hypnosis. In late 2006, I spoke by phone to a therapist who had relieved a woman's chronic pain on television; three months later she remained pain-free. My expectation was modest: the ability to switch to thinking that would change or dampen sensations when the pain became intolerable.

'Chronic pain is caused by a failure to forgive,' said the therapist, who happened to specialise in regression.

'But the pain comes from a nerve that was entrapped in an accident.'

'You'll need to forgive the person who caused the accident.'

'I slipped in a pool of water on a bathroom floor. Are you saying that I need to forgive myself?'

I rang another practitioner, a psychologist. He demurred. He didn't believe that persons distracted by pain made good subjects. Nonetheless, he offered to predispose me to post-hypnotic suggestion in two sessions, after which I should see how I went myself, with the aid of tapes.

On the day of hypnosis, he discussed the induction and deepening during which, as I reclined in a chair covered by a rug, my eyes, body and extremities

would become progressively heavy. He moved on to the therapeutic, or sugges-
tive, phase. He detailed the return. My eyes, he agreed, would remain closed
until he asked me to open them.

Oddly, I began to feel uneasy and delayed the induction with questions and a
conversation about the Bloxham tapes (with which the therapist was familiar).
When I could find no firm reason not to proceed, I prepared to 'go under'. But in
less than half a minute, my heart began to race and miss beats. The unease turned
to panic when I tried to say that I didn't want to continue, but my voice seemed
blocked: I'd been told I could answer questions while in a trance – but could I
initiate them? Oblivious, the therapist continued his routine of relaxation. Had
my blood pressure dropped, as he'd advised it might? I felt faint. Would I remain
incommunicado, heart fast, and perhaps even pass out, until I was counted back?
I mustered concentration and tried to drag 'I want to stop' from my mind to my
mouth. Finally, to my astonishment, I blurted the words out. The terminology of
hypnosis, identical to that of anaesthesia, had opened the subconscious mental
pocket that stored the Hong Kong Caesarean section.

'I think you're absolutely right to explore every option available,' emailed
Andrew. 'If we abandon hope then we might as well give up altogether. And,
especially with nerves, that is NOT an option. Remember Henry Cooper, to
whom a setback was only ever a setback, never a defeat.'[54]

'*Dolor dictat*,' I said, quoting the Romans.

Directly overhead, the builders hammered and staple-gunned the new apart-
ment's echoing floorboards.

*

The sounds of reconstruction were matched by those of the bare-eyed cockatoo on our neighbour's balcony imitating a telephone, repeating her name, berating the sparrows and tui that flew past her cage. Her wings had been clipped and the cage triple-locked ever since she escaped to a wire across the street, where, despite seeds and entreaties, she screeched until dusk and the arrival of an animal rescue team with a ladder. I wondered what she was thinking the day she made her bid for freedom? Why head for the busy road? Why bypass the dappled light of the ngaio in which heavy-winged kereru caught their breath? The brush of the pine? The soft heart of ti kouka? The kowhai's spring blaze buzzing with nectar-drunk tui?

*

Becoming an oyster

I opened the blank computer document that would become *Vivid Familiar* (2009), another collection of poetry.

Memory of the airship framework of the hollowed out upstairs apartment lingered. Notions of isolation, and of living in limbo, floated within reach. Ovid's *Metamorphoses* again came to mind. And a couple of lines from the tale of the escape of Daedalus and Icarus from exile on Crete wearing feather and wax wings:

> … So then to unimagined arts
> He set his mind and altered natural laws.[55]

An extended fantasy of liberation, less dependent on the precision of metaphor than on enigmatic fable and metonymy, started to take shape. I typed onto the screen:

> I was finished with geegaws
> and tyre tracks in the mud,
> with waiting for whales to surface
> and distinctive geysers to blow,
> with throwing myself from bridges
> only to swing by a rope
> tied to my ankles.[56]

A *sensitiva* – a spirit, a figment of feeling, a personification of the seat of sensitive power believed, in medieval psychology, to reside in the front of the brain – appeared at my kitchen window. She lifted the sash and said:

> 'Sell your car,
> cover your garden with potash;
> take east from the moon,
> west from the stars
> and wind from the breeze;
> confront the plain wood of your house
> and sun-strengthened corner
> with tableaux of stone and soft light
> at a mappable edge of the sea.'[57]

The figment 'waved a handful of basil and thyme which she chopped and softly shook in a tin'. Summoned an aerostat 'moored to a tripod on wheels' to the front lawn. Insisted that I leave now,

> 'while memory is less reflection
> than the sudden tripping of fragments.

The air is still delicately sentimental,
and the season has much
to recommend it.'

'Turn your pen outwards,' she encouraged,

'thicken your ink,
stroll for the sake of strolling
and sit to think.'[58]

During the summer of 2007, I put the poem aside while we moved into the upstairs apartment – accompanied, in my case, by foolish bending and lifting. A flare began to build. It continued, unrelieved, through the winter – a ball of burning, clenching tissue in and above my pelvic floor, a tumbleweed of pain with nowhere to go.

A specialist attributed new symptoms – swollen, reddened, burning fingers, and back pain provoked during showers – to reflex sympathetic dystrophy (RSD),[59] also known as complex regional pain syndrome (CRPS) and causalgia.

Unfamiliar with the condition, I asked, 'Do you mean the body's overloaded with pain?'

'In a nutshell,' he said, recommending the addition of anti-epileptic drug Neurontin to my regimen in order to further dampen the pain pathways.

But, as the pain intensified, a rebellion of brain chemistry rendered me sensitive to medications. The Neurontin caused the walls between rational and irrational thinking to break down and had to be stopped. I also discontinued the amitriptyline, on account of heart symptoms. Given morphine's disturbing hallucinations, I was reluctant to take opioids stronger than codeine, which even at an increased dose had little effect.

I thought longingly of the Bromptons Cocktail that I had once poured for terminal patients unable to tolerate morphine, in the 1960s – its combination of heroin (for pain) and cocaine (to assist clear thinking) had relieved not only pain but also fear and anxiety.

Could I make a case for laudanum, still available on prescription in the US and UK? Probably not: a pharmacist I phoned said, 'It's not even listed', and Google research showed that the drug of today was no longer a tincture of 'whole opium', but a 'denarcotised' product consisting principally of morphine.

'You're grey with pain,' said my doctor. 'This is a nightmare. I have cancer patients who are better controlled than you are.'

I went to bed for six weeks and lay flat, standing only to eat and drink. I took the example of Ivan Turgenev, whose life I was following. When pain struck, Turgenev, yet to suffer the final distress of his spinal cancer, became an oyster. 'As it turns out,' he wrote, 'one can go on living even when one is incapable of standing, walking and riding.' He continued, 'Look at oysters. They live like this. I have even come to the conclusion that it is quite all right being an oyster.'[60]

The pine, backlit by a white sky, was unwatchable. I ordered venetian blinds and lay with my back to the windows until they could be installed.

Daudet described unremitting pain as 'an infiltration': as '[finding] its way everywhere, into my vision, my feelings, my sense of judgement'.[61]

Aleksander Wat spoke of its 'mask of ugliness on everything, on all the beauties of the world'.[62]

Harriet Martineau knew it as 'a thick heavy cloud of care'.[63]

John said, 'I'd want morphine, *Band of Brothers* style, straight into the thigh.' And that if I were an animal in continual suffering, it would be kinder to put me to sleep.

Blinkered eyes open, sinuous legs webbed

I read obsessively about pain – in the traffic of the Internet, the witness of pain narratives, the idealisations of self-help manuals, the neurobiological, psycho-social and cultural examinations of pain published for a broad audience. Distraction had run its course.

When I couldn't sleep, I shared the experiences of fifteen New Zealanders with arthritis, whose plainly told stories were collected by fellow sufferer Mary Ciurlionis in *A Twist of Fate: Tackling Arthritis* (2003).[64] Those with the most severe form of the illness spoke about the fatigue, the multiple joint surgeries, the 'huge strain' on their families, days when they wanted to 'shout and scream' that they could not tolerate any more pain. Each concluded by emphasising their blessings, and the need to see the disease as a part, 'and only a part' of their lives. I was comforted by their camaraderie, but unable to adopt their positivism.

Was there a character in fiction who mirrored my predicament? 'It is writers,' David B. Morris suggested in *The Culture of Pain*, (1993) 'who have proved especially interested in understanding the place of pain in human life […] in creating – not just observing – the social and personal meanings we make out of pain.'[65]

But while there were any number of subjects believably portrayed in acute pain, states of sustained pain were hard to find. In *The Truth About Chronic Pain* (2004), Arthur Rosenfeld (not a sufferer) confirmed literature's absence of authors writing from the cliff face of this condition.[66] Lous Heshusius – who wrote about the 'hell' and 'depletion' of more than a decade of untreatable neck pain following a car accident in *Inside Chronic Pain: An Intimate and Critical Account* (2009) – also pointed out that 'little that conveys the depth and detail of day-to-day living in pain, as experienced and recounted by the sufferer, is available'.[67]

However, the travails of Ivan Ilych in Tolstoy's *The Death of Ivan Ilych* (1886) rang true. Indeed, the story of Ilych's journey into self-realisation through acute pain, which became chronic pain, then terminal pain, read like a template for writing a chronic pain narrative today.

Ilych falls. The acute pain he sustains passes to a dull ache. The ache turns into an intense and constant pain. Clinicians are mystified and prescribe random medicines. Ilych continues to work. He reads medical texts. Goes from doctor to doctor. Feels isolated, changed, irritated by the thoughtlessness of friends. Is swayed by a report of a wonder cure. Tries to think himself back into health. Questions the strength of his mind. Secretly takes medicine prescribed by a 'homeopathist'.

The pain becomes unendurable, inexpressible. Ilych is misunderstood. He longs to be 'petted and comforted'. Opium and injections of morphine do not bring relief. His wife becomes impatient. He lies in his familiar room, with his familiar pictures and furnishings, 'and the same aching, suffering body', and begins to moan. Weeks pass. He stares at the back of his sofa, reviewing his life, searching for deeper understanding of pity and forgiveness. At one point, he can say of pain, 'Well, what of it? Let the pain be.'[68] But the pain will not 'be', and before long, his moans become screams.

I marvelled at Tolstoy's genius in bringing the anguished body and mind of Ivan Ilych to life. Had he based the novella – written following his own spiritual crisis – on the suffering of someone he knew? Were his insights gained during the Crimean War at the Siege of Sebastopol, where he encountered pain as it really was? Where, as he wrote in *Sebastopol*, in the hospital in the Hall of Assembly, he saw seriously injured men who 'love to see a sympathetic human face' and 'talk about their sufferings' and 'hear words of love and interest'. Where he would have liked to convey his 'sympathy and admiration', but could find no words and was dissatisfied with those that did occur. Where a man in 'intolerable agony', asked how he feels, 'merely mutters: "There's a gnawing at my heart."'[69]

I wondered whether personal experience was the key to achieving narrative proximity, and how reliably a 'pain naïve' author might lift the bodily distress of fictional characters to the reader's imagination. Was 'being there' the reason Tolstoy could write, as he left the Hall of Assembly: 'the beholding of the clear sky, the brilliant sun, the splendid city, the church, the soldiers moving about, soon brings your mind back to its usual state of frivolity, petty anxieties, and absorption in the present alone'?[70]

I turned to literary non-fiction – to stories fixed in actual examinations of body and spirit, fate and necessity. The composer Douglas Lilburn articulated the way I was feeling at that time. Examining the turns of history and circumstance in *A Search for Tradition & A Search for Language* (2011), he cited the 'humanity as well as the technical brilliance and originality' of the music written by 'a post-war school of Polish composers'.[71] The 'crucible of European suffering', he wrote, 'formulated' their achievements. 'We don't inherit such things overnight, we must earn them. [...] And I suggest the true lesson of all of this is that human experience is the valid and essentially unique thing, be it in Warsaw, or, as Denis Glover said, in Johnsonville and Geraldine.'[72]

Essays, biographies and poetry of authors who'd lived through twentieth-century European and Russian suffering were piled on the chest beside the bed. In their measured intelligence – in their chronicles of endurance and awareness of what was possible, in the challenge and value of the moment and the notion that all else is history – I felt validated, and absolved of the need to rationalise and explain.

'Can literature save your life?' José Saramago was asked, after a serious illness.[73]

'Not as a medicine,' he replied, 'but it is one of the richest springs from which the spirit can drink. Perhaps it can't do great things for the body, but the soul needs literature like the mouth needs bread.'

Storks with ribbons

My reading also relieved me of the expectation that, sooner than withdrawing to the floor of the cave, I should pass beyond, or be greater than pain.

What does transcendence of pain mean? The phrase is everywhere, distinguished by mental images of a rising retreat by the soul to a place in the mind where freedom is found, or a grove in the shade of which one's body can rest. Does it imply saintly patience and inner peace? The state of intense and sustained concentration achieved by monks? Warlike defiance, confrontation and re-grouping? Submission? Survival? A reason for being?

'Pain has two senses,' C.S. Lewis said of the meaning of the word in *The Problem of Pain* (1966).[74] There is pain 'below a certain level of intensity', and pain that is 'synonymous with "suffering", "anguish", "tribulation", "adversity"'.

Transcendence of the physical toll and mental strain of chronic bodily anguish, I decided, is a consoling and uplifting myth. For those who have not known such pain, the myth counters witness of another's suffering and fear of one's own. For the afflicted, it offers suffusion of pain with literary, philosophical or spiritual meaning, and aspirations of stoicism and heroism. 'Pain provides an opportunity for heroism,' agreed R. Harvard.[75] In the appendix to Lewis's thesis, he says of his observations in general practice that 'the opportunity is seized with surprising frequency'.

The dark eyes of Isak Dinesen (1855–1962) and Frida Kahlo (1907–1954), synonymous with transcendence of physical pain, stared from the bookcase.

Isak Dinesen endured the effects of syphilis (incurred during her marriage) in its tertiary form, together with those of mercury and arsenic treatments. A fabricated encounter had enabled her to negotiate and seemingly rise above this ordeal. In 1915, in a hospital room, a fantasy she called the devil offered to 'transform everything that happened to me from then on into a story'.[76] Forty years later, she explained that, naturally, 'he [set] certain conditions for his assistance. And it is, I guess, from around that time I called upon him most urgently that I stopped recognising or taking physical pain into account.'[77]

Dinesen's spinal pain and gastric crises, problems with balance, numerous surgeries and malnourished state provided, observed her friend Aage Henriksen, 'the power and the means to go through another person's bones and marrow and to open up his inner world of dangers and unslayable hope'.[78]

Her suffering also enabled her to affirm publicly the positive role of fate in her life, to fashion rationalisation into belief, and to create a personal legend of strength in the face of pain. 'As my innermost nature teaches me, whatever is necessary, as seen from the heights and in the sense of a *great* economy,' she wrote, – 'is also the useful par excellence: one should not only bear it, one should *love* it. *Amor fati*; that is my innermost nature. And as for my long sickness, do I not owe it indescribably more than I owe to my health?'[79]

However, behind her public courage and among confidantes, Dinesen remained earthbound in her pain's progression, shedding veil after veil. In *Out of Africa* (1937), she recalled a story of misfortune she was told as a child, in which the victim's faltering, repetitive footsteps traced the outline of a stork. Dinesen's impulse to elevate her frailty was unmistakeable. 'I will remember [the tale] in the hour of need,' she wrote. 'The tight place, the dark pit in which I am now lying, of what bird is it the talon? When the design of my life is complete, shall I, shall other people, see a stork?'[80]

Frida Kahlo sustained serious spinal, pelvic, leg and foot injuries when the bus in which she was travelling collided with a streetcar. She was eighteen. Ahead lay chronic suffering, some thirty-five surgeries, amputation of her right foot and the close to fifty-five graphic autobiographical portraits of physical torment Diego Rivera called 'anguished poetry'.[81]

All the while, Kahlo bore open witness to 'grace under pressure', as Ernest Hemingway characterised courage. On canvas she confronted her reality, eyes staring, mouth set, and her tragic body – as seen by Carlos Fuentes – a symbol of Mexico, 'a country that has been made by its wounds'.[82] In company, she was an Azetc goddess, bright with ribbons, flouncing skirts and spectacular jewellery.

But her domination of pain was a brave act. Reading her diary, published as *The Diary of Frida Kahlo: An Intimate Self-Portrait* (1995), I was moved to find the extent to which her art and personal magnetism had masked fragility. The *Diary* was kept during the last decade of her life when her condition worsened, and, like Daudet's *In the Land of Pain*, it was not intended for publication. In confronting images and poignant, poetic streams of thought, Kahlo reminisces and mourns. She speaks to friends, the baby she never had, of her love for Rivera, the troubled interior and exterior of her body. On plate 41, entitled 'Yo soy la/DESINTEGRACIÓN' ('I am/DISINTEGRATION'),[83] she is set atop a classical column wearing a wide skirt. In this scene – perhaps reminiscent of her accident, at which time a steel spike passed through her pelvis – discarded body parts float alongside: the hand and eye of her art, a second head – her mental coherence, her resilient spirit – severed at the neck.

For myself, transcendence, if I choose to call it that, means patches of near normality in the transient lightness of lesser pain, when there's a lull in the trenches – 'when things have calmed down',[84] to apply Daudet's conclusion that pain cannot be verbally expressed in the moment of pain. Or, to extend Montaigne, 'when I dance I dance, when I sleep I sleep',[85] and when I'm in the sort of pain that Lewis places as synonymous with suffering, I'm in pain. Any suggestion that I appear to be 'coping', or 'managing', or even 'overcoming', merely indicates a persuasive pretence – an attempt to ease the burden of close observers and raise my sense of self worth. Like Aleksander Wat, I can take shelter in 'tiny boats of poetry',[86] but until they reach port the small crafts remain fragile, wind-tossed, at the mercy of the storm.

A lake without a silver foundation

Also on a bookshelf: Ruth Harris's *Lourdes: Body and Spirit in the Secular Age* (1999). Harris, a historian who travelled to Lourdes with an undiagnosed and uncertainly treated condition (now resolved), addressed questions as to why, in the new secular and scientific climate, the 'golden age' of Lourdes still prevails.

Touched but not converted by her experience, she examined the Sanctuary's historical and still crucial contexts; at the centre of her work was the 'omnipresent' and 'often inarticulate expressions of the body and of physical pain'. Pilgrims came to Lourdes, she wrote, because 'neither suffering nor its alleviation were easily contained within the defining power of language'.[87]

I studied a photograph of 'Procession of the *Miraculés*' (1897),[88] commemorating twenty-five years of pilgrimage. Thirty thousand sick and dying patients had arrived in a specially equipped, traditionally plain white train. Over 300 *miraculés* travelled in carriages painted papal white and yellow. The participants – in wide-shot a divided sea of black – were supported by companions and attendants, coach drivers, hoteliers and shopkeepers, nurses, nuns and priests – all speaking the same language, pain the lingua franca.

Today, as science quickens, and the philosophical, mythical and cultural appeasements that once imbued pain with meaning diminish, the language of suffering contracts. This, despite our living into older and older age and an epidemic of chronic pain as medicine prolongs lives as never before.

True, illness narratives abound as 'wounded storytellers' try to make sense of their suffering. Blogs detail personal distress. Illness forums and Facebook pages overflow with information and sympathy. Laypersons, demonstrating competence in medical language, download peer-reviewed studies, interviews, the mights and maybes of the latest research, even footage of surgeries in their field of interest. But with the words of 'sharing and caring' largely exchanged at a distance, sufferers continue to fill the clinics of counsellors; and the tangible assurances of complementary practitioners, chants of healers and trances of mediums are as necessary as they ever were.

In his 2012 article 'Is Facebook Making Us Lonely?',[89] Stephen Marche argued that the 'web of connections has grown broader but shallower'. He wrote: 'We were promised a global village; instead we inhabit a drab cul-de-sac and endless freeways of a vast suburb of information.' Concluding that solitude once enabled 'self-reflection and self-reinvention', and that 'connection is not the same thing as a bond', he reflected that 'we are left thinking about who we are all the time, without ever really thinking about who we are'.

'Can someone call me,' a young man on a pain forum pleaded. 'I need to speak to someone. I'm in a rough patch right now.'

Although the Age of Understatement has given way to an Age of Confession, outside medical science and cyberspace the language of pain is declining when it might be gaining its defining power.

What has been the effect, I ask from my vantage point, of the assertive climate of wellness, exercise, physical perfection, the righteous cry of health-care, and the replacement of strolling and seeing with jogging, speed walking and scanning? At this point I note the irony of living alongside a daughter who holds twenty-one New Zealand track, road and cross-country titles, a world ver-tical (stair racing) circuit title and two mountain running world championships, and has represented New Zealand every year since 1994; who speaks of the pain of pushing her body to its limits, building endurance, the power of the mind; who runs through tapes to applause, endorphin rushes and personal bests. The winter I was 'an oyster', she was a participant in the Blue Planet Run:[90] a non-stop relay of twenty athletes running 25,000 kilometres around the top of the world in ninety-five days to draw attention to the global lack of safe drinking water. She was wearing out five pairs of shoes running through sixteen coun-tries, testing herself in places like Siberia and the Mojave and Gobi Deserts. Praise for the pain of athletic endurance and other heroic overcomings of pain, observed David B. Morris in *Illness and Culture in the Postmodern Age* (1998), leaves 'a difficult legacy for chronic pain patients, who cannot surmount their affliction in a moment of glory, but must live with it unpraised and often unob-served day after day'.[91]

I also ask, at what cost have the enhanced outcomes and heightened expecta-tions of modern diagnostic and treatment protocols altered attitudes to pain? Short hospital stays and scant attention to rest and recuperation are now the norm. In clinics and wards, life-threatening events aside, impressions of indiffer-ence and presumptions of mere indisposition prevail. The patient as 'one who suffers' (Latin *patiens*, from *patior*, 'I am suffering'; Greek *paskhein*, 'to suffer'), is 'one who is under medical care or treatment' – a customer, a client.

While recipients of passing illness and pain fit the modern model without significant repercussions, for those struggling in chronicity's 'continuous cycling from damping to amplification of symptoms, from marginal functioning to dis-ablement',[92] the language of care and concern falters, and isolation and uncer-tainty deepen. I agree with the journalist Julia Magnet, whose forceful article in *The Sunday Times* (2003)[93] argued that nursing skills, now in decline, still matter. Magnet, who suffered from a chronic condition, had been admitted to a famous London hospital where, though sedated, she languished 'in pain and ter-rified'. Lamenting the decline in clinical expertise and the absence of the 'essence of nursing', she said of the 'uber' theoretical nurses who attended her that night (who, verbally, gesturally, personally, were rewriting communication of pain): 'Their training has robbed them of the language of compassion.'

'Pain has an uncanny power to throw us back on thinking styles absolutely basic to who we are,' observed David B. Morris in his Foreword to Lous Heshu-sius's *Inside Chronic Pain*.[94] Julia Magnet had reverted to journalism, Heshusius to research in academic mode. During the months when the pain was at its most remorseless, my reading was in large part influenced by the features of my formative years: childhood observations of pain, teenage experience of pain, my training as a nurse. The focus of my thinking – the sifting and distillation of each minute, each telling personal detail; the perception, as Jung puts it, of background processes – caused me to shape and contain events within the suggestion and essence of poetry and the intimacy of essay, memoir, biography.

I recorded each day of the insatiable season. I had the same ear for pain as a musician for perfect pitch. I thought of Nina Cassian's poem 'Pain':

> This is pain I told myself keeping vigil,
> This is how it hurts.[95]

Occasionally, a fine shining mist clung to the air, shaped by all who passed through it.

*

There was an additional problem: the fast-growing ghost gum that belonged to the watercourses, tin roofs and late pastel skies of Australia, that lamented our unsettled springs and nonsensical summers, was blocking the sun on our north-facing windows. We sawed a branch from the tree, but the gain was minimal and the raw patch on its trunk wept reproachfully for months.

*

Looking ahead

In 2007, as winter closed, Andrew came to inspect the new apartment.

We stood at a window overlooking the valley in what he christened my Raj Room (rattan furniture, large kentia palm, covered veranda), watching magpies swooping like kamikaze pilots full tilt at the pine. I pointed down to the garden, to the small sago palm that had belonged to my mother. Six years after she died I had lifted it from an indoor pot to free light and root spread. Within a season it shed its protective barbs and revolute leaves and etched itself in the earth. Now, nine years later, it was awakening to a strengthening frond and swaying acceptance of moss and small creepers. Andrew spoke of it often. I'd sent him a photo of the small plant putting forth a shoot, after his transplant.

We had long anticipated this visit – the cake and fine wine I'd serve, the Gregorian chants during which Andrew would smile and nod his head. That day, he was in a great deal of discomfort. The myeloma was, for the moment, quiescent, but the pain of nerve damage remained. He arrived at the door carrying his cane. Tried a selection of chairs for comfort. Settled stiffly on a sofa guarding his lower back. Sipped a cup of tea, but hadn't felt like a biscuit.

As his mobility and flexibility had slowly improved, and 'pain became a guide as to what [he] should and shouldn't be doing', the prospect of chronic pain had been a daily concern. 'Permanent pain relief is promised,' he wrote hopefully as the cancer went 'into abeyance, at least for the moment', and options for 'reconstruction' of his spine were explored.

'The ticklish subject of life expectancy' also came up. 'Myeloma is notorious in this regard,' he wrote, bringing me up to date on his latest oncology report, 'with an average life expectancy of three years after diagnosis. But mine is an exceptional case, it appears, and the possibility of an autologous stem-cell transplant, whereby all the bone marrow cells are removed, nuked and then put back in, was raised. This may increase life expectancy by up to ten years.'

In July 2006, following a particularly complicated 'bone marrow aspirate', and as the uncertainty of nerve damage took its toll, he observed that he was now 'resigning [himself] to experiencing pain of different kinds and in different places for a long time yet'.

A couple of months later, out and about again, he was 'reasonably confident that with time the pain [would] pass altogether. But the walks do remind me,' he said wistfully, 'how far I have to go to return to something close to normal. What I would previously have regarded as a prelude to a good walk, an easy amble before lunch, becomes the target in itself, and quite a hard thing to achieve by the end. Enjoyable though that walk is – being out in the wilds and the sun and wind – I become acutely conscious of what I have lost so suddenly, and wonder just how far I will be able to go towards regaining it.'

That afternoon, despite all, Andrew was looking ahead, seeing a naturopath.

I spoke of resignation and confinement to a sofa.

'Remember the sago palm,' he emailed when he arrived home, hoping I might 'gradually find that there is less to be resigned to!'

I too still had choices, none of them heartening.

Should I go the way of a pain pump, or intrathecal drug delivery system, which, implanted beneath the skin of the abdominal wall, delivers narcotics via a catheter into the cerebrospinal fluid close to the spinal cord? The direct route allowed for lower drug levels, meaning fewer side effects, including hallucinations, but had potential for catheter blockages, pump dysfunction, dosage irregularity, infection and leakage of cerebrospinal fluid.

What about neuromodulation: a spinal cord stimulator, implanted in the lower abdomen or buttock area, with leads to the spine to confuse the damaged nerve's incessant firing of pain signals, enabling the spinal 'pain gate' to close and stop the signals from reaching the brain? An invasive procedure, unwieldy 'hardware', an unreliable outcome. A pain specialist advised that while such units were usefully employed in a range of neurological conditions, the outcomes for pelvic nerve pain were mixed, and that my nerve's bilateral involvement meant I was unlikely to achieve the 50 per cent reduction in pain considered a success. There was a chance the pain would worsen following implantation.

A five-day intravenous ketamine infusion under either sub-anaesthetic conditions, or, if undertaken in Germany or Mexico, in a medically induced coma? High doses of the drug were said to 'shut down' a dysfunctional nervous system. In theory, one's system reset or rebooted itself when it was brought back to life. Hallucinations were promised. I read that a patient had awoken from a coma unable to walk and talk. Where I was concerned, resetting the system might achieve partial short-term relief, but was unlikely to remedy the pain of ongoing nerve trauma.

One day, I thought, when pain gives up its secrets – when inexact control of symptoms is replaced by precision relief that targets the mechanisms of transmission – the idea of living with intractable pain will make people shudder in the same way that surgery without anaesthesia now fills us with horror.

Falling to bits

Word was out that a surgeon in Sydney was about to become the Southern Hemisphere's first pudendal neuralgia and entrapment specialist.

In September 2007, three years after decompression in Nantes, I flew to Sydney, via Christchurch. The same rigmarole: standing on the domestic flight, lying flat on the international leg, semi-reclining across the back seats of taxis.

The surgeon understood the depth of the pain. 'This particular combination of neuralgia and myalgia is the worst possible,' he told John. He suggested a threefold approach: surgical clearance of the abdominal adhesions of past surgeries; bilateral cortisone blocks to calm the nerve; injections of botox into the pelvic floor to reduce muscles that had thickened through clenching in response to pain and hours of standing, and that were compromising the nerve. Desperate for relief, I agreed, despite my reservations about botox. The measures were speculative; the only certainty, uncertainty.

Following the interventions I was discharged to a rented apartment where a ferocious flare – a delayed effect of the nerve blocks – developed. A specialist from whom I sought advice on future pain management recommended daily methadone and, for 'breakthrough pain', liquid oxycodone (a semi-synthetic opioid similar to, and more potent than, morphine). The drugs should be started at paediatric doses and titrated up slowly to discourage hallucinations. He said firmly: 'You must say "The pain's unbearable, I'm not prepared to *bear* it any longer."'

Shortly before I was due to fly home, and with the new medications on hold, I was readmitted to hospital with increasing core weakness and a sense of impending collapse.

The symptoms had started the day after surgery. The anaesthetist who had called by was just leaving. As he shut the door, I registered an odd sensation somewhere near the pit of my stomach – a muffled clunk, as if a rock had hit sand. A dent in a dry lakebed flashed into view. I'd dismissed the event, keen to leave for the apartment. But over the next week I began to feel shaky. Insomnia set in. And my sensitivity to medications was heightened. The buprenorphine (semi-synthetic opioid) patch prescribed for the flare caused cardiac irregularities and had to be discontinued; and a racing heart and faintness after starting the antibiotic, keflex, resulted in admission to A&E at four in the morning. By day ten I felt as if I were melting inside.

In the ward, in the last cubicle before the fire escape, an endocrinologist outlined testing for Conn's Syndrome. I scrabbled in the locker for my notebook but found only a pen. John, sitting nearby reading *Moby Dick*, transcribed the specialist's diagnostic comments inside the book's front cover: 'Hypertension + hypokalaemia = primary hyperaldosteronism. ECG borderline. Nodule on adrenal gland?'

'It's uncommon,' said the physician.

'Of course it is.' John handed back the pen.

'It might explain her drug reactions.'

The ensuing debilitation went beyond fatigue. A plug had been pulled. My battery was flat. Even the sound of John in constant touch with his office, coaching a junior barrister through a case in the Court of Appeal, was taxing. How was I going to get home?

The full extent of my frailty became apparent one afternoon in the waiting room of the X-ray Department. A man on a cot-sided trolley was wheeled in and left beneath the blaring, wall-mounted television set. He became restless and agitated and looked around. Called for a nurse. Plucked at his sheet. Stared into the glare of the fluorescent lights. I stared too, unable to cross the room and assist him.

'Chassis intact, battery flat,' I wrote in my diary.

The investigations were non-conclusive. 'Is the anaesthetic responsible?' I asked, tremulous on the side of the physical cliff. 'The cortisone? The botox? Stress? A silent virus?' Heads were shaken. Five days later, a tentative diagnosis of 'de-conditioning' after six weeks' bed rest, a circumstance not likely to improve swiftly, was made. I returned to Wellington on the verge of profound depletion. Airport wheelchairs were necessary, even though I could not sit. In the absence of a lie-flat seat and with the plane full, I stood for the three-hour flight.

'You'll be right by Christmas,' said my doctor.

My freezer was stocked with celery

I had flown too close to the sun.

I barely left the house for over two years. There were days when I couldn't talk on the phone, even though my thinking was not affected. At times I felt too weak to breathe. The doctor, phlebotomist and hairdresser visited.

Is this 'some sort of exhaustion which is taking the form of a dangerous illness,'[96] Yury Zhivago wondered? He had been similarly debilitated following his escape in high winter from eighteen months' captivity in a partisan camp in a Siberian forest. This is 'an illness with a crisis; it will be like any serious, infectious illness'.

Is it the physical equivalent of depression, I puzzled? Has my overtaxed body shut down as an exhausted brain shuts down?

I set myself alongside Yury, who recovered in a season. 'I must be having typhus after all,'[97] he decided. 'It must be some special form of typhus which isn't described in the textbooks.'

The enforced inactivity reduced the pain. During especially acute waning, when my body seemed too spent to send pain signals to the brain, I experienced the unfamiliar, disorientating lightness of no pain. What were these new coordinates, this sublime state?

'Submit to uncertainty,' said the airship captain in 'Feathers and Wax',

> 'you are now lighter than your surroundings.
> Reassign with relief
> warriors taking tight steps and shouting,
> women jousting at the height
> of their powers,
> insignificant birds gliding
> until the last possible moment.
> Such is my record of care
> I once sailed as far as
> the organism-free air of the Arctic.'[98]

Meanwhile, the oxycodone produced hallucinations if not used sparingly, and in view of US Federal Drug Association publicity about methadone's potential for toxicity I did not start that drug.

A possible cause of the perplexing energy deficit appeared on the Internet, in 'significant debility' as a rare consequence of medical (as distinct from cosmetic) botox related to the spread of the neurotoxin distant from the site of injection. My immune system's in rejection overdrive, I decided. On board the blimp,

food had run low,
the rum had lost its bite,
and I longed for coffee
with a spot of milk broth
and the unrefined grain of a loaf
baked in a generous tin.

I yawned and stretched,
tired of standing at the telescope.
Tired of dreaming I hunted crickets
and wild pigs without success,
and netted seals for livers
which I ate raw
because I was too drained
to care,
because the night gasped
and blew through my skin,
I had lost my bright voice,
my freezer was stocked with celery,
and despite advice from the captain
that soon pliant stems would steam
beneath sepia suns
[…]
arrival at the dotted line
where the reef ran out
seemed as likely as a tartan rug
at a picnic covering a clump
of Scotch thistles.[99]

In 2008, Andrew entered a 'grim period'. My problems paled in comparison. But he rallied, and at the end of November he was photographed on Mt Kaukau, overlooking Wellington.

*

The tree feller arrived with a chainsaw and ropes to remove the cramped holly, lemonwoods and laurel bay from the upper lawn. At the end of the first day, the grass was thick with the sawdust of felled branches and trunks reduced to firewood. On the second day, the empty spaces were weeded and replanted with cream and crimson camellia and mauve agapanthus. In the fever of clearance, my mother's sago palm was lost. Thereafter, the newly visible ngaio bared its moss-speckled branches and assumed the shape of a fan. A ponga curl on the lower lawn could now be seen. And the pine appeared in clear view from the porch, where the *sensitiva* raised a restless arm, waved as the airship hovered and touched down, and called:

> About time.
> Breakfast's ready,
> coffee's served,
> thanks for the postcard.
> I've trimmed the tawa,
> harvested the karaka,
> boiled the kopata
> and split the kindling.
> A kereru has toppled the bird bath.
> The compost is stacked and smoking.
> The ti kouka flowers,
> gathers strength,
> pushes its heart upwards.[100]

*

The life

In January 2009, Andrew died. Still too debilitated to leave the house, I could not attend his memorial service. I read, and was moved by, his letters instead – the letters he had written with such clarity, compassion and courage, supporting me during his own difficult times.

In his last message, in December, he had awaited the outcome of his latest radiotherapy, saying, 'Pray for success!' He spoke of the 'consolation' of his garden, and of sitting in 'our light-filled room watching the sea and the hills, the birds and the clouds'. And of the growth of the life of the mind as 'physical capacity reduces', 'as if in compensation'.

He was keen for news of *Vivid Familiar*, which was nearing completion, and asked if I had ever thought of writing a memoir. 'No rush to reply to this,' he finished, 'why should there be?'

In April that year, the FDA issued a Black Box warning regarding the medical use of botox, confirming that, rarely, minute particles of the neurotoxin could leave the site of injection and enter the circulation, triggering severe health problems and even fatalities.

A couple of months later, I watched a television documentary about contemporary Russia.[101] A young man was interviewed in what was once a dismal communal kitchen. Asked how the Russian people cope with adversity, he replied: 'They cope by separating their Life and their Everyday Life. Their Life is something special. It's the spirit life, realisation, achieving through work, writing books, having relationships. The Everyday Life is shopping, cooking and eating, washing dishes. The Everyday Life is not important to the Life.'

I spent a second year indoors. Confined to the sofa, I fretted about muscle loss, reminding myself that the New Zealand pioneers had barely moved on cramped emigrant ships for three months; while the captains of epic voyages of discovery, infrequently in ports of call, did little more than watch the wind and plot courses for years at a stretch.

I paced the house in small increments, and figured that by walking two lengths over the course of a day I would equal a cabin passenger's 'constitutional' on deck and perhaps surpass the exertions of those travelling steerage.

I had researched the pioneers as I wrote a cycle of poems for *Vivid Familiar* that extended the theme of escape in 'Feathers and Wax'. The poems were prompted by my dual relationship with New Zealand as both home and a remote outpost that engendered a longing for elsewhere; they emerged as explorations of pain – the psychic pain of settler separation, dislocation, perpetual uncertainty; of the horses in the ships' holds.

Raised in the sway
and stiffen of broad-leafed trees

they had known light
and blessed darkness.

Now, they slept
with their eyes open

night to night,
and ate with their ears

simultaneously cleaving
and folding as if

amongst lions.
They saw no new dawn.

There was no stepping back.
Only wave spray,

and the ocean's halters and ropes
on their long pale bones.[102]

The depletion started to ease in small steps from the first to second lampposts. But my battery's cells still emptied quickly and were slow to refill, and there was no way of knowing if I would completely recover. The enforced rest placated the nerve, and the burning in my fingers lessened (indicating, perhaps, a resetting of dysfunctional neural mechanisms). But the pain was only containable as long as the 'halters and ropes' were not loosened.

Summer arrived. Holiday highways beckoned from the window. Everyone was out and about. Barbecue smoke wafted past.

I lay on the balcony making shapes of the clouds – a swan, in honour of Mallarmé;[103] a white bee, in obeisance to Neruda.[104] When I felt most confined, I visualised myself lacing my sneakers, pocketing the key to the front door and taking the track beneath the pine to the park. Here, I watched the caretaker trundle his paint dolly and mark out the seasonal sports field. On the best days, wind roared through the row of pohutaukawa trees bordering the croquet lawn, blowing spray from the fountain onto my face.

Am I isolated or solitary? I wondered. Have I been randomly confined, or gifted with seclusion?

In his last message, Andrew asked if I had considered writing a memoir. He hadn't mentioned this before. Did he mean I should write a pain narrative?

Cicadas thrummed. The cats hunted them down, scattering their translucent bodies on the carpet and batting them, alive or dead, with their paws. Wasps and white butterflies, attracted to the balcony clothes line's green and pink pegs, hid in pillowcases and sheets.

I had a recurring dream in which I walked towards a tarsealed horizon, pain and depletion free, only to find, as a car approached at speed, that my legs were too heavy to move.

One night I awoke breathless, my heart pounding, after struggling from a vehicle beneath the sea, hoping the power with which I burst through the surface was a promising sign.

*

A calm autumn afternoon:[105] should I walk to the park and circle the croquet lawn – ten minutes there and back, half the minimum daily 'yard time' for prisoners? 'Pacing, pacing,' I reminded myself, 'a front runner is not necessarily still in the race at the end.' I headed slowly up Salamanca Road. Turned right at the tennis courts. Passed the Rec Centre (squash, gym, pro-shop, physiotherapy). Took the narrow path to the wide green space. But the setting was not as I knew it. The edges of the croquet lawn were untrimmed, the centre was patchy, and a flamboyance of flamingos on the clubhouse veranda jostled a tubbed rose tree bursting with blooms painted red. 'We planted a white bush in error,' said the leader of a team of painters wearing hi-vis vests. 'If the Queen finds out we'll lose our heads.' Where was the caretaker with his rake and purple bucket of topsoil, his fleecy jacket, cheerful wave, measured tread? A 26-point croquet game was in progress. The participants stalked, swung and connected, roquetted, rushed and pegged out. 'Your ground's parched,' I told an out-player. 'Yes, it's threadbare, but it's also hard and fast – just as we like it,' she said, returning to the court and hitting a hedgehog, with her flamingo, through a playing card hoop.

*

5   The vendor of happiness

An interview with French novelist Alphonse Daudet[1] (1840–1897)

As the notion that I should write an illness narrative grew, I went in search of writers who, 'within the narrow bed of [their] flesh',[2] had found ways of speaking about pain. I wanted to delve into their daily lives and pertinent language: to hear about their challenges and interpretations of pain unblemished by societal niceties, to feel them walk off the page and into the room. 'As controversial as any evidence of shaping may be in a trauma text – and what text is not shaped? – part of what we must call healing lies in the assertion of creativity,' said Leigh Gilmore in *The Limits of Autobiography* (2001), considering the 'ability to write beyond the silencing meted out by trauma'.[3]

I booked a flight to Paris to interview novelist, playwright and memoirist Alphonse Daudet. Paris – *La Belle Époque*, the mystery of the Symbolists, the artifice of Decadents, the fleeting detail of Impressionism.

The interview took place on the morning of November 1897, in Daudet's first-floor apartment at 41 rue de l'Université on the left bank of the Seine. The family had shifted to the address only a few weeks previously in order to spare Daudet the climb to their fifth-floor rooms at 31 rue de Bellechasse – the home, in the same quarter, to which Madame Daudet would return to live after his death. In particular, I wanted to ask Daudet about his posthumously published notes, *La Doulou* (Provençal for *douleur*, pain), described by his fellow writer and friend Jules Hoche as a 'balance sheet of [Daudet's] daily misery'.[4]

I arrived time-lagged and, it is fair to say, nervous, carrying a polished paua shell in a box (with a leaflet showing the sea snail's point of collection on the New Zealand coastline). I was prepared for postponement. Daudet was *un homme fatigué* who directed his life carefully, day to day. For the past fourteen years, he had suffered from the progressive locomotor ataxia and severe nerve pain of *tabes dorsalis* – the phase of tertiary syphilis that destroys the dorsal columns of the spinal cord. Nonetheless, as an article in *New York Times* had reported following the launch, in May, of *La Fedor*, his latest novel, 'his genius triumphs over the excruciating nervous rheumatism which has crippled his lower limbs and even the opiates to which he has been obliged to have continuous recourse'.[5]

André Ebner, Daudet's secretary and friend, met me at the door and showed me to the Writing Room. He declared that the author had been at his desk dictating correspondence since eight and was in sound spirits awaiting my visit.

'You'll find he's part ebbing strength and part prodigious energy,' said Monsieur Ebner. 'As his body fails, all his efforts are concentrated on preserving his intellect. To that end, and to discourage brooding, he works, works, works.' Ebner knocked on a closed door. 'But we cannot discount the force of will and support of morphine with which he also opposes his suffering.' He glanced at the unwrapped box. 'I see you've brought him a shell.'

Daudet was sitting at his table in the light of a lamp with a stamped paper shade. 'It was the hour of intimacies and exchange of confidences,' he had written in the prologue to *Les Femmes d'artistes* (1889):

> The lamp shone softly under its shade, confining its bright circle to that intimate conversation, leaving in shadow the capricious luxury of the vast walls covered with canvases, panoplies and hangings and ending at the very top in windows, through which the dark blue of the sky entered freely.[6]

As I entered, Ebner at my elbow, Daudet turned, fixed his monocle and, grasping first the arm of the chair then the edge of the table, slowly stood. He wore an unbuttoned jacket of black velvet over a charcoal waistcoat and white shirt, and a floppy maroon bow tie which lifted the sombre apparel but accentuated the thinness of his chest and pallor of his face. He waved Ebner, who had moved forward to assist, aside, grasped his silver-tipped cane and walked forward, shakily but unaided, with the hesitant rolling gait typical of his ataxic condition. He was smaller and frailer than I had imagined, but an awareness of his own charm and once youthful capability was still apparent in his attentive gaze and lingering smile. I remembered Émile Zola's description of him in *Les Romanciers Naturalistes* (1881) as a young man, as 'handsome, subtly and nervously handsome, like an Arab horse, with an abundant mane';[7] and his own remark, made a decade before when, fencing with the foil, he fell, that while his mind had kept 'all the youth, vigour and drive'[8] of his best years, his body was 'a wet rag'. I was also reminded that he was so short-sighted that he had once talked for fifteen minutes to a rug on a chair, believing it to be Edmond de Goncourt.

He greeted me warmly, in the French manner. Politely accepted the paua shell. Gestured to a sofa beneath the window suggesting the light would assist with note-taking. I said that, as I was unable to sit, I would stand against the wall. Concerned, he pressed me for details. I summarised my predicament (heavy fall, marble floor, damaged nerve). He shook his head. Murmured sympathetically. Insisted I recline on the *méridienne*. Observed that since sitting was almost as natural as walking, I must be greatly inconvenienced.

'Even more natural than walking,' I said, pointing out that babies sit before they walk.

'Just so.' He looked at me thoughtfully. 'Do you attend the theatre and dine out? Ride in cabs? How do you write – do you employ a secretary? Nerve pain, you say? If Jean-Martin Charcot, my neurologist, were still alive I'd urge an appointment. His successor at the Sorbonne, Fulgence Raymond, might see you. Ebner will send a letter of introduction.'

Daudet's eldest son, Léon, had written in *Alphonse Daudet: A Memoir* (1898), 'My father's welcome is always pleasant. His kindly air is in no sense a mask.'[9]

The interview immediately focused on pain.

I had intended to open by reviewing, with Daudet, details of his life and writing career. He was born in Nîmes, son of a silk manufacturer who suffered financial ruin during the Depression following the Revolution of 1848. He had an unsettled childhood, and an adolescence and young adulthood marked, in the words of his brother Ernest, by 'wretchedness, dangerous escapades and unwholesome distractions'.[10] Despite his reputation as a sensualist with a propensity for affairs, he remained happily married and devoted to Julia Allard (author of *Impressions de nature et d'art*, 1879, and *L'Enfance d'une Parisienne*, 1883), his intellectual and creative companion. The couple had two sons, Léon and Lucien, and a daughter, Edmée. As an author, he had produced poetry, novels, plays, musicals, memoirs, newspaper serials, chronicles, children's stories – more than forty popular works that also appealed to a literary readership. Read widely in translation in England and America, he was favoured as a French Dickens (Daudet knew and admired Dickens but decried his influence), and as a Gallic Mark Twain 'with a flavour of Cervantes' (it's said his larger than life Provençal character, Tartarin, of *Tartarin de Tarascon* (1872), and subsequent Tartarin novels, was inspired by *Don Quixote*). His first publications were a collection of poetry, *Les Amoureuses* (1858), and *La Double Conversion* (1861), a short story in verse. And his most lasting works were *Le Petit Chose* (1868), a partly autobiographical novel of which the first section is related to his own boyhood; *Lettres de mon moulin* (1869), evoking scenes of life in Provence; and both *Contes du Lundi* (1873) and *Contes et récits* (1873), primarily patriotic tales related to his experiences during the Franco-Prussian War. He was especially remembered for his Tartarin series, and for *Numa Roumestan* (1881), which contrasts meridional and Parisian life. Although commonly associated with Naturalist Realism, his most memorable works are described as 'delicate transpositions and subtle evocations of human suffering'.[11]

I had also anticipated setting parameters regarding discussion of syphilis. This might include his infection, at age seventeen, by a *lettrice de la cour* (a woman employed by the court of Napoleon III to read aloud from recently published works); the dormancy of his disease (apart from episodic insomnia, mood changes, visual disturbances and pains thought to be 'rheumatisms') until the onset, at age forty-five, of full-blown *tabes dorsalis*, also known as neurosyphilis; his fear that the *tabes* would progress to paralysis and the dementia known as general paresis. I was anxious to ascertain the necessary level of discretion, for, despite the societal prevalence of syphilis, the disease was not named in *La Doulou*, or in any of Daudet's writings, and his biographical profiles deferred to descriptive variations of a disabling and painful spinal condition. Of course, there would be no mention of his son Léon's subsequent development of the disease.

But, as Daudet settled in his chair, the purposeful mood of the room changed. Heavy rain, threatening since dawn, started to fall. The light dropped, shadowing and relaxing his face. The windows became foggy. The coal dwindled to ash, its remnants glowing in the grate. And, as we conversed – Daudet taking time to fill his small pipe, stroke his beard and sift through papers in order, I assumed, to facilitate my note-taking, or alert me to the weight of a phrase or a silence I was expected to consider – I became aware of a shift beyond the lamp with the stamped paper shade to the lightness of relief, birdsong, a sunny nook in the garden – to a place of the poppy, perhaps?

DE MONTALK: How should I address you – Alphonse? Daudet? Alphonse Daudet?

DAUDET: Please, call me The Vendor of Happiness[12] – this is how I should like to be remembered.

DE MONTALK: Even though you're in pain? Do you speak allegorically – how would someone who suffers, sell happiness?

DAUDET: I intend no allegory. I refer to the happiness that arises from *conforter* in Old French: to solace, to help, to strengthen.

DE MONTALK: Rather than the luck, fortune or chance of *hap* in Middle English?

DAUDET: Exactly.

DE MONTALK (*after a pause*): Are you in the present or past? Here or there? Informal or formal?

DAUDET (*amused*): I am wherever the past and the present meet, wherever there's a garden or cagnard [wind shelter] and the unalloyed joy of baring one's back to the sun. I travel imaginatively: as you can see, I'm limited by my illness. I stand at this window and roads appear to me, as escapes from my pain. I tread paths soft with simple herbs. I hear broom popping. I stroll into the distance. I listen and remember. On turnpikes, Léon calls, 'Papa, Papa, watch out for the little stones!'

DE MONTALK: As a vendor of solace, how would you dispense your comforting wares?

DAUDET: I would reach out to everyone and gently gain their confidence. In the case of the sick, like an understanding physician I'd examine the psychological response, mark its outline as I might a wound on the skin and follow its fluctuations, all the while reassuring the suffering one with the passing parade of his contemporaries! This appeal to the ego is failsafe! Then, I would gradually produce a picture of a constrained but a nevertheless worthwhile future, in which the patient consoles and supports himself by comforting others. Placing my aims beyond myself in this way enables me to evade Fate to some extent.

DE MONTALK: Has pain been your Fate? You've said that in the first half of your life you knew misery, and in the second half pain. Which has predominated?

DAUDET: The pain of *tabes dorsalis*, certainly – the incessant physical agony.

DE MONTALK: The fatigue, the weakness, the unsteady gait?

DAUDET: Those too – *les souffrances*.

DE MONTALK: The visceral symptoms, real and false?

DAUDET: Notably the misleading bladder tenderness, which was the beginning of the terminal phase.

DE MONTALK: A damaged nerve playing games?

DAUDET: An illness testing me, gathering strength, wearing me down.

DE MONTALK: Despite the offerings of prominent neurologists such as Jean-Martin Charcot and, from Harvard, Charles-Édouard Brown-Séquard?

DAUDET: I can date each aspect of my pain's progression – each ghastly surprise, each teasing remission.

DE MONTALK: I have read and reread your pain notes, *La Doulou*.

DAUDET: But these are unpublished. They're still in my drawer – in draft form! How can this be?

DE MONTALK: You are where the past and the present touch. I am between the present and the future. *La Doulou* was published by Madame Daudet in 1930, and in 1934 and 2002 appeared in separate English translations.

DAUDET (*shifting in his chair*): *Vraiment*?

DE MONTALK: The first translation was made by Milton Garver, a professor of French at Yale. It's entitled *Suffering*, and includes a commentary and notes by Monsieur Ebner.

DAUDET: The title's appropriate, Ebner has seen to that. He – like his father, who was my first secretary – knows as well as anyone that when I say 'I'm in pain', what I mean is 'I'm suffering'. What of his commentary?

DE MONTALK: He says that you contemplated your suffering with 'lucid pity'.[13]

DAUDET: If you can't pity yourself, who can you pity?

DE MONTALK: And he says that this pity, by which I assume he includes empathy, was apparent in your dealings with other sufferers, and in your writing generally.

DAUDET: The second translation?

DE MONTALK: It was made by the English writer Julian Barnes. It's entitled *In the Land of Pain*: 'The street carriages passing at a gallop. Lamalou in winter. In the land of pain.'[14] Barnes's focus is pain, Garver's is suffering. For instance, in Barnes's book you're a 'band of pain',[15] while in Garver's you're 'an orchestra of suffering'.[16] Take, too, the opening dialogue. 'What are you doing at the moment?' someone asks you. 'I'm in pain,' says Barnes.[17] 'I am suffering', translates Garver.[18]

DAUDET: An unlikely social exchange.

DE MONTALK: Yes. I find that the borders quickly close at mention of untreatable pain.

DAUDET: Unless you're speaking to someone with exactly the same problem. How you warm to such a person, how you insist he tells you every last detail!

DE MONTALK: The 'pain diary', as the small book's been described, was edited for publication in France by your family. The original manuscript has disappeared. The work in English has been reviewed as 'harrowing'; as 'terrifying … dry, cold, helpless'; as rendering pain 'in images that because of their modest particularity have rarely been equalled'.[19] A friend in severe pain for a year turned away from it. I understood why. The grind of untreatable pain weakens one's mind.

DAUDET: Mist against bricks.

DE MONTALK: It heightens awareness of fear.

DAUDET: I shake if I see my wife or one of the children lean out of a window.

DE MONTALK: It fosters acceptance of death.

DAUDET: To be free of pain...

DE MONTALK: Nonetheless, I found your explicit descriptions of agony and desperation validating. Like supporting shadows, they lent me a strange comfort and strength. Were the notes compiled to console others as well as yourself?

DAUDET: When I learned I'd have this condition forever, I started writing about it in order to counter the pain and temper my fear – to assuage 'the fierce necessity of confessing myself',[20] as Léon used to say, by raising suffering to the light, and inspecting it. Not just my own plight, but also those of the sufferers I met at the spas. From an early age, it was my habit to record life, as I observed it, in notebooks. I've always believed that fiction should be the history of people who will never have any written account of their lives. More recently, I've stopped studying myself in order to give comfort to others.

Charcot encouraged me to sketch medically. He'd say of a patient, 'Daudet, you should relate to this, I took some notes, I'll give you the details later.'[21]

DE MONTALK: Charcot of the barbaric Seyre's suspension treatment at Lamalou – the specialist who may have been able to help me!

DAUDET: He had faults. His death four years ago – a heart attack – was a great loss to neurology. But he was an unrivalled diagnostician. As for the beam and harness affair, it was designed to extend the spine and slacken the joints of ataxics.

DE MONTALK: An extreme form of 'traction'.

DAUDET: He imported it from Russia. He didn't operate the Lamalou apparatus himself. He didn't consult at the spa, and I'm not aware that he ever went there. Keller, the hydrotherapist, carried out the treatments in the spa room – in the evening when no one was around.

DE MONTALK: Edmond de Goncourt witnessed the spectacle. He found the sight of patients hanging in the shadows beyond description.

DAUDET: I instantly remember the grimness. I hang for four minutes, the last two of which I'm supported only by my jaw – causing terrible pain in my teeth. In front of me the small dark Russian writhes and moans and lifts his arms in the air. As I'm lowered to the ground and relieved of the harness, pain explodes in my sinews and bones. I kneel on all fours waiting for the fire in my back and neck to subside and the melted marrow to congeal so I can be helped to my feet. I subjected myself to thirteen sessions, not stopping until I vomited blood – the intense stress, I imagined. The fruitless search for relief.

DE MONTALK: Including the disagreeable injections of guinea pig liquid?

DAUDET: Indeed, and infusions from bulls' testicles when the guinea pig extract ran out. And the numerous trips to spas, which I visited to cure what were believed to be symptoms of rheumatism – even though, increasingly, I felt that something was forever faulty inside of me and I wouldn't be able to take my body for granted any more. In 1885, when the pains became relentless and the unsteadiness and sense of myself in space worsened, I finally mustered the courage to consult Charcot – the ultimate classifier. I told him, 'I've been saving you up for last.'[22] He gave me a direct diagnosis. Shocking, but necessary. One needs to know the worst. He prescribed gold chloride[23] and advised the hot baths at Lamalou. For bouts of extreme pain there was morphine, which he recommended keeping below a certain dose and switching the times it was taken.

DE MONTALK: To prevent addiction.

DAUDET (*shrugs*): One succumbs.

DE MONTALK: There's no option.

DAUDET: Are you a user?

DE MONTALK: No, the hallucinations are too disturbing. I take liquid oxycodone, synthesised from a different part of the poppy; it's more potent than morphine and produces fewer side effects.

DAUDET: Hallucinations?

DE MONTALK: Some, but they're less threatening.

DAUDET: Tincture of opium?

DE MONTALK: Laudanum's no longer available.

DAUDET: Curative spas?

DE MONTALK: Where I come from, convalescent resorts are few. Tell me about Lamalou.

DAUDET: From the time of Charcot's diagnosis I went yearly. I immersed myself in the waters up to my neck reading my old friend Montaigne.[24] He was sensitive to others' physical suffering. I sat on a stone bench inside the bath in the opaque yellow water, reading and eavesdropping and remembering dramas and remarks for my notes.

    At night, in the hotel, I read about Livingstone in Central Africa. The plodding monotony of his journey. The constant checking of air change and altitude. The grasslands and swamps. The preoccupations with cooking pots. The supplies, slow to arrive. All quietly providing *mis en scènes*, locations, through which my imagination could roam.

DE MONTALK: The travels of Sir Richard Burton work in the same way for me. I savour his tribulations as much his exotic locations. As Shakespeare says in Romeo and Juliet: 'One pain is lessened by another's anguish!'[25]

DAUDET: Ah! And as they say in the Midi, the land of the sick: 'The illness of a neighbour is always a comfort and may even be a cure!'[26]

DE MONTALK: Lamalou-les-Bains – I hope to go there. I have a pamphlet. Healing waters first revealed during mining in the eleventh century. Muddy pools used by peasants in pain, their clothes impregnated by sulphur. These days, there's a twenty-one-day thermal treatment for rheumatoid, neurologic and traumatic conditions for which application can be made for insurance support on the recommendation of a doctor.

DAUDET (*between pauses*): Lamalou. The Institution. The hotel's roughcast walls. Concerts and plays. The smell of wood fires. Potted lemon trees in the courtyard. Ataxics shuffling to and fro, performing their three-steps-and-a-hoppolka. Subjects to study. Patrons who share the same pain – no longer loners with odd illnesses, dismissed as hypochondriacs, considered sad but boring. Subjects also to avoid – in the dining room, gummy mouths ruminating, eyes glued to their plates, casting furious glances when their dishes are carried in late; and in the latrine, side by side, sharing their distressing evacuations, lit by the same gas jet ring...

DE MONTALK: In *La Doulou* you describe pains in your legs, bladder and waist. Rats gnawing at your toes with razor teeth. A blade repeatedly thrust into your little finger. Intolerable flashes of pain in your heels and the soles of your feet. A pocket knife twisting beneath your big toenail. Muscles ground beneath the wheels of a wagon.

DAUDET: The worst was the pain I call the breastplate – a continuous, hideous spasm in my ribs, hoops of steel crushing my lower back. The terror. The panic.

DE MONTALK: It had you in its grip for months. You couldn't undo the straps. You couldn't breathe.

DAUDET: Tabetic pains vary in type and intensity.

DE MONTALK: They typify the caprice of nerve pain.

DAUDET: After one cruel night I wrote: 'Crucifixion. That's what it was... the torment of the Cross: violent wrenching of the hands, feet, knees; nerves stretched out and pulled to breaking point.'[27]

DE MONTALK: The same night you imagined Christ and the two thieves conversing about pain.

DAUDET: Intimations of agony floated to and fro. I don't recall what was said. I took a spoonful of bromide, salty, bitter. Sometimes I wonder if Flaubert struggled to find the right words because of the enormous quantity of bromide he ingested.

DE MONTALK: Then you had several days of peace in the hot, cloudless June weather.

DAUDET: A brief peace, broken by my need for bromide with its side effects of depression and memory loss, and the chloral, which leaves me tired and on edge. Before I returned to morphine, from which I wake in the night in a vacuum with no sense of time and place, with no sense of myself as a person, with no ideas.

DE MONTALK: With only, as you have written, 'a sense of EXTRAORDINARY moral blindness'.[28]

DAUDET: Morphine – the only true analgesic. The unpredictable rages it provokes, the interference with my writing and dreams. It makes me unkind to Julia and the children.

DE MONTALK: Side effects – no drug of relief is without them. Yet you've also said that morphine makes you talkative, takes you out of yourself.

DAUDET: Morphine *has* helped me to function. Without it, who knows what I would have become?

DE MONTALK: Marcel Proust – Lucien's friend – recalls you self-injecting. He writes about this in *Contre Sainte-Beuve*, a collection of notes published in 1954, like *La Doulou* more than thirty years posthumously.

DAUDET: Young Proust, ah yes. And Sainte-Beuve[29] – he had an affair with Hugo's wife. At Hugo's funeral I struggled to sign my name in the book, in the presence of other mourners.

DE MONTALK: Proust refuted Sainte-Beuve's contention that one can only understand the work of an artist by understanding the artist's biography. He believed the hidden self, the inner biography, the experiences processed and stored in the memory – the song *within* an author – was of greater importance.

DAUDET: Sainte-Beuve suffered much hidden pain in retirement. Like you, he was unable to sit and had to write lying or standing. His doctors were unable to diagnose the problem. People would ask after his back, but as far as we knew his back was sound. After his post-mortem, it was rumoured the pain had been caused by the stone.

DE MONTALK: I have to wonder – about the stone.

On the subject of morphine, and Proust's recollection, he writes that during a discussion on courage you retired, without explanation, to an adjoining room. He later learned your pain had intensified. When you returned, your brow was perspiring as if in the wake of a struggle, but your breathing was easy, calmed by victory.

DAUDET: He remembers correctly.

DE MONTALK: Proust was in awe of your courage. His own suffering, he says, was of no consequence by comparison. He describes you as 'the poet whose approach turned pain into poetry, as iron is magnetised when brought near a magnet'.[30]

DAUDET (*making a sweeping motion*): Supposition and long-windedness bothers me. One needs to pass through theory and into the picture.

At this point, as if prompted, Daudet excused himself and, with the aid of his cane, left the room. A door opened and shut, further down the hall.

I took the opportunity to look over the table where he wrote very slowly and revised, revised, revised. 'I am never satisfied with my work,' he had confessed earlier. 'My novels I always used to pen myself. I could never dictate a novel. However, lately, I've relied on my family's assistance.'

In the wake of the family's recent move, the floor was cluttered with small boxes tightly packed with hard-backed jotters, canvases beneath dust covers, plants growing in copper holders. And the workspace was piled with papers and books, of which I listed the yellowed (sulphur-stained?) pages of Montaigne, whose reassurance and advice he was never without; Pascal, the master of style;

Tacitus, whom he translated one page at a time; Schopenhauer's dark 'arguments and picturesque aphorisms'.[31] There were also Rousseau, whom he defended against those who railed against sexual transgression; Napoleon on campaign; undertakings in Africa; a mission to Madagascar; an expedition to the North Pole.

Here, I thought, he keeps his disease on a lead. Here, he hides his pain beneath a table.

After a brief intermission, I heard a door shut and the halting sound of Daudet's progress along the hall – reminiscent of the far off sound of Philoctetes approaching the stage, crawling, dragging his festering foot and leg. 'To reach this armchair, to go across the waxed floor of the corridor,' Daudet had written of his worsening pain and ataxia, 'requires as much effort and ingenuity as Stanley used in an African forest.'[32]

He entered the room, assisted by Ebner, carrying a pillow, which he offered as 'a little extra height for your head.' His forehead appeared moist. 'He observes rather than imagines,' writes the author and critic Edmund Gosse. 'And he does this... as a "realist", as one who depends on little green books of notes, and docketed bundles of *pièces justificatives*.'[33]

I positioned the pillow. What would Daudet observe about me: my bobbed hair, travel trousers, shoulder bag and corduroy jacket? He took the shell from its box and held it to the lamp. Turned it this way and that. Smiled. Propped it against his pipe. Watched it gleam blue, silver and green.

DE MONTALK: Can we revisit the notes you made about the sufferers you met at the mineral pools? Léon writes that their subtlety and completeness astonished Parisian physicians. He describes you as recording the 'secret wretchedness of men, women and aged men [...] discreetly, with the wisdom of a physician-poet'.[34] 'Entire lives,' he says, 'are summed up in a few lines.' He quotes you: 'Misers turned to spendthrifts. Violent men become timorous.'

DAUDET (*running his hand through his hair*): As I say to Léon, 'Poetry is deliverance.'[35]

DE MONTALK: Léon – who published over forty books including a second memoir, *Quand vivait mon père*, in 1940 – makes the point that while scientific knowledge of pain fills but a few pages, the observations of pain made by a poet may be infinite. Was *La Doulou* intended as a work of poetry or fiction?

DAUDET: Neither. I envisaged an honest confession – *dictante dolore*, with pain dictating – of moving through pain and disability towards death. But, writing as a husband and father, I was reluctant to express the unsettling thoughts and longing for death that illness provokes, to compare suffering as the lynchpin of a family, with suffering on one's own. I wanted to leave no suggestion of complaint against those I loved. Goncourt and I discussed a work of fact incorporated within fiction. I doubt I'll write it now.

DE MONTALK: The 'terrible and implacable breviary',[36] to quote Léon, appeared instead. The text frequently calls for poetic form:

I struggle to sleep
without chloral.
Behind my closed eyes
the earth splits.
Chasms open right and left.
Short naps turn
into nightmares
of vertiginous skidding,
sliding,
crashing into the abyss.
When the garden awakes.
The blackbird's song
patterns the pale window.

DAUDET: I wrote only poetry in the beginning – until I gave in to prose, working for newspapers in order to make a living.

DE MONTALK: Why did *La Doulou* not take the form you envisaged?

DAUDET: Julia thought it might be interpreted as a curtain fall on my writing life. She influences all my compositions. There's not a page published on which she has not scattered flecks of her fine bright mind.

Daudet stopped and blew his nose. I remembered *Les Femmes d'artistes* and the paragraph in which he writes of his marriage:

I love my wife with all my heart. [...] Marriage has been for me a port with calm and safe waters, not one where you tie your boat up to a ring on the bank at the risk of rusting there forever, but one of those blue coves where you repair sails and masts for new excursions to unknown countries.[37]

DE MONTALK: Was Julia also concerned that writing about pain, in addition to living it, would bring you down? Or that making your ailment public would harm your reputation?

DAUDET: Not once, neither at the doctor's, nor the spa has the disease been given its real name. Mostly, I'm held to have 'rheumatisms'. More formally, I have a disease of the bone marrow, or a degeneration of the nervous system – which is, of course, accurate.

DE MONTALK: Could your contemplation of suicide have been a factor? Julia begged you to think of the children.

DAUDET: Above all, I didn't want to worry her. I didn't want to worry any of my family. I took the view, as I told Ebner, that 'Suffering is nothing – the difficult thing is to avoid making those one loves suffer.'[38] Not that they're always taken in.

DE MONTALK: Ebner quotes you saying just this. He recalls an occasion on which Julia entered your study as you were sharing your pain with a friend. Your body was slumped, your head was bent, your 'loins' were being tortured, you said, as if with a hot poker. Upon seeing the doorknob turn, you quickly stood, smiled and replied strongly, in response to her question, that all was well.

DAUDET: Pain soon becomes mundane to onlookers, even those closest to us. Compassion fades. I attempt to keep my ordeal to myself to protect others, and as a matter of pride – in order not to see tedium in their eyes.

DE MONTALK: What of those who suffer alone – who have no family or friends with whom to share their anguish?

DAUDET: For me, the easiest way to be in pain is to be alone, like a mole in a burrow, free of explanations, expectations, the limitations I place on my family.

DE MONTALK: I have a photograph of you and Julia,[39] taken five years ago in the garden of your country house at Champrosay. You sit on a slatted seat. Julia stands alongside, holding a folded parasol. You tilt your head, and feign interest with a half-smile. Your face seems pallid, even in black and white. I sense fragility. For some time, you'd been finding writing a challenge – a test of will and endurance?

DAUDET: By then my writing had become a daily exercise of effort and will-power, of binding myself to the fixed moment at which I'd seat myself at the table and challenge my illness. I felt my life was effectively over. I lived instead through my novels.

DE MONTALK: These challenges have resulted in some ten publications and plays since 1885, when *tabes* declared itself and the pain became almost constant. What have been your motifs during the twelve years of greatest pain? I've listed: adventure, reminiscence, satire, romance and the pitfalls of divorce, jealousy, studies of the stage, the purifying effects of true love in *La Fedor*, and contrasts within families in *Soutienne de famille*, to be published next year. These topics seem to be consistent with your pre-*tabes* oeuvre, written from the heart of humour, sadness and 'living fact'. To which work do you feel closest?

DAUDET: Of all I've written – and since I'll always love the South – *Lettres de mon moulin* remains my favourite book. I write according to my surround-ings. For some ten years now, I've been mostly surrounded by Paris.

DE MONTALK: And by pain: except that physical distress as a theme doesn't feature. It has been said that something of the natural energy and allure of your writing has been absent since *Sappho* was published in 1884.

DAUDET: One has only to imagine the torture of living within a wall that is gradually tightening, adding one constraint to another.

DE MONTALK: Do the distraction of writing and the impetus of responsibility – of maintaining your place in the family – help to hold back the wall?

DAUDET: My responsibilities and anxieties as a father and head of a household are certainly an incentive to keeping me on my feet. As is comparison with the less fortunate – with sufferers for whom financial hardship and a lack of warmth, food, wine and affection are added to their misery.

DE MONTALK: In a conversation with Léon, in his first memoir, you keep return-
ing to the 'alliance between pity and pain'[40] – an alliance seen in your
writing, in poignancy arising from pity for human misery, as much as in
irony prompted by your observations of absurdity. Are your acts of pity in
daily life a manifestation of compassion through pain?

DAUDET: Living in pain can isolate people, and cause them to lose touch with
the reality of the wider world. Self-pity can then become overwhelming. I
remind myself that there are heavier burdens than mine. In this way, I have
pity left to expend on others. I advise sufferers to concentrate on 'active
pity' rather than 'useless fears'. You'll be aware that many philosophers
dismiss pity as a product of weakness.

DE MONTALK: In *Much Ado About Nothing*, when Antonio speaks of self-pity as
shameful, Leonato rejoins there has never been a philosopher who patiently
endured toothache![41]

DAUDET: If one has never been cold or hungry, or otherwise suffered, one cannot
imagine, or speak about any of those things.

Something else to consider is that, for the person in pain, the torment is
always new. But to family and friends – even those who by nature are most
compassionate – the witness of suffering can become a stale habit. I say to
the sick: Don't try to convey your pain to those who cannot imagine it, find
distractions, wrestle to the end.

DE MONTALK: You've written of the difficulty of shouting to your children
'Long live life'[42] when you are 'ripped apart by pain'.

DAUDET: True. The Stoics championed the benefits of constantly exercising
one's energy. I, however, recommend exercising the imagination – if one is
so gifted. I suggest piling up one's sufferings to form a mountain from
which the beauty and grandeur of the climb can be appreciated. In this way,
inconsequential hardships fade into the background, and everything else
falls into its natural place. Had I not been afflicted, I might have inflated my
view of myself as an 'Author', becoming prey to the petty rivalries and
hollow vanities of those who write. Naturally, I still have weaknesses, but to
some extent I've been purified – by the climb.

DE MONTALK: You've reminded me of the actress in *La Fedor*, who squanders
her life in wild living. She comes to know one ideal love – a love by which
she's purified, but at the cost of her art and her life.

Léon suggests that your thinking, like that of Pascal, became purified by
the courage needed to endure pain – as a result of which you reached a ter-
restrial serenity though pity. He writes that 'great pain leads to either mean-
ness and belligerence, or pity' and you 'chose the second way'.[43] He sees
your will to work and contribute to family life as standing amidst your lit-
erary achievements. Does pain leads to moral and intellectual growth?

DAUDET: Only up to a certain point.

DE MONTALK: Beyond which?

DAUDET: It steals your energy and sours your life, and you must decide whether
to take the path of bitterness or pity.

DE MONTALK: Léon also writes – in *Devant la Douleur*, published in 1916 – that in the face of continuing pain, even medicine seeks to escape. He insists it's important to combat this withdrawal. In this respect he's calling for a rhetoric of pain. What are your thoughts?

DAUDET: Just that there is nothing customary about pain. Each pain is individual and fluctuates, like a performer's voice, according to the auditorium's acoustics.

DE MONTALK: *La Doulou* seems to be as much about your search for language as about voicing the pain experience.

DAUDET: This has never occurred to me.

DE MONTALK: You say, 'We should have a term to define the crisis through which I am passing.'[44] Also, that no words, only screams could 'render' the torture. And you speak of a note you have scribbled as 'unexpressive and secret' having meaning 'only for me, for I have written it in one of my cruel indispositions'.

DAUDET: Part of you slides out of sight if you are unable to communicate your pain.

He shaded his eyes with his hand. I asked if we had spoken for too long and offered to leave. Daudet shook his head emphatically, stretched his left leg, straightened in his chair. I continued cautiously, aware that he counselled and instructed regardless of discomfort.

DE MONTALK: I am interested in your dual relationship with pain.

On the one hand, you personify pain with a capital P, refer to it as 'the most despotic and possessive of Imperial hostesses',[45] lament the endless days when the only part of you that's alive is Pain, invite it to be your 'philosophy', your 'science',[46] a travel destination.

On the other hand, you objectify pain with graphic and uncompromising descriptions.

DAUDET: Yes, like many writers, I have a dual disposition. There's an authorial Me who observes, sees into things and describes. And a responsive Me who weeps, struggles and suffers. Even as a child I was aware I had two sides.

DE MONTALK: Your stark accounts alongside moments of deep understanding illustrate a duality of watching and feeling.

DAUDET (*leaning forward*): I'm extremely myopic, as a result of which I feel and listen to people, landscapes, wherever I might be in the world, as much as I look at them.

DE MONTALK: Just as you gauged the mood of the sick at Lamalou, in the Hotel Mas's little garden – where you reassured the nervous, comforted the despairing and let everyone glimpse the possibility of a positive outcome.

DAUDET: Hope on the scaffold of loss. I met with the distressed and shared their martyrdom. I told them that their doctors don't know any more than they do, and many know even less than they do. I found our conversations consoling – while soothing others I soothed myself.

DE MONTALK: I'm trying to write about pain. I'm finding this difficult, even though English comprises over one million words![47] I identify with what you describe as the 'bitter disproportion between what my pen determines and what my mind has conceived'.[48]

DAUDET: Physical pain, unlike most illnesses, is slippery. Its expression can only be guided by style – style as a state of intensity.

DE MONTALK: The greatest number of things in the fewest number of words.

DAUDET: Some people possess the innate gifts of taste and tact that constitute style, and instinctively choose the right words. But minds of that sort are rare.

DE MONTALK: Specificity. Refinement. Imaginative prompting. *La Doulou* – a decade of pain on small pages.

> Sounds from the shower –
> tiled walls echoing
> voices,
> water;
> the precise click
> of foils
> from the practice room;
> the deep sadness
> these absences cause me –
> the physical life
> I have lost.

DAUDET: Impressions. Flashes of light and colour. Music. The juxtaposition of colours and sounds. All these are important. Remember, too, Pascal, who wrote: 'Let no one say that I have said anything new; the arrangement of the subject is new.'[49]

DE MONTALK: Edmund Gosse describes you as an impressionist painter.

DAUDET: When I was London, two years ago, we met at dinner –

Daudet paused, interrupted by a tap at the door. I turned, hoping to see Julia, but no one entered.

DAUDET: After dessert I described the Nîmes melon harvest when I was a boy – the white marketplace, the masses of fruit, the morning light… Are you comfortable? We should talk on.

DE MONTALK: I'm fine, but I don't want to tire you.

DAUDET: I come to life in the presence of strangers. I can even appear to be in perfect health. I want to know more about your country with its limitations on convalescence, and about the future with its cure of syphilis and restrictions on opium. I wonder which of my works are still read. Tell me about the book beneath your notepad.

DE MONTALK: It's a work of science fiction set in a bar, where there's a law that says joy shared is joy increased, and pain shared is pain lessened. The patrons include a vampire and a talking parrot – and Time Travellers who must pay cash for their drinks![50]

DAUDET: It reaches a long way into the future.

He stopped. Rubbed his thighs as if distracting his pain. Clasped his thin hands. Stared at the paua shell. Looked towards the door.

Postscript

A month after this interview, on 16 December 1897, Daudet, aged fifty-seven, died during an evening meal with his family. He was chatting and sipping soup when his head fell back and his breathing became laboured. He was laid on the carpet. Doctors arrived and pulled rhythmically on his tongue (the mode of resuscitation briefly in practice) for over an hour, to the distress of Julia and her mother, Léon, Lucien and Edmée. When this failed, 'faradisation of the dia-phragm' – the intermittent application of an electrical current to the midriff – was attempted. The cause of death was reported as apoplexy.

A few days earlier, Daudet had attended a dinner in memory of Honoré de Balzac. As he returned home in his carriage, invigorated, he remarked to Léon, 'Such love fests are indispensable. They whip the spirit up, they beautify things. By exchanging ideas we penetrate each other's brains. We see the same fact and the same event appreciated in all kinds of ways in accordance with the character and the habits of different men.'[51]

I lay on my side facing the ghost gum. A kingfisher had made its home in a cavity in the trunk.[52] The hollow was set in soft, discoloured timber, recalling last year's amputation of a sun-blocking limb. I watched the bird come and go, flashing its deep green and ultramarine feathers. Between sorties, it perched on the lip of its dark space, calling *kree, kree, kree*. The opening to its south-facing chamber would be exposed to Antarctic winds in winter – as a kingfisher, native to New Zealand, would know. Did this lapse suggest the nester was a gum-loving Australian cousin, drawn to familiar surroundings despite the climate? Or was it a northern hemisphere variant with an injured sense of the earth's tilt and rotational axis? Had a mythological Halcyon decided to lay her eggs in the security of a tree, rather than a nest floating on a solstice sea?

6 The consolator

An introduction to English social theorist Harriet Martineau (1802–1876)

Essential chronology

1802	Born at Norwich, the sixth of eight children,[1] to Unitarian parents with progressive beliefs regarding the education of girls.
1818	Hearing fails; also senses of taste and smell. Deafness precludes employment as a governess. Begins to write on themes of divinity and religion.
1826	Father dies. Family suffers financial hardship. Martineau advances her writing, supplementing her income with needlework. Takes on social causes.
1832	Moves to London. Becomes a self-supporting author and political and social commentator. Enjoys commercial success and literary lionisation.
1834–36	Travels in America.
1839	Collapses, suffering from pelvic pain and exhaustion.
1840	Seeks solitude for five years in a Tynemouth lodging house.
1844	Publishes *Life in the Sick-Room: Essays By an Invalid.*
1845	Recovers health. Moves to Ambleside in the Lake District.
1846	Travels in the Near East. Social and political activism gathers pace.
1855	Relapses into permanent illness and seclusion at Ambleside.
1876	Dies at Ambleside 'after diligent, devoted, suffering, joyful years'.[2]

And now may be our time for taking a new growth through pain[3]

I am outside 57 Front Street, Tynemouth – once the lodgings of Harriet Martineau, novelist, journalist and prodigious social theorist. This is the brick Georgian guesthouse to which Martineau, prostrated and in pain, was driven nine miles from her sister's Newcastle home to solitude and stillness to die. In fact, she was immured here, from 1840 until 1845, in two first-floor rooms, before recovering and moving to the Lake District, where she remained in good health until relapsing into permanent illness ten years later. During her initial seclusion, the prolific, popular and today largely forgotten author wrote *Life in the*

Sick-Room: Essays by an Invalid (1844) – a memoir-treatise of consolation and support for fellow sufferers and advice for the untroubled. She was well placed to sympathise and advise. She endured persistent, frequently severe, undiagnosed pelvic pain and backache; episodes of depression; debilitation so encompassing that she was unable to venture beyond the upstairs landing. She passed her time at Tynemouth alone, watching from a window, reading, reflecting and, pain permitting, writing in a prone position on a specially adapted sofa.

I was introduced to Harriet Martineau while researching Florence Nightingale. I had begun to realise there were degrees of chronicity less transcended than managed, and had seen, in Nightingale's enquiring and writing through three decades of illness and pain, a model for a meaningful life. Nightingale (who, twelve years after *Sick-Room* was published, would return from the Crimean War with what has been retrospectively diagnosed as chronic brucellosis) had read Martineau's recently published memoir, and was refuting the writer's view that as the body loses strength, 'the stronger the conviction of an independent and unchangeable self'.[4] Persuaded that Martineau was worth pursuing, I sent for *Sick-Room*, described by its author as 'a record of the thoughts and emotions belonging to the peculiar and ill-understood condition of protracted disease, in sharp contrast with the ways of healthy people'.[5] A preliminary reading of the book showed that, behind Martineau's tendencies to empathetic effusion, Christian piety and moral instruction, lay a grounded account of suffering and a practical approach to dealing with it. At the time of my reading I had been immersed in the psychosocial and cultural entanglements of illness beliefs and behaviours and was ready to re-engage with a thinker who wrote in the personal moment of pain.

Martineau's lodgings comprise a small living room – overlooking the village market, the river mouth, Northumbria's rolling grasslands and the coastline's long golden sands – joined to a bedroom in the house next door by an opening cut in the wall.

Martineau, in person, is a woman of forty-one, of medium build, maybe five feet six inches tall, with wavy brown hair parted in the middle and coiled at the back. Her features are regular, and her eyes, which are light – between grey, green and blue – convey an expression of steady enquiry. She wears a tight-sleeved dress with a ruffled neck, lace at the wrists and a decorative bow above a loosened waist. She walks awkwardly, leaning forward as if anticipating or warding off a spasm, her hand supporting her lower back. Seven years previously, in America, she attracted adjectives like affable, unaffected, womanly and courteous. The New York diarist Philip Hone had found her not, as anticipated, 'a little too blue to be agreeable',[6] but rather an engaging conversationalist, given to laughter. Hone's assessment was shared by many of her literary acquaintances in London. 'She pleased us far beyond expectation,'[7] said Thomas Carlyle, who was not noted for tolerance, after meeting her for the first time, adding that despite her deafness she spoke readily and was 'really of pleasant countenance'. John Stuart Mill, however, dismissed her as a gossip, Robert Browning as conceited, and Hans Christian Andersen, to whom she was introduced at a garden party in London, as so talkative that he had to lie down for the rest of the afternoon. Nevertheless, there was general agreement as to her thoughtfulness, generosity and independence as a single woman. She valued her self-reliance so much so that the death, in 1827, of her fiancé (a young clergyman who suffered from depression) appears to have been tinged with relief. Her strong will, she later decided, aged twenty-four, 'combined with an anxiety of conscience, makes me fit only to live alone'.[8]

She opens the door to a maid carrying a coal bucket. The girl stokes a low flame, sweeps an ember from the hearth and places a nightdress and bed jacket over the fireguard to warm; her movements are deft and economical. The ideal attendant, in Harriet's view, should not jar the sofa, delay meals, neglect comforting routine; like the perfect nurse she should demonstrate 'no fear in her tread, no reserve in her eye, no management in her voice'.[9]

Harriet approaches the bay window and swivels a floor-mounted telescope. On the foreshore, two boys tease a smaller boy. They pull off his coat. Roll it into a ball. Throw it back and forth. Harriet knocks on the window. Raises the sash. Beckons and waves her arms. The child's coat is thrown into the Tyne, and the teasers race away. Rain spatters the pane. Her sense 'of being too weak for the ordinary incidents of life,' says Harriet to the maid, 'is strangely depressing – it evokes a scrupulous need for fairness, a heightened sense of responsibility and an absurd restlessness to set everything right.'[10]

Life quickening along its course[11]

Harriet Martineau's ordeal by pain and fatigue began at age thirty-seven, in London, in the early summer of 1839. Ignoring intimations of general malaise and nervous exhaustion, she escorted an invalid cousin to Italy on vacation. She attributed her symptoms to a demanding publication schedule, a dysfunctional liver (no, she did not imbibe), responsibility for her older brother Henry who had joined her household and *was* drinking, and the stress caused by her mother who was confused, going blind and wandering in the streets. In accordance with Martineau's tendency to travel less for pleasure than purpose, the trip to Italy was to include visits to the settings of a number of Shakespearean plays, and a research trip to the fortress cave on Mt Jura, in France, where the African slave leader, François Dominique Toussaint Louverture – the subject of an intended novel – had been imprisoned and died.

She collapsed in Venice with severe pains in her abdomen, back and legs. A local physician, whose gynaecological examination she declined, diagnosed a prolapsed uterus and cervical 'polypous tumours'. Nonetheless, she recovered sufficiently to continue to tour for a time. On returning to England, her condition worsened. She moved to Newcastle, into the care of her sister and brother-in-law doctor, where the Venetian physician's diagnosis was upheld and she underwent minor surgery for removal of the benign polyps.

Less than a year later, her pain unrelieved and her debilitation increasing, she supposed her condition to be terminal (an opinion not medically shared) and retired to seclusion in Tynemouth to await a lingering death. Not that she over-played her condition: Thomas Carlyle, visiting in 1841, found her confined to a sofa, but as 'brisk, alert, invincible as ever. There is a kind of prepared com-pleteness in Harriet,' he writes, 'which does honour to nature and the Socinian formula. In all my travels I have met with few more valiant women.'[12]

An appeal to the whole mind of society[13]

At the time of her sequestration, Martineau was financially secure and enjoyed a literary reputation in both Britain and America: she was, as the *Dictionary of National Biography* would remember her, one of the 'lions' of the day.

Her first book-length publication, *Devotional Exercises for the Use of Young Persons* (1823), comprised fourteen essays reflecting her youthful Unitarian con-cerns regarding such subjects as Habitual Devotion, Benevolence, the Goodness of God, the Uncertainty of Worldly Enjoyments, and the Value of Time. *Exer-cises* was followed by numerous articles, largely concerned with religion and her developing interest in social and political issues, of which 'Letter to the Deaf',[14] an empathetic advisory drawing on her own loss of hearing (opening 'Dear Companions' and closing 'Your affectionate sister') appeared in *Tait's Edin-burgh Magazine* (1834). Some twelve titles, also pertaining to social concerns, were produced; of these, her literary success was marked by the twenty-five well-received book-length tales published monthly as *Illustrations of Political Economy* (1832–34) and *Poor Laws and Paupers Illustrated* (1834).

After a two-year trip to America in 1836 – undertaken to assess the country's treatment of its underprivileged population – she released *Theory and Practice of Society in America* (1837), *Retrospect of Western Travel* (1837) and *How to Observe: Morals and Manners* (1838). She was by now thirty-six.

A three-volume novel of middle-class life in the country, *Deerbrook* (1839), appeared in the spring prior to her collapse in Venice, following which, newly invalided, she completed *The Hour and the Man* (1840), a novel based on Tous-saint L'Ouverture, and *The Playfellow* (1841) – four individually published, semi-instructive stories for children. She held that her fiction, like her non-fiction, should demonstrate possibilities for human improvement – a 'Victorian analogue to "socialist realism"',[15] remarked R.K. Webb in *Harriet Martineau: A Radical Victorian* (1960).

Life in the Sick-Room was set down between September and November 1843, after Martineau had brooded over the project for four days. Such was the fever of her belief that society should be appraised of the realities of chronic illness that she was barely aware she was writing. 'I needed to pour out what was in my mind,' she says in *Autobiography*, noting that the memoir 'went off like sleep [...] – so strong was the need to speak.'[16]

The work was published anonymously in January 1844 (Martineau, with a high public profile, guarded her privacy), and sold out by the end of the follow-ing month. Recognised almost immediately as Martineau's work – on account, perhaps, of the fluid, conversational and educational style for which she was known, or because word of her isolation in illness had travelled – the volume was welcomed by invalids and generally admired. The *Dublin University Magazine*'s assessment that it was a 'wise and thoughtful book – the offspring of a lofty mind',[17] typified the many positive reviews. The qualitative response was characterised by the pathologists of the *British and Foreign Medical Review*[18] who noted the writer's significant pain, but also pointed out her morbid self-consciousness, which they viewed as peculiar to women and those culturally inclined: an observation not lost on Thomas Carlyle, who wrote to his wife that Martineau 'has clearly shown in her *Life in a Sick Room* [*sic*] that to accept more sympathy than one's accurate due is a turpitude little short of stealing a purse'.[19]

Some supposed that the unnamed patient to whom Martineau addressed the work was her reclusive correspondent, Elizabeth Barrett. But Martineau firmly rejected the rumours, insisting that she spoke to each and everyone who suffers. If her words, she opens,

> should have the virtue to summon thoughts which may, for a single hour, soften your couch, shame and banish your foes of depression and pain [...] I may have the honour of being your nurse, though I myself am laid low.[20]

She situates the displacement of long illness in ten essays on such subjects as 'sympathy', through 'nature', 'temper' and 'death', to 'becoming inured' and the 'power of ideas'. She shares the indescribable dread that grips her as the pain escalates; the alternation of hope and hopelessness; the soul-sickening desertion of reason. She confesses to seeking out newspaper reports on starvations and other horrors abroad, in order to lighten her mind while awaiting the relief of an opiate. She despairs of the avoidances by and misunderstandings of the healthy and recalls the ache of confinement to a couch while others took long walks or simply sat 'upright upon chairs'.[21] She speaks of the silent message of congratulation she offers on hearing of another sufferer's death.

She balances her lot by defining protracted suffering as a rite of spiritual awakening. Solitude is seen as a bestowal of privacy and contemplation – an opportunity to develop ideas and measure the depths of one's soul – and bouts of severe pain, as allowing, on departure, a joy that those not in pain rarely experience. To the question of whether there is 'one idea with more potential than any other' in protracted illness, she replies: 'it matters infinitely less what we *do* than what we *are*'. She continues:

> If we cannot pursue a trade or a science, or keep house, or help the estate, or write books, or earn our own bread or that of others, we can do the work to which all this is only subsidiary, – we can cherish a sweet and holy temper, – we can vindicate the supremacy of mind over body, – we can, in defiance of our liabilities, minister pleasure and hope to the gayest who come prepared to receive pain from the spectacle of our pain; we can, here, as well as in heaven's courts here after, reveal the angel growing into its immortal aspect [...][22]

This thought prompts heartfelt and vivid reflection on the torment of the poor, who are denied the necessities of life without the respite of inspiring ideas, and a plea to readers to supply the destitute with food, warmth and the means of kindling their inner illumination.

As to optimum invalid living conditions, she stresses the need for a sick-room close to nature so that growth and movement can be sighted, since it is not the beauty and scent of a bloom that the confined person longs for but the vitality of vegetation. A wide and varied view is also advised: Martineau believes that her insights as 'a prisoner' are heightened as much by her lodging's leavening outlook as by the singularity of the sufferer's vantage point for philosophical vision – for gazing 'into the mirror of events'.[23] The art of seeing as an act of visionary perspective, she claims, is special to long-sequestered patients; it is a gift of pain and illness. 'We lie on the verge of life,' she writes – attuned, with the aid of a telescope, to shifts in the landscape and activities in the village – 'and watch, with nothing to do but think, and learn from what we behold.'[24]

I must write on for every day of my life[25]

In 1845, Martineau's pain and depletion abated, and she left Tynemouth for Ambleside in the nearby Lake District. She attributed her improvement to a course of mesmerism, also known as 'animal magnetism',[26] initially undertaken to lessen her dependence on opiates. Her enthusiasm for what she hailed as a new natural law resulted in the publication of her 'Letters on Mesmerism' in the *Athenaeum* (1844). Named after the Viennese physician Franz Anton Mesmer and a forerunner of hypnosis the therapy, which was often associated with somnambulism, depended in essence on the transfer of invisible healing magnetic, or 'universal', fluid from the fingertips of the mesmerist to the patient. This fluid, or energy, Mesmer believed, was a life force through which the constituents of the universe were interconnected. When the force was blocked in living beings, illness resulted. Animal Magnetism, writes Mesmer (in an apt explanation of the state of being and expression of pain), is comparable to a sixth sense, and, as such, it has to be felt to be understood. Just as one cannot explain colour to a person blind since birth, so understanding magnetism requires 'inward' feeling or seeing.

At Ambleside, she had a home, The Knoll, built in the vicinity of Matthew Arnold and William Wordsworth (who died in 1850), and established a small, two-acre farm, from which she donated produce to neighbours in need. So complete was her recovery that she hiked and climbed in the District, for up to six miles at a time, eliciting comments on her 'brown-complexioned health'.[27] From the autumn of 1846 until the summer of 1847, she travelled with friends to Egypt and Palestine, riding a camel to Mt Sinai and Petra, and a horse to Damascus – resulting in three volumes of *Eastern Life, Present and Past* (1848), and occasioning some doctors to conclude that she had imagined her pain.

Ten years after her 'cure' by mesmerism, the pain returned, permanently. Although less intense and relentless than before, its reappearance, together with fatigue and alarming cardiac irregularities, caused Martineau, now aged fifty-two, to confine herself to Ambleside.

In the beginning, as at Tynemouth, she expected to die. Her palpitations, breathlessness and faintness, which she was convinced were due to enlargement and weakening of her heart and would prove fatal, were dismissed by clinicians. Cardiologist Sir Thomas Watson, comparing a compromised heart to a slightly cracked china jar, 'which, if carefully handled, may remain long unbroken',[28] concluded that 'in Miss Martineau's case there was no such obvious rift, and I therefore affirmed to her that her life was in no immediate danger'.

Despite her condition, Martineau's output for the next fifteen years (until six years before her death, in 1876) was sustained and wide-ranging. Demonstrating acceptance and resolve, she produced her two-volume *Autobiography* (written in 1855, published after her death), 1,500 or so *Daily News* leaders (1852–1869), book reviews, and pamphlets and articles pertaining to politics and social issues including abolitionism, matrimony, population control, feminism and nursing education. Her non-fiction publications included works as diverse as *A Complete Guide to the English Lakes* (1855), a free translation and commentary on *The Positive Philosophy of August Comte* (1853), *British Rule in India* (1857) and a series of weekly articles collected in *Health, Husbandry, and Handicraft* (1861). Stirred by her correspondence with Florence Nightingale (with whom she corresponded from 1858), by Nightingale's seminal *Notes on Hospitals* (1859), *Notes on Nursing: What It Is and What It Is Not* (1859), and by developments in the care of the sick, Martineau also established herself as an authoritative voice on health. She challenged medical knowledge and practice and advised on matters of public health, including the advancement and professional standing of nursing. ('This little book of Miss Nightingale's is a work of genius,'[29] she enthused in her review of *Notes on Nursing*.) In all, in both sickness and health, Martineau composed thousands of editorials, articles and reviews, and over fifty pamphlets and books. Of her literary accomplishments she wrote in her pre-emptive obituary, prepared in 1855 and filed by the *Daily News* until required in 1876:

> Her original power was nothing more than was due to earnestness and intellectual clearness within a certain range. With small imaginative and suggestive power, and therefore nothing approaching genius, she could see clearly what she did see, and give a clear expression to what she had to say. In short, she could popularize while she could neither discover nor invent.[30]

Seeing 'clearly what she did see' included her disavowal of religion in view of Christian superstitions succumbing to science – a distancing that caused her to reject *Sick-Room*'s piety. Considering the memoir in *Autobiography* a decade after its publication, she abhorred the 'moaning undertone', and 'crude, if not morbid' thinking that resulted in

> the solicitudes, regrets, apprehensions, self-regards, and inbred miseries of various kinds, which breathe through these Sick-room essays, even where the language appears the least selfish and cowardly.[31]

Although she accepts that the truth of the essays, written from the heart, is not in doubt, she declares: 'I should not now write a sick-room book at all, except for express pathological purposes.'[32]

Nonetheless, Maria Frawley, writing in *Invalidism and Identity in Nineteenth-Century Britain* (2004), finds that Martineau's memoir 'still stands as a defining moment for a genre of invalid literature'[33] as the form developed in the era's commonplace books of confession, consolation and assistance. 'Never again,' notes Frawley, 'would a nineteenth-century British author deem it necessary or desirable to analyze chronic illness in so extended a manner' – a probing which, within the routines of a sick-room, enabled, if not empathy with her condition, recognition of the everyday surroundings it inhabits. *Sick-Room*'s 'great strengths', says Gillian Thomas in the *Dictionary of Literary Biography*, arises from Martineau's 'ability to generalize and derive insights from her own experience'.[34]

It is indispensable to our peace of mind to be alone when in pain[35]

With invalidism in vogue, rumours circulated that Martineau was beset, if not by hysteria, by neuroses or hypochondria; that, despite her activism and productivity, like other invalids without accurately diagnosed illnesses (Florence Nightingale, Charles Darwin and Alfred Tennyson included) she cultivated an indisposition of convenience and myth in which to work; after all, Darwin was said to have commented that although ill health had obliterated several years of his life, it had benefited his work by saving him from societal distractions and time-consuming amusements.

Yet, as Martineau had demonstrated before her illness, and during the decade when her pain was quiescent, she worked just as resolutely *outside* a sick-room as she did in quiet monotony within one. Of the subjects she discussed during mesmerism, biographer R.K. Webb observes that she spoke 'a great deal about suffering, about pressing ahead without stopping for it'.[36] What her invalidism *did* provide, she repeats, was a perspective, impossible for those in good health to appreciate. Central to that perspective was her view that passing pain allows occasional recognition of life's truths, but suffering for years brings proof. This frame of mind appears to have been compensation, rather than a reason, for her lasting seclusion. Speaking through *Deerbrook*'s disabled governess, she indicates an awareness of the insights gained in confinement even before she retreated to Tynemouth – reminding her readers that Lord Byron was unable to write poetry on Lake Leman, but had to wait until he was within four walls.[37] Supporting that outlook were her ability to adapt to and make the best of her circumstances, and her history of connectedness to 'fellow feeling'. The latter facility, which went beyond the general perception that empathy and moral responsibility were the concern of women, was evidenced in what can best be described as a drive to alleviate and promote understanding of suffering in all its forms: physical, emotional and social. This preoccupation, together with her remarkable resilience, almost certainly had roots in her youth – in particular, in the distress and social disruption, during her adolescence, of encroaching deafness, loss of smell and taste, adjustment to using an ear trumpet, and attunement, if not to isolation, then to solitude. Additional psychological conditioning is found in her reliance on observation, the need to establish 'rules' by which to negotiate life (presenting 'a pleasant self', turning 'every sigh into a smile'[38]), in her attitude towards Stoicism and martyrdom, and in the 'most beggarly set of nerves'[39] she describes as her birthright. She recalls, in particular, the trauma of her neighbour and childhood friend Emily's leg amputation (by Martineau's doctor uncle, as it happened):

> I was naturally very deeply impressed by the affair. It turned my imagination far too much on bodily suffering, and on the peculiar glory attending fortitude in that direction. I am sure my nervous system was seriously injured, [...] after my friend E. lost her leg. All manner of deaths at the stake and on the scaffold, I went through in imagination, in the low sense in which St Theresa craved martyrdom; and night after night, I lay bathed in cold perspiration till I sank into the sleep of exhaustion. [...] The good side [...] was that it occasioned or strengthened a power of patience under pain and privation that was not to be looked for in a child so sensitive and irritable by nature.[40]

She relates, too, her concern for Emily Cooper's parents' minimisation of their daughter's lameness, thereby adding to the child's suffering. And she recalls the hours of play she forwent as Emily's companion, concluding that her own 'self-denial which I never thought of refusing or grumbling at, must have been morally good for me'.[41]

We must rise, sooner or later[42]

Harriet Martineau died, aged seventy-four, of heart failure. 'Her last years,' writes R.K. Webb, 'must have been deeply distressing. Her poor health really made work impossible.'[43] Her heart and lungs were strained, her legs were oedematous and her abdomen was enormous, causing painful complications necessitating a return to opiates. Despite her difficulties, she turned brightly to anyone who came through her door with a fortitude that had been forged in childhood and moulded in the sick-room, where she assimilated the difference between reading 'from the clear print of assertion or observation' and gradually learning from personal experience, 'when every line is burnt in by pain'.[44]

Speculation about her condition was finally settled by her post-mortem, which proved that, far from exaggerating or imagining her symptoms, she had been genuinely and disturbingly ill. So widespread was literary and medical interest that the pathologist's report was made public in the *British Medical Journal* in 1877. The report stated[45] that Martineau had been afflicted with 'a vast tumour', a pear-shaped, fluid-filled cyst, with a circumference of thirty inches at its largest part, attached by a pedicule to a small, normal uterus. The cystic tumour had caused the lifting of her liver into her chest 'by pressure from below'. Her intestines had also been displaced upwards. And her 'diaphragm was much arched, by which the cavity of the chest was much diminished'. This meant, writes the examiner concerning the severity of Martineau's unsubstantiated heart symptoms, there must 'have been considerable interference with the action of both the lungs and the heart from pressure'. The abnormal positioning of the affected ovary, close to the uterus, suggested that the former, as it grew, had slowly been forced through the left-sided fallopian tube, 'attended with much suffering' analogous to the protracted 'passing of gall-stones or of calculi through the male urethra'. The slowly growing ovary had also caused the uterus to be displaced painfully downwards, pressing on her pelvic organs. The ten-year relief of her distress, from 1845, coincidental to the course of mesmerism, was explained by the gradual mechanics of the tumour's enlargement resulting in release of the uterus upwards, into a (temporarily) less confined space.

Had Martineau's tumour been diagnosed (a doctor had raised this possibility at Ambleside as her 'girth' increased), removal would not have been an option: England's first ovariotomy, performed in 1857, two years after her condition permanently reasserted itself, was denounced as murder, and another twenty years would elapse before the mortality rate dropped to an allowable level. Nor would Martineau have found relief in Europe, where renowned Paris neurologist Jean-Martin Charcot (physician and friend of Alphonse Daudet) would doubtless have subjected her to his ovary compressor – a heavy leather belt designed to push a pointed metal device, progressively tightened against the 'hysterogenic' zone of the ovary, over three days.

Today, the brick building in which Harriet Martineau lodged at Tynemouth is a bed-and-breakfast establishment, named after her. Martineau House displays Harriet's pleasant, patient face in a wrought-iron frame above the front door, and recalls her as 'one of the great social reformers of the 19th century'. It offers a Big Geordie Breakfast, including a Martineau Sausage (consisting of pork spiced with red onion, rosemary and sage, made by an award-winning Northumbrian butcher)[46] and a Harriet's Hamper Lunch (with organic bread buns, a selection of patés and a choice of pie or quiche) packed in a willow basket with a picnic rug provided. Special mention is made of the sweeping views from the bay window in what is believed to have been Martineau's bedroom.

*

The arborist had returned to prune the holly and laurel bay – fast approaching their pre-coppiced heights. 'How's your pine?' He clipped carelessly, as if cutting a hedge. I'd expected a degree of shaping, a trim: the use of secateurs rather than tree toppers. 'It still rocks like crazy in the wind; I'm on alert each time there's a gale.' I raked the ghost gum's incessant leaf drop. 'Too much movement in that canopy and tons of tree will come down.' He parted the cluster of spidery leaves encircling the holly with a practised hand, and plucked and ate a couple of its small orange projections. 'It's a kawakawa, or pepper tree, your garden's filling up with them. The fruit spikes are delicious – a spicy blend of black pepper and pineapple. Want to try one? The whole plant's edible – roots, bark, fruit. You can brew it to make a tonic. Chew it if you've got toothache. Māori plugged up their wounds with its leaves during the Land Wars.'[47] My rake made small piles of the aromatic gum leaves, also said to be medically beneficial. 'It's been nibbled, it looks like a weed, what else is it good for?' The tree surgeon shrugged. 'Asthma, high blood pressure – you name it. Use it in poultices to relieve arthritis and neuralgia.'

*

7 Observatory

A narrative poem set in Harriet Martineau's sick-room[1]

On 16 March 1840, Harriet Martineau, her pain rising and her strength ebbing, entered the stillness and solitude of Mrs Halliday's Tynemouth guest house expecting to die.

Tynemouth, September 1843

1.
Harriet rests her pen.

Each day, she thinks, the light
and shade of the landscape,
the inescapable gaze of the sky.

She blots the page and surveys
her lodgings:

her bedroom, where the curtains
remain closed for days;

her living room, ordered by
writing,
reading,

needlework,
the *faux* tortoiseshell horn
she cups in her palm
and holds to her ear,

the mounted telescope
that beckons heaven
and beguiles the river mouth's
myrtle leaf tide,

the breezy tree
on the wall
easing her longing
for foliage,
unmet by the haven's
only exposed
'scrubby little affair' – [2]
a sycamore barely altering
season to season,

Euclid's geometry of
postulations,
common notions,
and lesser angles
of perspective.

She pulls her sleeve over
her thumb and shines
the blotter's plated casing.

Her steel nib clinks.

Four years' pain,
patience,
piety
and compliance with divine tuition
have called for authorship:

a *solatium* for fellow sufferers
paused in a cleft of bed
and soft chair,
praised for their obliging quietude
while withering
further into silence;

a parabolic mirror
for attendants and friends
who have known only
passing storms.

She wipes her pen,
rearranges her cushions,
places her notebook
on her knee and stares
at the ceiling.

The normally diligent maid,
having swept the carpet
and shaken the drapes,
has missed a cobweb.

Filaments of silk and dust sway.

Harriet narrows her gaze
but sees no spider
biding time
in a draughty gap
or dark corner.

She winces,
slowly shifts into a prone position
on her adapted sofa,

makes a note
to turn her losses
into gains,
embrace her role
as 'a pioneer
in the regions of pain
[and] make the way
somewhat easier, –
or at least more direct
to those who come after.'[3]

A robin alights on the flower box,
bare, but for the promise of crocuses.

Half a potato,
a small portion of poached game
and yesterday's leeches
in a jar on the sideboard
await collection.

She raises the window,
sprinkles crumbs for the bird,
brushes a sluggish wasp
from the neck of her dress
and sighs.

Everything has been tried –
warm baths,

internal infusions,
anodyne lotions,
belladonna plasters,
iodine ointment,
tonic pills,
ergot of rye,
surgical removal of the polypous tumours –

but only opiates
(at a low dose to defer dependence
but sufficient to ease
conversation with guests)
have brought relief.

Above the hollow
where the prior once
sun dried his fish,
cows graze into winter.
Along the ridge,
the windmill and colliery wagons
intermittently mark time.

Across the river,
on the beach,
a girl holding her skirt
pursues a runaway ball
and a couple of boys
chase a kite.

'The delight of a happy mood
of mind,' says Miss Young,
Deerbrook's lame governess
sewing at a sunny window,
her face turned to the breeze,

'is beyond everything at the time; […]
but one cannot recall it:
one can only remember that it was so. […]

The imagination is a better
medium than the eye.'[4]

Harriet swivels her telescope,
trains her lens on the sand,
on the children's effortless shadows.

2.
She centres a leaf
on stretched linen,
smoothly in stem-stitch,

adds a petal
in straight-stitch
to prevent puckering –

another embellished pillowslip
for Mrs Chapman's anti-slavery bazaar in Boston.[5]

The jug on the dresser jolts,
imperceptibly.

Harriet's fingertips
on the wall
feel
footsteps,
a silence of enquiry
and reply,
the door closing,
shoes on the stairs,

as if sensing music,
her back pressed against
her sister's piano,
mingling pleasure and pain –
for what are
aching and throbbing
but vibrations?

Yellow or gold?
Shine, or secure finish?

Now, she holds a selection
of skeins to the light,

lays them alongside
the petal's white rays,

settles on the solid
cotton of gold

and, dot by dot,
shades the centre of the daisy
with French knots.

Overhead, Ary Scheffer's *Christus Consolator*[6]
enhaloed,
robed,
his palms open to the woman
weeping for the child
she has laid at his feet,

the man about to end his life
with a dagger,

the exile holding fast
to his wanderer's staff,

a soldier of the Polish uprising[7]
dying,
sword blunt,
cannonball silent,
body draped in his country's flag.

The print – without colour
but every bit as real
as the original –
radiates the solace
of centuries

as she hums hymns
of submission,
clings to the comfort
of sweet childhood tunes,
searches for charms
in the darkness,

and, when night
has faded and morning
is slow to break,
crawls beneath Milton's
'Insuperable height of loftiest shade,'
into the green calm
of 'Cedar, and pine, and fir,
and branching palm'.[8]

She averts her face:
redemption seems distant,
and contribution to life's spectacle
is the only honour she finds
in crossing the deep river's
rickety bridge.

An envelope with a foreign stamp
slides beneath the door.

A rare letter from Henry,[9]
financed abroad
with his hip flask
to Port Nicholson, New Zealand,

where he hitches his horse
to a post at high water mark
on Lambton Quay,

and ambles about his general store
in a dusty apron
polishing tin-ware,
trading blankets and brass
and weighing potatoes

a dart throw
from the Union Jack
fluttering in a cold southerly wind
above Barrett's Hotel?

Has he lapsed?

Is he happy in a land
without swans,
listening to the hoot
of a strange owl,
tending cabbages
in a salty patch
only yards from a beach?

She passes her needle
through a loop
on the underside of the fabric,

pulls the knot tight
and reminds herself:

'It is what we *are*
that matters,
not what we *do*,
that counts,'[10]

whether hidden by flax
at the watery edge
of the earth,

or in a sick-bed
behind a tapestry screen,
head inclined,
newspaper loosely in hand –

laudanum-sticky bottle
within reach,

counterpane
all concealing –

smiling
and implying
that an invalid's recess
is bread and fireside
warmth for the soul.

3.
She's aflutter.

Thomas and Jane Carlyle
have arrived, unexpectedly,[11]

interrupting a thought
that past pains
are as evanescent
as past pleasures,
and all that remains
are impressions –

causing her hand
to hesitate
between pen,
earpiece
and a bunch of late roses.

Thomas, beset by his stomach,
requests a glass of warm milk
sweetened with honey,

lights his pipe,
sits without speaking,
glances at the radiant
Consolator on the wall,

says (of her proposed memoir):
'Take care not to sound
like a "female Christ"
announcing "Look at me;
see how I am suffering!" '[12]

and asks for a plain biscuit.

Jane, still recovering
from last night's cruel headache
after sighting the four
moons of Jupiter
when she should have been resting,

peers through the telescope
but is distracted
by the unbounded glare
of the sea.

Harriet confesses
she imagines her mother
lost in London,
falling over bannisters,
floating from cathedral spires,

and Henry,
cheeks strangely red
on the deck of the *Arab*,
crossing the equator,

before directing her trumpet
to the shortcomings
of the Dundee Steamer
in bad weather,

heavy rain in the night
on Sunday,

an oppressively hot afternoon
on Monday,

the tempest induced
by a neighbour's howling dog
and talkative parrot,

two afternoons at Sunny Bank
with the Donaldsons,

the house at Kirkcaldy
'full of sumptuosities,
of flunkies,
and all sorts of superfluities',[13]

Jane's sadness
beneath her heart

and the He and Him
of her father,
outside whose door
she lay the night
He was dying,

Thomas's desire
to shut down his senses,
sleep like Epimenides
for fifty-seven years
in a cave
and awaken a prophet,

his manuscript,
mistaken by Mills' maid
for waste paper,

his identity,
pointing this way and that,

his call from the hall,
'There's a *gude* time coming!'[14]
as he and Jane leave,
chairs out of place,
books and cushions
scattered like papers.

4.
She stifles a yawn.

Such a night she's spent
gathering thoughts
on sympathy for invalids,

searching for a shared mood
and inflection,

ideas scratching
like a broad nib
on grained paper,

or pouring like watered ink
from an unstoppable bottle
staining the table,
doily
and damp cloth.

Such discomfort,
tossing from side to side,
pillows flat,
mattress lumpy,
legs tangled
in September's hot sheets;

turning from the scourges
of unuttered enquiry,
promises that pain
doesn't last
and fantasies that long-suffering
builds endurance
enabling transcendence,

to the clear-eyed consolation
of the friend
who declined to conjure
a favourable outcome
because she saw no signs
of recovery
and none likely,

to the wisdom of the guest
who had proffered

neither false protests
nor hopes,
but simply pressed her hand
and said, 'Yes',

to the silent spirit
of François Fénelon[15]
who pressed a finger
against his lips
and slid his doctrine
of Quietism
from the shelf,
reminding her to
'Listen awhile for the small
voice within.'

Truth is crucial,
she says, her voice rapid and low.
It rests the weary,
appeases the intellect
and gratifies the spirit's need
for all that is honourable.

Let visitors say
the patient is wan,
nurses declare
the medicine bitter,
doctors confess
painful treatment,
friends admit
imminent death,
attendants remonstrate
if praise is delayed
or their sleep interrupted.

She closes her work basket,
re-ties her wrapper,
gets heavily to her feet,
places the completed pillowcase
in an ironing pile,

brushes her hair
(decidedly brown),

pinches her cheeks
(unquestionably pallid),

stills the white curtains
flurrying and billowing
in the mirror.

Her maid sets down a tea tray
and decorates the pot
with a red brocade cosy.

A kindly, matter-of-fact servant
or nurse,
she decides,
creates less anxiety
than the most compatible friend.

She butters a fruit scone,
leans on the sill
and watches her leisurely neighbour
stroll down the lane,
hands on hips,
to tend the cow
and feed the pigs.

A dreamy door
opens and closes.

A window, narrowed
by wall-papered roses
and stifled by chimneys,
jostles with the height
and width of her once
London street.

Pain for life
on her shoulder –
its caprice,
its plunder,
its craving habit –
crowds the candle.

She rubs her eyes,
dips her pen
and writes:
'I descend into the deep.
How *shall* I bear this for five minutes?
What *will* become of me?'[16]

Her hand is even and neat
but the lines look heavy.

She reaches for
her lipped ink bowl,

mixes dense black
with medium blue,
saturation
with shading,
feathering
with flow

and refills
her cut glass well.

The sea's summer sheen,
steadied by rocks,
lights up the room –

ballast for winter storms
when, right before her eyes,
so close she can see
their mouths move,

men, miles off course
praying to be saved,

lash themselves
to tilted masts,
their arms barely shifting,

their life boats
breaking up,

the tug boats,
steaming and straining
in the swell,
running impossible lines to the beach.

8 An imago[1]

A contemplation of Polish poet and intellectual Aleksander Wat (1900–1967)

The very principle of pain and existence[2] – principium individuationis

I happened on Polish poet and intellectual Aleksander Wat in 2008, in *Polish Writers on Writing* (2007);[3] this was during the time I was preoccupied with the poetry and non-fiction of Central and Eastern Europe, with writers whose histories had been 'cut through by sudden lightning',[4] whose 'streets and attics' had been 'places of deportation, war, humiliation and pain'. The book had arrived in the post and I was scanning its contents. Wat, whose contribution was a personal essay entitled 'Diary Without Vowels',[5] was introduced as the author of the posthumously published memoir *My Century: the Odyssey of a Polish Intellectual* (1977) – a contemplation of totalitarianism regarded as 'one of the great documents of our time'.[6]

His essay, dated Berkeley 17 November 1964, had been written during his residence at the University of California; I immediately saw that his subject was the 'convoluted tangle' of severe chronic pain, and that he spoke with much bitterness. 'No one, no one but Ola,' he stated without preamble, and with a soon to be familiar directness,

> understands anything, anything at all about my illness or about my difficulty writing. They see how I complicate everything: my thoughts, my life, my fate.[7]

He continued:

> It's a puzzling thing – to go on about sickness, which to me is a fascinating theme and the mother of philosophy, something that Novalis[8] understood best of all – it is an astonishing thing to what extent people who are not suffering lack even the most elementary understanding of what constant, chronic physical pain is, pain lasting years, *la maladie-douleur* [pain-sickness].[9]

I read on, still standing at the table where I'd unpacked the parcel. Wat scrutinised those who, incapacitated by the pain of common ailments, were mistrustful when they heard he had suffered from the equivalent of toothache for twelve years with only rare intervals of relief. Are they so limited by their own passing indispositions, he asked, that they can't conceive of someone conversing, engaging in conceptual discussion and even laughing in a state of significant pain?

He bemoaned the insensitivity of friends who, having known about the burning pains in his face for years, declined to imagine what he might be enduring, and conveniently referred to them as migraines. Naturally, he concluded, 'the necessary condition here is experience of one's own suffering'.[10]

He lamented the humiliation caused by the practical assistance he received, not to lessen his suffering, but rather to placate 'the unfortunate *emmerdeur*, who for base reasons isn't in control of his own life', and the suggestion that his request for understanding stemmed from a plea for pity.[11]

The essence of 'incurable and chronic pain sickness', he wrote,

> with which one can live, but to which one can't become accustomed, is its suffusion of the intelligence and the whole social behaviour of the sufferer; so when people look at what I do, write and say, not seeing in me what is modified by sickness, they create in their minds a model of Aleksander Wat that I can't tolerate in my friends, which is humiliating to me. So more and more often I respond with only a wave of the hand. I insult those who are most concerned about me, and against my nature I wall myself up in misanthropic silence. And in this way my diabolical sickness can torture me all the better, raising up blind walls around me.[12]

I was captured by Wat's avid clarity. There was something elating and reassuring about his candid dissection of the 'monotonous terrain of long suffering', the unapologetic honesty of his 'misanthropic' response, his exposure of the scepticism, knowing asides and false positivity that negated his pain and trivialised his despair; the idea that a writer 'modified by illness' can be caught in a paradox in which their facility for writing suggests he or she is not really ill.

The lethargy of mid-afternoon lifted. The trees outside the window, weighted with morning rain, rustled. The sodden camellia blossoms on the lawn regained their pinkness.

I read the essay a second time: listening more closely to his restless voice, to the suggestion that political, spiritual and moral turmoil intensified his distress; reflecting on his need to justify and explain his physical suffering, and on the toll that his pain-laden cerebral cortex – in which his thinking was either frenetic or dogged by a barren somnolence – took on his writing.

I especially pondered over what he described as his 'nightmare of mental galloping like a void in the night',[13] his reference to being imprisoned behind 'blind walls', and what I found to be the perplexing significance assumed by such common descriptions of pain as 'diabolical' and 'torture'. Was this fervid patterning, I wondered, related to his self-acknowledged manic-depressive way of thinking, or to his contradictory personal history?

A quick check revealed that he was born Jewish, but converted to Christianity. Espoused Marxism, only to be tormented by guilt as the reality of 'the demonic bond' that was communism became apparent. Survived the ordeals of World War II, fourteen prisons and multiple near-fatal illnesses, only to succumb to pain.

When I went in search of Wat, I found that he was not widely known in the West.

At the time of writing the essay at Berkeley aged sixty-four, in exile in France since age fifty-nine, he was the author, in Polish, of only four published works: *Me From One Side and Me From the Other Side of My Pug Iron Stove* (futurist poetry, 1919); *Lucifer Unemployed* (experimental short stories, 1927); *Poems* (winner of the prestigious Nowa Kultura Prize, 1957); and *Mediterranean Poems* (1962).

Furthermore, although much of Wat's unpublished writing – including his autobiographical work *Diary Without Vowels*, in which the pain essay of that name was collected – had become available in Polish after his death in 1967, his work in English translation remained limited. I obtained *Mediterranean Poems* (1977), which arrived via a library in Virginia stamped 1978, having never been issued, *With the Skin* (poetry, 1989), *Lucifer Unemployed* (1990) and *My Century* (2003).

My Century, available in English since 1988, integrates autobiography with Wat's evaluations of Central and Eastern European history between 1919 and 1943. The work comprises a series of interviews with Wat recorded at Berkeley by Czesław Miłosz, himself in exile since 1951 and in 1980 to win the Nobel Prize for Literature. However, the recordings were discontinued prematurely on account of Wat's worsening pain, and the project languished during his lifetime. Regardless, Wat's mobile associations of memory, analysis and philosophy gives voice to 'the whole weight of reality',[14] as students at Berkeley described his poetry: a reality weighted, perhaps, not only with Wat's decade of physical pain, but also by what he refers to as his early psychic awareness of pain.

'I was always healthy,' he told Miłosz, 'though I may have had a certain philosophy of pain right from the start':

> The philosophy of pain – that's an old story in literature; beginning with the Romantics, if not Pascal, the greater part of literature is dominated by it, right up to the present day. Pain or despair. Only the costumes change.[15]

I started to ask myself if Wat's life events had not only encoded his writing, but also dominated his response to pain. If his belief that a poet's biography is the price 'paid for the poem, paid in his own flesh and blood',[16] explained the state of crisis evident in the essay he had written at Berkeley. To what extent had Aleksander Wat also absorbed the pain and despair of Poland?

In the cool fall air[17]

2003. Warsaw in autumn. Not the warm golden weeks of late September for which Poland is famed, when the sun glances sideways and Arius, at its brightest, is directly overhead, but November, as the last skylark departs and ankle-deep leaves and sharp air take the breath.

The slip: jetlag at six in the morning, water on the floor, a shudder in midair, the crash onto my back; able, after cautious testing of fingers, toes, limbs, to be levered by John to my feet.

Paramedics. The click and hum of the hotel lift. Subdued light in the lobby. Swing of the solid front door. And, from the ambulance, jolting and swaying en route to the Clinical Hospital of the Infant Jesus, the landmark outline of the *soc-realizm* Palace of Culture and Science – 40 million bricks placed by 3,000 Poles and over 3,000 imported Soviet builders between 1952 and 1955 – a monument to the forced Stalinisation of Poland.

*

WAT: *I was also in the Infant Jesus Hospital.*

*

Aleksander Wat, the familiar voice in my head. The ghost with a broad brow, dark eyes and modest moustache, always stylishly clad – cuffs, links, hat, whatever's the fashion. He was admitted following a stroke on 14 January 1953, the day that Stalin initiated a new purge alleging his doctors had plotted to poison him.

*

WAT: *I waited three days before agreeing to admission.*

*

The hospital was an orphanage in the 1770s. Today, the Clinical Hospital of the Infant Jesus is part of Warsaw's Emergency and Trauma Centre. It has kept its original name, despite the political climate.

*

WAT: *Everyone was gripped by fear, anticipating the latest purge. Stalinism was the realization of Marxism-Leninism – the practical result.*

*

John and I are ushered along corridors with high walls and wooden benches. I have an impression of grainy half-light, film footage of Soviet hospitals, scenes from Solzhenitsyn. The Uzbekistan clinic in *Cancer Ward*, Kostoglotov to Dontsova: 'No sooner does a patient come to you than you begin to do all his thinking for him.'[18] The camp dispensary in *One Day in the Life of Ivan Denisovich*, Vdovushkin to Shukov: 'Why didn't you report sick last night? You know very well there's no sick call in the morning. The sick list has already been sent to the planning department.'[19]

Workers (orderlies, cleaners?) in white coats and caps stare from doorways with unabashed curiosity.

'*Dzień dobry.*'

'*Dzień dobry.*'

We wait. My passport is examined by a nurse.

'Stefania? Potocka de Montalk?'

'Part Polish, part French.'

She takes me to an X-ray room where I undress in front of an uncovered ground-floor window and edge, unaided, onto a table. Radium, plutonium, the atomic bomb; discoveries used in the treatment of cancer. Marie Curie: the first woman to be awarded the Nobel Prize, to teach at the Sorbonne, to be awarded the Prize for a second time; the mustard frontage of the house in which she was born, in the Old Town, close to the hotel – its two-roomed museum, Marie dressed in black, the curious luminosity of her face.

We wait again.

'The window in the X-ray room was bare,' I whisper to John. 'At the same height as a busy footpath.'

'People here have seen more than you could ever imagine,' he replies.

An industrious bucket and mop: another inquisitive onlooker.

I recall a previous trip to Poland: to Auschwitz-Birkenau; the 900-year-old Wieliczka Salt Mine, still operational, with its chest sanitorium 135 metres down; the cottonwoods scattering their snow-like seeds in Łazienki Park; the scarf I bought in the Nowy Świat that I wore straight from the counter through parks and neo-classical palaces, children playing descant recorders in doorways, reflections moving in and out of the trees like tramlines in autumn.

A doctor, traditional in white, methodical and thorough, looks and listens. Since three lower ribs are implicated, he wonders in English if I've incurred adrenal bleeding, ruptured a kidney or damaged my spleen and advises bed rest for two days. I tell him I will recognise the symptoms. He sits at a small wooden desk and writes a prescription for painkillers. Says, 'You have a famous Polish name.' Unlocks a little tin box on a chain with a key from his pocket and extracts his signature on a stamp. Reaches for an inkpad. Endorses the script. Re-locks the stamp in the metal container. Hands me his phone number and says, 'Call me at once if you start passing blood.'

*

WAT: *I felt as if my skull and body had been smashed by a tank: a tank painted a drab olive or khaki green – inferior Soviet quality control meant colour variations batch to batch. The diagnosis was a tongue-testing thrombosis arterieae cerebelli posterior inferioris.*

*

Wat's stroke had produced piercing pain on the left side of his face and right side of his body, as well as nausea, hiccup, laryngeal spasm, photophobia, vertigo, headache and double vision: symptoms collectively known as Wallenberg's Syndrome. When he attempted to stand he fell to the left. If he lay down, he felt that he and anyone else in the room would fall and the walls would collapse.

In the ward, despite the severity of his condition, he was subjected to indoctrination by loudspeakers from early morning until ten at night. He found the most tolerable instructions to be those related to agriculture (including the potentially useful conversion of refuse into compost). The worst were the 'optimistic songs or choral howlings and recitations, and the very worst – the sports news, which, to make it more intolerable was broadcast late in the evening',[20] setting everyone up for insomnia. He would later write of the blaring intrusions in the poem 'Dreams from the Shore of the Mediterranean, Third Dream' (1962),[21] composed in exile, in France:

[…] By the way,
is it possible to make one's own psychoanalysis while sleeping?
Once I succeeded.… In the 'Siberia' of the Warsaw neurology
clinic, where the epileptic Y*** kept jumping up
and throwing his arm wildly. *Tu-les*, they howled then
outside the window. Old M***'s death rattle came from above his
hanging jaw, a withered Ramses, he will die in the morning
under the loudspeaker which will splutter sweet
cream of wheat for the hog
and a plump watch will scratch her unsleepy behind
bandaging with her other hand that unruly
jaw. But you are with me, now nothing can
happen to us.

After a couple of months, he was moved to the Hospital of the Ministry of Health. Shortly before his transfer, Stalin died. That day, 5 March, when his wife Ola (Paulina Watowa) came to visit she found a small, hushed crowd of doctors and nurses at the entrance to the ward and thought they were mourning her husband. The ward was turned into a chapel of grief. Candles were lit, flowers were brought in and a large photo of Stalin was trimmed with black crepe. Wat scribbled 'AT LAST' on a calendar and then tore out the page, to be safe.

*

Lying down is painful, so I sleep in a chair. I read Władysław Szpilman's memoir *The Pianist*, formerly *Death of a City*, published in Warsaw in 1946; the book was banned during communist domination and out of print until 1998. John, never far from Dickens, reimmerses himself in *Bleak House*. People are sympathetic; everyone knows someone who's bruised their back or broken a rib.

The intermittent pelvic pain, diagnosed as ischial bursitis, hints at a return. 'Bones mend,' I think. 'Muscles and soft tissues heal. Pain passes.'

After two days I move gingerly around the city. The air's misty, minus one degree Celsius. We walk to the Church of the Holy Cross where the urn containing the ashes of Chopin's heart is sealed in a pillar; there's standing room only at the service. We also spend an afternoon in the 600-year-old Castle. After the failure of the World War II Warsaw Uprising in 1944, German sappers laid dynamite in the tens of thousands of holes they had bored in its stripped walls. The crystal, gilding, parquet and marble have been faithfully recreated, and the tapestries and treasures, spirited into safekeeping, are in place once again.

I buy a woollen hat from a woman wearing several coats in Castle Square, and a series of postcards depicting the scale of the city's demolition, and the speed and accuracy of its rebuilding. Of Warsaw's razing following the sixty-three-day failed Uprising, poet and insurrectionist nurse Anna Świrszczyńska writes in 'The Last Polish Uprising' of 'the hour'

> When the place where a million people had lived
> became the emptiness of a million people.[22]

*

WAT: *Imagine this: pain heightened by concentrated thinking or writing for more than fifteen minutes; a rare condition, consistent with damage to the central nervous system.*

*

Wat slowly recovered, but the biting, searing, radiating nerve pain in his left face and right leg, and the tendency for discomfort elsewhere in his body to be amplified, did not abate. Nonetheless, he believed, as he left the Ministry of Health hospital with Ola, that pain, with which he was not unfamiliar, eventually ceases or at least settles at a liveable level.

In 1954, Soviet officials gave him permission to travel to Stockholm to consult foremost neurosurgeon Professor Olivecrona. The professor diagnosed atypical Babinski–Nageotte Syndrome, a rare complication of the stroke. 'A tiny injury,' writes Wat.[23] A clot 'in the medulla oblongata on the very path to the still mysterious thalamus'. Surgery in the injured area – instrumental in the transmission and integration of pain sensations – was not advised, owing to the risk of paralysis, auditory and visual damage or impairment of mental faculties. Olivecrona predicted that the pain would lessen in seven years. 'From this sickness,' said Dr Hartwig, a physician in Poland, 'you can escape – only by the window.'

11 November: Independence Day.

We join the crowd assembling in Piłsudski Square before the Tomb of the Unknown Soldier: Warsaw is commemorating Poland's restoration as a democratic nation in 1918, following 123 years partitioned between Germany Austria and Russia. The country had suffered over a century of resistance, rebellion and disappearance from the map of Europe. My great-great-grandfather, Count Józef Franciszek Jan Potocki, was sentenced to death by Tsar Nicholas I for his role in the 1830–1831 uprising, and sought exile in France, where he took the name Potocki de Montalk. In 1868 Józef's son, Joseph Wladislas Edmond (beset, it's said, by inheritance difficulties), emigrated to New Zealand.

Warsaw also remembers: World War I; The Polish–Soviet War of 1919–1921; World War II, during which Poland lost 22 per cent of her population, the greatest percentage of all countries involved including Germany and the Soviet Union; forty-four years' post-war Soviet domination; the Solidarity trade union movement which, supported by the Roman Catholic Church, brought about the collapse of the communist regime in Poland in 1989 and the subsequent weakening of Soviet Eastern Block governments.

Sun. Music. Everywhere, red-and-white flags, stylish young women in long belted coats, elegant older women wearing fur, men in windbreakers with children on their shoulders. The army marches past. Strong boots pound the ground. Poland's resilience in the face of repeated foreign occupation is palpable.

Shivering hurts. I stand on the periphery of the commemorations to avoid being jostled.

*

WAT: *The eminent professor was wrong.*

*

The following day, still in Warsaw, a policeman cordons off a blanketed form beneath a bush in a park, checks his watch and records his findings in a ring-bound book resting on the roof of his car.

John and I recall a friend who emigrated from Soviet Poland, and, despite having served with the Israeli armed forces, still panics at the sight of a police officer.

We speak of another friend who emigrated from Russia. Her father, a surgeon, was sent to the Gulag after returning from a World War II concentration camp, his capture by Germans deemed to be an unwarranted surrender. The summer her parents visited us in Wellington they asked, in translation: 'Is your house warm in winter? The walls are so thin. There is sky at the tips of our fingers.'

Acrobatic birds – white specks on blue – search for air currents, circle and float, rise higher and higher.

John reminds me of the dream I once had in which I tripped and fell, and, falling, thought, 'I might die, how can an incident this trivial end my life?'

All this and much more[24]

*

WAT: *My quest for the root cause of my unresolved pain was endless. Was some sort of genetic predisposition responsible? The disunity of an unemotional father and over-reactive mother? My physical asymmetry, as pointed out by portraitists? My manic-depressive tendency as a youth? War? Political pollution? In the end I settled on supernatural castigation and had Padre Pio, the stigmatic, perform an exorcism in Italy – with bitterly disappointing results.*

*

Aleksander Chwat (he took the name Wat as a writer) was born in Warsaw of liberal Jewish-Polish intellectuals, the youngest of seven children. His paternal and maternal ancestors included Jewish scholars and commentators and a Rabbi. However, his father, influenced by Kierkegaard, declined to regulate his family's religious decisions. Consequently, and despite Yiddish as the preferred language at home, the essential sway of Polish Roman Catholicism, and the pious example of their Catholic family nurse, the Chwat children grew up as atheists and socialists. Recalls Wat, in *My Century*: 'I had total freedom at home. I was already a Darwinist by the time I was a six- or seven-year-old brat.'[25]

As a child and an intellectual prodigy, Wat read widely in German, Russian and French. He studied philosophy and logic at Warsaw University. And he wrote poetry, although not in the 'spoken language' of the newly formed Polish *Skamander* school, named for the journal that published their work. The Skamander poets believed in 'the sanctity of a good rhyme, in the divine origin of rhythm, in revelation through images born in ecstasy and through shapes chiselled by work'.[26] But Wat's preference was the cultural and intellectual nonconformity of Dadaism, and the syntactically liberated language of futurism. With Poland recently independent after more than a century of partitioning, literary expression was expanding, and the duty of writers to patriotism was easing giving poets the freedom to write, 'And in the spring, let me see spring – not Poland.'[27]

There were broader political associations. Wat came of age in the wake of World War I's atmosphere of chaos and nihilism; and in the aftermath of heavy fighting in partitioned Poland where Germany, Russia and Austria had formed the Eastern front. He absorbed the idealism of the Russian Revolution, the rise of the Soviet Union, and debate about the necessity of far-reaching political and social changes in Europe. Just as sections of the academic and literary communities in the West embraced Marxist theory and moved to the left – unclear as to the consequences of classless socialism in practice and the true extent of Bolshevik terror – so too did Poles, Wat prominent among them. For the 'young Polish literati of the 1920s', writes Marci Shore in *Caviar and Ashes: A Warsaw*

Generation's Life and Death in Marxism 1918–1968 (2006), 'communism was cosmopolitan, avant-garde, sexy.'[28]

*

I take a photo of John in Castle Square beside King Sigismund's Column, twenty-two metres high. 'There's too much backlight,' I say. 'I'll use the flash – you'd better look to the side.'

Within walking distance, the Palace of Science and Culture, nicknamed Stalin's Syringe, impales the indigo sky. Not even the autumn sun softens its outline. The structure's reach, once unmatched in Europe, has been overtaken by sixteen European skyscrapers and some one hundred and eighty-six buildings globally. The dedication to Stalin has been removed from the lobby, and the forty-three floors of stolid space – engineered to emote grandeur and political power – are now occupied by offices and shops, as well as museums, theatres and exhibition halls. But while the viewing terrace on the thirtieth floor offers the best views of Warsaw because, as Varsovians say, 'It's the only location from which the structure cannot be seen,' it catches a cold wind not felt on the street.

*

In keeping with his teenage 'philosophy of pain', Wat's first book, *Me from One Side and Me from the Other Side of My Pug Iron Stove* (1919), was, as he puts it, a narrative of 'authentic despair, an entirely ungrounded horrible despair'.[29] An extended prose poem, *Iron Stove* tells a story of the disintegration of civilisation, and also of self. In the final stanza Wat reveals it is he who burns in his stove's accusatorial chamber. The tale of diabolical torment, temptation, disease and suicide might be described, writes Tomas Venclova in *Aleksander Wat: Life and Art of an Iconoclast* (1996), 'as a journey through a Dantesque or Brueghelian hell with no paradise in sight':[30] a purgatory in which, Wat writes in the poem, 'Girls die on the white sow thistle of the horizons'[31] and 'At midnight it is always necessary to place your head under the dazzling, yes! dazzling knife of the guillotine.'[32] The poem's disturbing images and hallucinatory flights of association, suggestive of a racing mind, confirm not only the force of Wat's preoccupation with world pain, but also with futurism's 'free words'.

> By day, I sleep.[33] By night, I sneak into sickly back streets [I am] very radiant, very radiating. When it is already late I fall on my back in gutters and hide my rumpled and blind face in the dazed humps of lanterns.

Parts of the book were declared blasphemous and censored, and critical response was guarded. A notable exception was the assessment of prominent writer and artist, Stanisław Witkacy, who asserted in *Iron Stove*'s only comprehensive review that the long poem was a work of genius.

However, Wat's second publication, *Lucifer Unemployed* (1927), comprising a collection of nine concentrated paradoxical parables scorning civilisation, was released to acclaim. Suddenly, Wat assumed the status of literary star. He was hailed by Vladimir Mayakovsky as 'a born futurist',[34] journals in Poland and abroad sought his essays and stories, and his financially rewarding Russian, French and English translation commissions earned him high praise.

A year after *Lucifer* was released, he married Paulina (Ola) Lew, a drama student. Leaving the ball at which they had met, Wat called across the street to a friend: 'Have you seen what good fortune has come to me? Such a beautiful girl – and she wanted me.'[35] Ola, also Jewish, shared Wat's political and literary inclinations. Theirs would be an enduring love. Recalling forty years together, Wat speaks of Ola's binding loyalty and love. It was Ola, he makes clear, who protected him 'against the temptations of conformism',[36] who tirelessly supported him through sickness and despair. Ola's memoir, *All That Is Most Important*, written after Wat's death, begins: 'All that is most important in my life is linked to Aleksander.'[37]

But Wat's literary rise was to be brief. As Polish Marxism strengthened and Dadaism and futurism were abandoned as 'bourgeois decadence', members of the communist avant-garde of the early 1920s confined their writing to popularising the new ideology. *Lucifer* and *Iron Stove* would remain Wat's only creative publications until *Poems* (1957) and *Mediterranean Poems* (1962). In 1929, faithful to his intellectual mission, he founded and edited the influential (and barely legal) communist journal *The Literary Monthly*. Ola joined him as typist and general administrator. Three years later, the *Monthly* was closed down by Polish officials and Wat, although not a registered member of the Polish Communist Party for fear his intellect would cause 'infection'[38] within the 'communist church', was imprisoned for three months. After his release he was subjected to ongoing Polish surveillance. Nonetheless, he obtained the literary editorship at prestigious publishing house Gebethner and Wolff, and held the position until Germany's later invasion of Poland in 1939.

Between 1932 and 1939, Wat's allegiance to communism faltered. News of the death sentences handed down at the Moscow show trials, reports of Soviet collectivisation's unsustainable quotas, and rumours of the annihilation of millions of peasants by famine in the Ukraine filtered through. Then, as the decade drew to a close, Stalin, suspicious of double agents within the ranks of Polish communism, disbanded the Party in Poland and had its members executed or dispatched to the Gulag. Wat, by now dominated by the ominous clouds of Soviet and Nazi extremism, confessed his fear that Ola, Andrzej, who had been born in 1931, and he 'would die horrible deaths, that Poland would go under'.[39]

*

I'm required in Kraków for a filmed TV interview, following the publication of *Unquiet World* in Polish translation. I sit with the book in the Café Bristol, revising. At the next table, the marking and passing of a manuscript, pipe smoke, coffee, the mysterious spoken music of Polish.

The director has expressed interest in *Unquiet World*'s chapter on the Katyn Massacre of 1940. Geoffrey Potocki's *Katyn Manifesto* (1943), a pamphlet self-published in London, was the only statement of the truth in English about the Katyn Massacre until after World War II. The truth was that the murder and burial of more than 5,000 Polish officers in the woods at Katyn, discovered by the Germans in 1943, had been carried out by the Soviets, by then Britain's ally. Moreover, the officers had been part of a larger group of over 15,000 Polish officer prisoners of war and Poland's elite intellectual and professional population taken from Soviet concentration camps, hands tied behind their backs, and individually shot with a bullet to the base of their heads. Although a public issue in Europe, both the scale of the atrocity and its perpetration by Soviets were dismissed by Britain as rumour. Potocki was accused in the House of Commons of threatening relations between the Allies, arrested by Special Branch on a 'trumped up' blackout charge, and imprisoned for two months before being ordered to an agricultural camp in Northumbria.

I'd been aware of 'Katyn' since first meeting my cousin in the late 1960s. Given his eccentricity, I'd regarded his account and claim of a cover-up with scepticism until the USSR finally admitted responsibility in 1990. Five years later, British intelligence reports, sealed for fifty years after the war, confirmed the British Government's complicity. 'This is obviously the most convenient attitude to adopt,' officials had stated, 'and, if adopted consistently enough will doubtless receive universal acceptance. [...] Any other view would have been most distasteful to the public since it could be inferred we were allied to a power guilty of the same sort of atrocities as Germany.'[40]

In Poland, the massacre and its cover-up remains a potent symbol of Soviet oppression – of the silence, indeed the lie, imposed for forty-nine years on Poles unable to enter the truths of their loved ones' deaths on gravestones and publicly grieve.

Memorials to Katyn have been erected worldwide. The previous year, John and I had stood at Warsaw's stark, haunting Monument to the Fallen and the Murdered in the East. The nearly two million Poles who were deported to Soviet camps between 1939 and 1953 are remembered, in bronze, by a rail truck filled with Roman Catholic crosses, Orthodox Christian crosses, Stars of David and Islamic crescents reminiscent of Eastern Poland's religious and cultural diversity – and by a section of railway track, its sleepers inscribed with the deportee's points of departure and arrival, Katyn among them.

*

WAT: *To think I once gathered, without knowledge of pain, at the Café Ziemiańska in Warsaw with Skamander, futurist and unattached poets passing from table to table, and in summer sat out in the garden sipping strong, bitter tea, watching Ola stir chocolate into her coffee.*
To think we didn't see that we were attempting to cure the sickness of nihilism with the metastatic cancer of communism.

*

Poland's pain. Invasion by Germany. Occupation by Soviet Russia. The imposition of foreign ideological extremism, twice over.

Wat's pain. Political. Psychic. Physical.

'Trauma is never exclusively personal,' writes Leigh Gilmore in *The Limits of Autobiography: Trauma and Testimony* (2001); 'it always exists within complicated histories that combine harm and pleasure along with less inflected dimensions of everyday life. Remembering trauma entails contextualising it within history.'[41]

Wat told Miłosz:

> I was political when it was time to be a poet and a poet when it was time to be political. My illness is a result, an expression of my anachronism.[42]

He also said, of intellectual endorsement of totalitarianism in Poland and abroad: 'In fact, communism arose to satisfy certain hungers.'

> One of those hungers was a hunger for a catechism, a simple catechism. That sort of hunger burns in refined intellectuals much more than it does in the man on the street. The man on the street always had a catechism: he replaced one catechism with another.[43]

On 1 September 1939, Germany invaded Poland from the west. Seventeen days later the Red Army, in contempt of peace treaties still in force with Poland and without any formal declaration of war, moved in from the east. In Warsaw, the Gestapo, with Wat's name on its list, began to round up members of the intelligentsia.

Wat, Ola and Andrzej, aged eight, joined the early exodus to Lwów in eastern Poland (today Lviv in Ukraine), soon to fall to the Soviets. They fled from one city of fear to another. Warnings of Poland's imminent dissolution and the threat of denunciation were ever present. At the Polish-language Soviet newspaper where Wat found work and a misspelling of Stalin's name could mean death, Wat lived with the terror that his proofreading would be less than perfect. So menacing was the climate of treachery that refugees from Warsaw, Jewish and non-Jewish alike, Aleksander Wat's younger brother and a sister among them, stood in long lines seeking permission to return to German-occupied Poland; two of Aleksander's brothers and their families, relatives of his mother and father, Anusia Mikulak, the Wat family's nanny, and Ola's parents and sister would die in Nazi concentration camps.

Anticipating arrest, terrified for Ola and Andrzej, Wat played the Soviet game. He re-established his socialist leanings, acknowledged Stalin's wisdom, spoke out against pre-war Poland, declaring the autumn of 1939 the last such season of autocratic Poland's oppression. Of the assailed, once vibrant and cultural city of Lwów, he announced that 'the observer is struck by the mental state of those who frequent the cafés – joyful greetings, sparkling eyes, an unrestrained tone'.[44] Sweating profusely in a public act of self-criticism, he confessed that his former concerns and the reported terrors of the Soviet system were wrong. He abhorred himself. Later, he would say, 'Poland was undergoing a tragedy, and there I was taking the grand tone.'[45] His role in the propagation of 'the lie', as he described communism, would torment him for the rest of his life.

His arrest came quickly. In January 1940, he was accused of being one of a group of 'depraved persons'[46] posing as 'revolutionary writers' and held under harsh conditions in a Lwów prison. He was interrogated continuously day and night as a Trotskyite, a Zionist, a Catholic and a Polish nationalist. Subjected to five days in a punishment cell open to the mid-winter weather, he paced cease-lessly without sleep to avoid freezing to death. Word circulated that Polish citizens judged to be resistant to communism on account of their education and social standing were being deported. Three months later he learned that Ola and Andrzej had been crammed into a cattle truck and sent on a gruelling 9,000-kilo-metre, three-week journey to hard labour in Soviet Central Asia.

While Ola made bricks, chopped manure for fuel, ground grain and battled starvation on a state farm in southern Kazakhstan with Andrzej, Wat was trans-ferred, by way of a series of Soviet jails, to Moscow's Lubianka Prison, and thence to incarceration at Saratov. Unlike his cellmates, and because the purpose of his interrogations was Soviet understanding of the Polish leftist mind-set, he was spared torture. Nonetheless, his malnourished state became critical and he was hospitalised, near death.

One night, in what might have been the hallucinatory effects of hunger, he interpreted the sounds of an anti-aircraft alarm as 'vulgar laughter'. When the mirth was followed by an image of hooves and the smell of brimstone, he believed he had encountered the devil. An awareness of God's presence fol-lowed, and Wat was overcome with a profound feeling of peace and spiritual unity.[47] He converted to Christianity; in his mind, perhaps, was the devotion of his family's nurse, and the constancy of his Catholic Ukrainian cellmates, with whom he had recited the Rosary in Lwów's Zamarstynow Prison. He had no way of knowing that Ola too had converted, during her ordeal on the Kazakh Steppe. In 1953, Wat and Ola would be privately baptised in a Roman Catholic ceremony in Warsaw. Their conversion does not appear to have been influenced by anti-Semitism, despite their concerns before the war. Wat was attracted to Christianity, writes his biographer Tomas Venclova, not by the Church's teach-ings or history, but by his identification with the figure 'of the suffering Christ'. In this sense, says Venclova, he 'saw the Crucifixion as an archetype of the dis-tress of countless peoples under totalitarian rule', and Christ as 'an archetypal image of Jewishness'. In Wat's own words: 'Jesus, as the Jewish son of Mary was for me then – and always – a Jew – a Jew from alpha to omega, the highest incarnation not only of the Jewish psyche, but also of the Jewish fate.'[48]

Released from Saratov in November 1941, in the amnesty for Polish prisoners that followed Germany's invasion of Russia, he set out, supported by a fellow Pole he met on the train, on a journey of some 3,000 kilometres in search of Ola and Andrzej, also recently freed. Such was his emaciation and debilitation that a doctor who treated him en route warned that he had less than two weeks to live.

*

We take a train to Kraków. On boarding, John, laden with luggage, is accosted in the corridor by pickpockets as I walk on ahead to secure a compartment. I miss the scuffle, the shouts and the quicksilver departure of the three men who weren't to know that John, a Scot, carries his wallet deep in an inside pocket.

*

The family was reunited in March 1942 in the Kazakh capital, Alma-Ata, into which Polish refugees from the Gulag were streaming. They met in the wretched room that Wat had taken on the outskirts of the city, a room bare but for the narrow plank that constituted his bed.

'And they arrived,' he says in *My Century*. 'Andrzej looked like a child from the Warsaw ghetto. He had the beginnings of tuberculosis, a corpse's skull.'[49] Ola, who was in her thirties, 'looked like a sixty-year-old woman'. She was 'completely ravaged', in rags. A few feet from Wat's plank, on a table, lay the scarlet-fever-spotted body of the householder's baby son who had died during the night. Ola recalls a wooden hut, 'stuffy and filthy'.[50] Aleksander, aged forty, last seen young, strong, hair dark, eyes large and shining, is remembered as an old man, 'grizzled, thin exhausted'.

They lived as best they could, dependent on contacts. At one time Wat made a meagre living translating Russian and inspecting schools for the local delegation of the London-based Polish government in exile. He was constantly fearful, pressured, subjected to questioning by the NKVD (the interior ministry of the Soviet Union, which included the secret police) about the possibility of his colleagues' anti-Soviet activities.

In early 1943, his heart weak, still suffering from scurvy and the other effects of the starvation he'd incurred as a prisoner, he was ordered by Soviet officials to move his family to the desert settlement of Ili in southeast Kazakhstan. 'At the slightest wind the sand rose as a dark rusty cloud,' Ola writes of Ili, and 'in the zenith of summer the heat reached 50 degrees'.[51] They barely existed for three and a half years, working as odd-job labourers, surrounded by criminals, dirty sand, patchy weeds, hovels of mud and cow dung, and stalls selling, to the 'richer' inhabitants, 'pieces of fat mutton speckled with flies'. Bouts of dysentery, pneumonia and typhus repeatedly brought Wat close to death – and burial in a cemetery where the bodies were scavenged by dogs.

Soviet persecution continued. An NKVD Passportisation campaign to force Polish nationals in Kazakhstan to accept Soviet passports began. Despite his health, Wat instigated mass resistance. Exposed, he and Ola were imprisoned. In jail, the pressure to sign up was brutal, resulting in suicides. Ola, who sustained a fractured rib, writes that the nights were filled with torture and terror; that the 'walls of the prison seemed to vibrate and tremble with human suffering'.[52] Finally, she complied, accepting a Soviet passport on a piece of cheap paper. Wat refused and was transferred to a common-law prison in Alma-Ata, where he was locked up with the jail's most violent criminals in the expectation he would be beaten into submission. He was spared when his proud conviction and bearing earned him the respect of the ringleader.

'Aleksander was even more haggard now,' Ola recalled after visiting him. 'The skin on his face had gone grey.'[53] Of his release, after three months, she remembered his shaved head, his eyes blazing with rebellion, and the aura of one 'who has the sense of freedom of being true to himself, who is determined both within himself and in his actions'.

In 1946, Aleksander, Ola and Andrzej made their circuitous way back to Warsaw. Poland was 'utterly' spent. Writes Neil Ascherson: 'The land had been drenched in blood; the forest turf bulged with mass graves. It was not only the Poles who had been slaughtered. Their country had been used as the site for the extermination of six million European Jews.'[54]

Ola immediately saw, in the devastation left by Germany and the gathering shadow of the Soviet Union, that Poland faced a bleak future. Like 'two halves of a cracked nut,' she writes in her memoir, 'the old life and the new life now approaching would not merge'.[55] Three years later, the coalition government was overtaken by Communist Party monopoly. Years of strict Stalinism followed. The newly formed Polish Writers' Union declared Socialist Realism – with its stated aim the promotion of socialism and communism – to be the sole direction of Polish literature.

Wat went to work as Chief Editor at the State Publishing Institute. He recoiled from the political and literary environment, spoke out against communism, was ostracised and classified as hostile. In 1953, arrest pending, he suffered his stroke.

*

The train to Kraków races over the flat lands of Poland, strategic terrain of invasion: horse-drawn artillery, armoured cars, the Wehrmacht's panzer divisions, the Red Army's T-series tanks, the barbed wire of the Third Reich's prisoner-of-war, labour and extermination facilities – more than 400 camps. On either side, farms and small woods slide by. Left, east. Right, west. Sovietism's 'Work is an Honour'. Nazism's 'Work Makes You Free'. Poland, in Wat's words, 'caught in that scissors'.[56]

In the neighbouring east, between 1932 and 1933, five million, possibly up to eleven million, Ukrainian peasants died slow deaths in the *Holodomor* – extermination by starvation – at the hands of Stalin, within their country's cordoned borders.

In the west, at Oświęcim an hour out of Kraków, between 1942 and 1945, an estimated one and a half million of the Holocaust's six million Jews were systematically murdered at Auschwitz-Birkenau, Hitler's largest camp of mass extermination. From 1940, Auschwitz, and later Birkenau, was also a place of terror and death for Poles; political and religious prisoners, homosexuals and gypsies from other Nazi-occupied countries; and Soviet prisoners of war.

We had visited the Oświęcim State Museum the previous year. En route, spring blossoms, villages and the tour guide's announcement of a house painted blue to indicate the presence of a marriageable daughter; and a conversation about blue as an insect deterrent, and laundry-blue as an inexpensive means of colouring lime. At Oświęcim, as the coach pulled into the car park, a hush. Brick buildings. The shadows cast by those buildings, despite the brightening of daisies in the grass. Concrete. A cool sun. A feeling of dread. A sense of duty. An immeasurable echo of silence. That evening I had no words for my diary. I left the terrible details in the *Auschwitz Birkenau Guide-Book*. Railway lines. Unloading ramps. Watchtowers. Faces photographed from three angles. Barracks. Punishment cells. Gas canisters. Crematoria. The Wall of Death. The medical experimentation block I could not enter. A bale of hair cloth. A child's name and address on a suitcase.

*

The lips [...] walked into and out of[57]

*

WAT: *Living in pain parallels the falsities of life in a totalitarian state. Neither states behave according to functional norms. They both suppress language and distort or confiscate disclosure of truth. Each would be easier to bear if not for its linguistic disguises ...*

*

In the relative thaw that followed Stalin's death, Wat, in the face of three decades of creative silence, turned again to poetry. 'We [...] had a respect for him as an intellectual power,' says Miłosz, 'but we didn't expect [...] his being reborn as a poet.'[58] Miłosz was of the view that Wat's poetic revival between 1957 and 1967, when his pain worsened by the year, verged on the 'miraculous'.

'One turns into a poet,' writes Wat in 1963, the year before he went to Berkeley,

> when one ceases to be him: when one comes back to the state of primeval consciousness of a six-month old infant, just a receptacle for voices which do not come from us, although they are in us.[59]

What of the role of pain in Wat's reawakening? Did its primitive power – the 'aversive intensity'[60] that Elaine Scarry describes as 'becoming in work *controlled discomfort*' – unleash poetry's 'primeval consciousness'? Was the condensed strength of the form best suited to expression of strong pain? Were its meditative pace and focus on particles, rather than paragraphs, of language, easier to manage than prose, when he was in pain? Miłosz confirms Wat's difficulty in sustaining long works of prose, pointing to poetry as a 'more pliable instrument'.[61]

In *My Century*, Wat attributes his absence from poetry – notwithstanding the period of his influence by Marxism – to acquiring a liking for editorship: for analysing and reordering and taking charge of the work of others. He tells Miłosz that he considers poetry 'a state and not a fact, the highest value in literature and language'.[62] He wonders how to define it; speaks of its 'consolation' and 'highest fullness'; and applies to poetry St Augustine's remark about time: 'When no one asks what it is, I know what it is; if someone asks me, I don't know.'[63]

He also recalls his realisation, in Lubyanka Prison, that poetry was and always would be the prism through which everything he experienced was reflected; that his life

> had been a constant search for an enormous dream in which my fellow crea-
> tures and animals, plants, chimeras, stars, and minerals were in a pre-
> established harmony, a dream that is forgotten because it must be forgotten,
> and is sought desperately, and only sporadically does one find its tragic frag-
> ments in the warmth of a person, in some specific situation, a glance – in
> memory too, of course, in some specific pain, some moment. I loved that
> harmony with a passion; I loved it in voices, voices. And then, instead of
> harmony, there was nothing but scraps and tatters. And perhaps that alone is
> what it means to be a poet.[64]

Restricted, reduced at times to negotiating pain line by line, Wat's literary output – essays, memoirs, philosophical meditations, poetry – was at its most prolific during the last fourteen years of his life. Frequent reference is made to his pain in ironic and paradoxical writings, and in narratives edged with humour. For those scored by pain sickness, he writes in *Diary Without Vowels*, there is a need to sanctify pain, but there is also a need to mock and humiliate it.[65]

'The borderline existence of an incurably sick man,' notes Venclova, 'was as conducive to writing in Wat's case as in Proust's (a comparison he was aware of)'.[66] Wat explores this connection as a patient, in France, in the hospital Saint-Mande, in his 1956 poem 'Before Breughel the Elder':[67]

> Work is a blessing.
> I tell you that, I – a professional loafer!
> Who bedded down in so many prisons! Fourteen!
> And in so many hospitals! Ten! And innumerable hotels!
> Work is a blessing.
> How else could we deal with the lava of fratricidal love towards our
>   fellow men?
> With those storms of extermination of all by all?
> With brutality that has no bottom, no measure?
> With the black and white era that does not want to end,
> endlessly repeating itself *da capo* like a record
> forgotten on a turntable,
> spinning by itself?

The pain behind Wat's writing was severe, almost constant, incurable. There was no transcendence of such pain. There were only brief breaks in the 'endlessly repeating' storm.

It would appear that Wat claimed the subject of pain partly in writerly confrontation, partly because suffering remained at the forefront of his thinking, and partly because he was a poet of Eastern Europe. 'What in the West is a mere diversion or at best a confession from the Freudian couch,' explains Tomas Venclova in his 1986 essay 'Poetry as Atonement',[68] 'is in the East a matter of life and, not infrequently, of death. In the West poetry abides largely on the college campus; in the East it tends to turn up in the prison camp.'

In Wat's poem 'In the Four Walls of My Pain',[69] the totalitarianism and physical pain in which he was locked, in which his body was also his prison, meet:

> The four walls of my pain
> have no window no door.
> I only hear – the guard
> pacing out there and back.
>
> His heavy faceless steps
> mark empty survival.
> Is it night still or now dawn?
> Darkness has become my four walls.
>
> Why does he pace there and back?
> How can death's shadow find me,
> when my cell of pain
> has no window no door?

They meet again in 'Here There is No Space No Will',[70] in his statement of mental desolation:

> Here there is no space no will
> only not-time, non-will
> not-nothing, non-form – mirage and stone –
> anti-matter of the brainwashed hollow.

These verses appear in *Scraps of Paper in the Wind*, published posthumously in Polish, in a cycle alongside poems written in France entitled 'In a Hospital', 'A Lullaby for a Dying Person', 'A Night in a Hospital'. In *Scraps of Paper*, Wat equates his life in incurable pain with life imprisonment. 'A Night in a Hospital' tells of darkness filtering the intrinsic blackness of pain, and of the nightingales singing for his death.

Wat's reflections on pain as a poet were as uncompromising as his thoughts as an essayist. He sought, writes Alissa Valles in 'A Wound Like a Mouth',[71] 'to talk back to the wound, to make the wound talk'. His persistent concern was the want of compassion, caused, as confirmed by Valles, in 'the clutch of contradictions' surrounding his experience of pain: by 'not only psychic aversion but intellectual doubt as to the reality of something one cannot perceive directly, and a spiritual conviction (or conditioning attributed by Wat to Christian culture) that pain can and should be transcended.' The 'wound', he believed, could not be persuaded to speak; but in circumstances of tolerance and acceptance (of acknowledgement of the toll exerted by pain on his life) it might whisper, paving a way to greater understanding.

In speaking to this 'wound' he limited his use of metaphor, viewing it as a 'dead end' because, as he explains in *Diary Without Vowels*, 'anything could be equated with anything and, precisely at that point, the very act of equation loses its value'.[72] Like Pasternak, he tended to forgo the implicit comparison or similarity of metaphor in favour of the contiguous approach of metonymy:[73] the play on mutually enforcing associations, the art of indirectly describing something by referencing or linking it to objects or ideas around it. In essence, he distinguished metaphor, as a figure of the imagination, from metonym as of the senses and memory, or, as Roman Jakobson suggests, 'the projection of the poet's being onto reality, which then appears as an endless chain of the lyrical person's suggestive states'.

His poem 'A Bit of Mythology'[74] *associates* his coexisting states of physical suffering and creativity with the torment of Hercules' shirt.

> I am not a Hercules,
> nor is Ola a Deianeira,
> my enemies are not centaurs.
> But I'll never get rid
> of the shirt of Nessos.
> It pours lead into my veins,
> it etches in its slow fire
> the outline of lymphatic's, the design
> of nerves.
> It grinds the living tissue,
> crushes the bone, squeezes the brain.
> To wring out a bloody sweat
> words words words.

Wat's metaphoric grinding, crushing, squeezing and wringing of pain is explicit, visceral. But equally if not more powerful are this formal, elegant poem's less explicit *associations*: the 'bloody sweat' of the wine press of pain that is producing the poem; the 'words, words, words', as originally spoken by Hamlet who, in the shadow of imprisonment, insanity and death, is asked by Polonius what he reads; the perpetually tormenting shirt of Wat's unshakeable suffering – the garment which, as Venclova notes, by metonym or contiguity 'becomes a figure for skin'.[75]

And yet, in the end, if one has not experienced the extended invasion and occupation of such pain, do Wat's similarities of metaphor and the associations of metonym convey more than an *impression* of his suffering?

The starless black veil of Veronica[76]

*

WAT: *For a time, I might have been a guest in a mansion in which I walked through a cruciform hallway into orchards of apples and plums; from which I strolled along avenues of chestnuts and pines; to which I returned, as if to my homeland, in the recognisable evening.*

*

All the while, Wat, with permission to travel abroad for treatment – facilitated in part by his history with *The Literary Monthly* – was taking trips with Ola to Italy and France. In 'A Song for My Wife'[77] he describes his fifty-sixth birthday, in a harmoniously furnished rented Menton house, surrounded by the scent of violet wisteria, with camellia in bloom at the kitchen door. He sings, even though 'there is pain in every breath':

> I have visited more than one hell,
> I have run through more than one country,
> I was never so glad
> as here, in this winter camp of birds,
> under this pink rock,
> over this green wave…

In 1959, a visit to France developed into permanent exile, mainly in Paris, supported by editorships, translations and literary grants. That year, he sent word from a writers' retreat at La Messuguière – near Grasse in southern France, where he and Ola spent their winters, within sight of Corsica on a clear day – that he could not have dreamt of more perfect circumstances.

At the retreat, he composed the two long narrative poems, 'Songs of a Wanderer' and 'Dreams from the Shore of the Mediterranean',[78] that Venclova believes are among his best work. Here, in appeasing climate and light, he summons sufficient concentration and strength to examine his psychic and physical challenges:

> Using both hands, my senses in rapt attention, gently,
> you see, doctor,
> I always carried before me, like a lantern, a cage
> made of young reeds
> and a butterfly circled in it, whose name I don't know.
> Not so much white as woven of light, only the ribbing
> was thick, not transparent. I say 'lantern' for indeed it illuminated
> the road before me. […]

Miłosz, principal translator of Wat's poetry into English, comments on the narratives of Wat's life as implied in his late poetry. He sees these narratives as linked to Wat's biography, as a transposition of personal experience into wider reflections of human destiny.

Wat's worldview, believes Miłosz, in addition to the influence of physical pain, was marked by his love for but one woman; his study of philosophy – principally Schopenhauer, Nietzsche and Marx; and by his being Jewish, yet having been raised apart from Judaism.[79] There was also his obsession with communism. Russian communism, continues Miłosz, is a phenomenon of which the West has only a superficial understanding. Consequently Wat, in the last part of his life, like Orwell, felt compelled to make its reality plain. Miłosz adds that he saw the threat of communism as essentially 'linguistic' – as one of 'domination by changing the meaning of words'.

Established in exile in France and burdened by his association with communism and the guilt of having been 'a seducer', Wat re-embarked on his ultimate goal – the search for a philosophical means of interpreting Soviet communism.[80] He harboured a sense of moral responsibility for all who had suffered under the system. Pain permitting, he filled hundreds of pages of a manuscript with the working title 'Some Strokes for a Future Portrait of Stalin', completing all but three chapters. He believed that his profound distaste of the subject, and especially of Stalin, caused him to develop eczema over his entire body. He wrote in 'Songs of a Wanderer':[81]

> I prattle. Grow muddy with drinks. Covered
> with sweat, yes, sweat, eczema, mycosis.
> My clothes are filthy. No fragrant oils
> from Grasse will help; not all the perfumes of Araby
> can clean them. Nor
> will the breath of my little sister mimosa under the window
> undo anything. […]

In 1962, he delivered a paper on the 'Relations Between Literature and Soviet Reality' in Oxford, where seminar members from the Centre of Slavic and East European studies at the University of California invited him to come to Berkeley.

Kraków. In 1038, the capital of Poland. Named after the livestock and virgin-devouring dragon in a cave dating from the Stone Age beneath Wawel Hill. Built and rebuilt following Tatar invasions. Home to the teenage Joseph Conrad, who remembered it as that 'old royal and academical city'. Home, too, to Czesław Miłosz and poet Wisława Szymborska, also a Nobel Laureate (1996). During Nazi occupation, Kraków avoided the level of destruction of other Polish cities. However, a heavy toll was taken on its cultural heritage following World War II, when the Soviet-imposed regime constructed steel mills nearby to punish the resistance of the 'reactionist social classes' of old Kraków to communism.

The taxi ride from the station is bumpy. John asks the driver to slow down over the cobblestones. 'An accident in Warsaw,' I say, bracing myself, gripping the front seat.

At our hotel, formerly a Czartoryski palace, a shoot for the feature film *Long Weekend* is taking place: a young couple meet on a TV blind date show and spend a weekend in a luxurious hotel in which a legendary poet is also a guest. We check in and progress to our room between takes.

Unquiet World is in the bookshops today. John goes off to find a copy while I meet Maria, its translator. 'I thought they were here to film you,' she jokes, dodging equipment and electrical leads in the lobby.

'Do you still think Potocki's cast a spell on me from beyond the grave? Do you think he's responsible for my fall?'

'I can't be sure,' she laughs. 'I just hope he approves of my translation.'

In the café lined with marble busts, a waitress brings afternoon tea. I ask her about the figures. 'Kraków intellectuals who used to gather at the Professor's Table for morning coffee,' she says, confirming that Krakówian scholars from Jagiellonian University continue the tradition.

*

WAT: *Our hopes were high as we prepared to leave the gentleness of the Mediterranean Sea for the elemental force of the Pacific Ocean.*

*

Wat embarked upon his residency at Berkeley in December 1963 in a state of elation. His pain – distracted by travel, his warm welcome, the prospects of collegial engagement and the mild Californian winter – was tempered for the first time in eleven years; the ache of his registration as a stateless person in Paris, in May, was also alleviated.

But the reprieve rapidly became marred by uncertainty. He had difficulty adjusting to American academic life: unlike that of Central Europe with its deference to intellectual debate, it proceeded without intensity. This caused Wat to misinterpret his colleagues' absence of enthusiasm for lengthy conversations as indifference, even ostracism. Moreover, his halting English hampered communication with all but the small number of associates fluent in Polish and Russian – few of whom were alert to his personal and political history. Affronts predating Berkeley started to surface: Miłosz's hurtful equivocation in Paris regarding Wat's status as a poet to a visiting American;[82] Miłosz's condescending instructions, regarding his conduct at Berkeley, that he was not to present himself as a scholar, since 'scholars are those who don't know how to become writers', and he was not to consider – and most certainly not to canvas – the feasibility of staying longer than one year.

Wat became stressed. A discomforting sense of obligation hovered; and the possibility that pain would overtake him and, despite the privileges of time and financial assistance, he would fail to be all that he had committed to be.

The fine balance of his life, sustained in France and Italy, began to shift. Although his public demeanour suggested otherwise, the years of unremitting pain had left him physically and mentally frail. His finite social reserves quickly became depleted. He began to experience panic attacks, feelings of inadequacy, the suffocation of self-judgement. Unresolved concerns asserted themselves – his Jewish-Christian identity, life in the void of immigration with its dearth of shared history and cultural intimacy, the long shadow of his association with communism. He was unable to sleep. Upon asking Miłosz which aspects of his behaviour were incorrect, and receiving advice that he should simply be himself, he wondered 'if it's just my nature and naturalness that repel people here'.[83]

In 1964, as winter turned to spring, he entered an especially intense and prolonged pain flare.

Elżbieta serves dinner. She and Antoni live in the hunting lodge of Antoni's former family home on the outskirts of Kraków. During Soviet times, when prohibitive taxes and confiscations were imposed on grand residences, Antoni's father retained the lodge and developed the property as a specialist mushroom farm. Today, many of these homes are being returned to their owners and restored.

We dine on pike – large and loricate-like on its platter, sprinkled with paprika and parsley. According to folklore, the bones of its head, if dismantled correctly, will resemble the cross, three nails and hammer of the Crucifixion. On the wall are historical treasures including weaponry from the Siege of Vienna in 1683. We're told of a ceremonial Ottoman tent captured by an ancestor during the Siege which, following an inheritance dispute, was shared, solemnly travelling back and forth between family members in a carriage.

I sit stiffly at the table, immobilising my ribs, laughing only lightly, picturing Elżbieta going to considerable trouble to find the right fish, rummaging in freezers, checking the market, speaking to poachers, choosing one from the live catch – the one fed the correct grain, from the correct harvest, from the correct quota – and returning the remainder to the river for another occasion, eyes closed, spines strong, fine bones still intact.

*

WAT: *The pain took hold, as if sensing victory. I was engulfed. A higher dose of Percodan [the trade name for the semi-synthetic morphine, oxycodone, with aspirin added] brought little relief. I couldn't eat. I lost weight. Some days I barely moved between bed and chair. I was convinced that even if the fire could be quelled, this time there would be no regeneration. Ola and I talked about committing suicide together – after everything we'd been through. She suffered with me. She couldn't live without me. I wrote in my notes:*

I grew old many years ago, yet only here, in America, after short weeks of a second youth, did I become an old man – here on this American soil. And

I'm mortally tired every evening – this fatigue never abates, and yet it is only in the evening, around eight o'clock, that I pray stubbornly and fervently not to wake up in the morning.[84]

*

Part of the agony of severe chronic pain is not knowing for how long an exacerbation will be endurable – or if it will end. Wat's pain was a major and debilitating consequence of nerve damage. Poorly understood today, such pain was even more poorly understood then. Resistant to standard pain medications, including opiates, Wat's damaged nerve cells and central nervous system were hypersensitive, bombarded indiscriminately by pain signals, leaving him exhausted and swinging between periods of relative quiescence and uncontrollable pain.

Also part of Wat's chronic neuropathic arsenal: dismissal of the invisible pain by onlookers. This caused him to be sensitive to impatience, disinterest, a falsely sympathetic response; to become hyper-vigilant, and, like a weakened animal alert to predators, to creep away into isolation and hiding. Heightened by pain, Wat's 'sensitive antennae' – his 'uncommon ability to observe people'[85] – as marked by Miłosz at Berkeley – undoubtedly magnified his sense of collegial mistrust and sense of cultural and intellectual displacement.

He writes in *Diary Without Vowels* that until recently 'even medicine […] saw *maladie-douleur* – as the pain specialist Professor Leriche called it – as a symptom of hypochondria, hysteria, over-sensitivity, imaginary sickness, delusionary pains'.[86] Wat's rare damage within his thalamus – his sensory relay station – predisposed him not only to dysfunctional sensory reactions to touch and temperature, but also to fluctuations of emotion. The latter played into the hypochondria confusion, strengthening rumours circulated by his political adversaries in Warsaw that his pain was imagined, psychosomatic.

It was the nescience of others and scarcity of insightful compassion that prompted the writing of the essay 'Diary Without Vowels' – which Wat completed at Berkeley some nine months after his pain started to intensify.

'The Greeks pitied, the Greeks identified with the victim of a tragedy,' he writes, 'but did they sympathize, did they have compassion?'[87] Thus it is, he continues, that one friend of

> rare goodness, delicacy of feeling and vast understanding […] when he received my desperate letters, must have nodded his head, both in pity and irritation, understanding nothing, or what's worse understanding wrongly while another friend who is so far from understanding the complexities arising from the cultivation of poetry in our times, only looked on and understood, with his Jewish heart.

The essay would form part of the work of 150 pages (written between October 1963 and May 1965) titled *Diary Without Vowels* and released posthumously in Polish by Ola. According to Hebrew tradition, Wat had composed the text without using vowels. In her publisher's note to the work Ola looks beyond the coded 'clusters of consonants' to a testimonial to Hebrew literature, believing 'the harsh, hoarse, crushed words [to be] both a symbolic and a very concrete expression of his state at that time'.[88]

Wat's Berkeley colleagues saw his health was disintegrating and urged him to rest. But rest was impossible with his thesis on communism to write. Communism – 'a demonic, pathogenic factor'[89] – was the rationale for his exile, where it was putrefying within him; it was the mystery against which he had tested his true qualities. Yet how could he proceed while he was incapable of controlling his thoughts? – one day they took flight, the next they were mired in mental stasis, and with each manic and depressive interlude his pain intensified.

An extended residency was offered, with an opportunity to record a spoken memoir in Polish. Wat cautiously agreed. He was finding that concentrated conversation modulated his thinking. He would attempt a chronicle of the epoch he had witnessed – not a retelling of political events, but a work that would decipher the stories beneath the surface of those events.

The tape recordings were made by Miłosz, who listened 'spellbound' to Wat's narrative. Undertaken in response to pain, they became both Wat's pain therapy and the summa that pain had prevented him from writing.

'I quickly realized,' writes Miłosz, 'that something unique was transpiring between us.'

There was not a single other person on the face of the earth who had experienced this century as Wat had and who had the same sense of it as he. This has nothing to do with cruelty of fate or history, for an enormous number of people were more grievously afflicted by it than he was. No, what matters here is a cast of mind, […] not only was Wat a member of the intelligentsia, but he was also an intellectual, educated in philosophy, and his Jewish origins made for a valuable shading, one that provided him with a certain distance on Polish ways; moreover, he was a member of the [socialist realism directed] Writers' Union for many years, and, further, he was a poet.[90]

My interview is conducted in a bookshop, said to be Europe's oldest. During World War II, the Matras at 23 Main Market Square, owned by Wat's former employer publishing house, Gebethner and Wolff, doubled as a literary salon – a convention still in place. Last spring, Carlos Fuentes signed copies of his new book, *Inez*, and opened his entry in the visitors' ledger with '*A Matras, Catedral del libro*'.

The director arrives with a crew of three. She and I sit at a table beneath the framed photographs of writers. She asks, 'What sort of man was Potocki, and what were the most important aspects of his life?'

I speak uninterrupted for some time about his difficult childhood, his extraordinary obscenity trial at the Old Bailey, his imprisonment in Wormwood Scrubs, his robe-wearing life as a poet, pamphleteer and pretender to the Polish throne. Maria is also filmed, standing in front of a bookcase, speaking about his

English translation of Mickiewicz's poetic drama, *Forefathers*, published in 1968. *Niespokojny świat* (*Unquiet World*) is positioned for shots of Potocki as a young man, and, at the age of eighty, his photo and mirror image on the cover; and of the chapter headed 'Katyn'.

Afterwards, Maria and I are instructed to stroll under the porticoes of the 700-year old *Sukiennice*, or Cloth Hall, and in the direction of the Palace of the Rams – a Potocki property from 1822 until World War II, not returned to its owners until 1990 after the fall of the Soviet regime. A TV news item and a short documentary for a national 'culture' programme will be 'cut' from the footage.

That evening, Maria joins us at the hotel for the Kraków television news. We watch ourselves stroll around the Market Square. In the interview, my answers in English are slow and faint beneath a rapid Polish voice-over.

*

WAT: *Each time I sat down with Miłosz and his machine, I felt as if an act of exorcism was being performed. The taping took place between January and June 1965 in our Benvenue Street apartment. I sat in a deep chair. On cold days Ola, who joined many of the sessions, covered me with a rug. If she wasn't staying she left the next dose of Percodan in a cup; in the interests of lucidity, I deferred taking the drug for as long as I could. Writer Richard Lourie – then a self-described 'twenty-five-year-old American innocent'[91] – who would translate Ola's transcriptions, was an occasional observer.*

*

There were thirty-nine recordings in all, each lasting an hour and a half and resulting in two thousand pages of typescript.

The third taping started with a discussion of *The Literary Monthly*. Wat spoke of his notion of communism as 'a demonic bond whose fruits are being felt only now, in my illness', and suggested that they talk about pain.[92]

Miłosz said, 'No, no', declining, perhaps, to deviate from their central objective (a historical memoir), or uncomfortable, like so many, with discussion of personal pain. At this point, he might have asked Wat why, with all his force of intellect and creative imagination, he was unable to describe the actuality of his suffering to his colleagues and friends.

Wat insisted: 'But the devil behind my illness is the devil of communism.'[93] So the conversation was steered in the direction of his early philosophy of pain, world and personal, and his leap towards 'social transformation'.

Returning to the *Monthly*, Wat declared it the *corpus delicti* of his degradation, 'in communism, by communism'.[94] He told Miłosz that it wasn't until he was incarcerated in communist prisons that he fully realised the implications of communism. From that time on, he said, whether 'in prison, in exile, and in communist Poland, I never allowed myself to forget my basic duty – to pay for those two or three years of moral insanity. And I paid, and paid.'

They talked about the difficulty of walking away from communism when it is part of one's idealistic youth. Wat said:

> I committed the most motley acts, but I didn't join the party. [...] I knew that if I were a member of the party, I would be surrendering my mind. When the majority outvoted me, I would have to accept the majority opinion. And I didn't want that.[95]

Shortly afterwards, he told Miłosz he was in a lot of pain and suggested they put off the sociopolitical and psychological motivations for his promotion of communism until next time.

Trees, love, death, all that is immutable from the beginning of creation[96]

*

WAT: *My mind was embattled, a city under siege, but intact nonetheless.*

*

In July 1965, the Wats returned to Paris. They rented a comfortable apartment in Antony, a southern inner suburb. The flat opened onto a large balcony, covered with a red awning, overlooking lawns, flowerbeds and poplars. Miłosz accompanied them, in order to conduct further interviews, but had to leave before the project was complete. The recordings were continued with someone else but as Wat, in pain, responded less favourably to Miłosz's replacement, they were abandoned.

Wat continued to write. He worked on poetry and the early draft of a novel, and on recollections not covered by *My Century*; the latter were published after his death in *Scraps of Paper in the Wind* and contained, writes Venclova, 'many pages of Wat's best prose'.[97]

In Poland, the press was disparaging. Wat's inclusion in an anthology of Polish poetry published in France provoked an angry 'How diluted is the book by the empty talk of that malingerer! (He feigned sickness so as to make the naïve People's Poland pay for his and his wife's long stays abroad, and finally "chose freedom".)'[98]

During difficult nights, when pain prevented him from writing, he whispered the words of poems into a tape recorder. In poems composed by day, the chirruping of their small bird, Macius, in its cage would be heard on the tape.

As the pain rose, so did his psychic anguish. Trapped in the *Pug Iron Stove* of his mind, he reviewed the remove and isolation of exile, his support for and failure to foresee the ways of totalitarianism, the prospect of death in a foreign land, his hope (unfulfilled) that he would be buried in Israel, in a Christian cemetery.

To view Wat's physical pain as secondary to his mental torment is to underestimate the exhaustion, distortion of thought and what he describes in *Diary* as the 'mask of ugliness on everything, on all the beauties of the world' that can accompany intractable bodily suffering.[99] Pain magnified his existential anguish, which in turn magnified his pain. It is conceivable that, free of pain's control, his resilient spirit – manifested during his imprisonments, and in the resolve with which, despite illness and debility, he not only resisted the Kazakhstan Passportisation but also tamed the prisoners charged with beating him into submission – may have curbed his remorse and self-rejection. Before the onset of intractable pain, he had been both the unflinching 'arrow' and 'target', remembered in the poem 'Japanese Archery',[100] written in Paris in 1963:

> The hand tells the bowstring:
> Obey me.

> The bowstring answers the hand:
> Draw Valiantly.

> The bowstring tells the arrow:
> O arrow, fly.

> The arrow answers the bowstring:
> Speed my flight.

> The arrow tells the target:
> Be my light.

> The target answers the arrow:
> Love me.

Now, three months before his death, he mostly sat in silence, staring into space or watching Ola move from room to room. Absented from the dreams of hope that feed men in exile (Aeschylus), his thoughts actively turned to suicide, to leaving Ola. Ola, who had written from a *kolkhoz* on the Kazakh Steppe as they waited to be reunited in Alma-Ata: 'You did not leave me for even a moment. You were pulling the oxen on the drag-rake with me, and when it seemed to me that I would fall – you and Andrzej called out that you needed me.'[101] He writes:

> I must endure that death in the same way as I have endured the hardest trials of my life: all my life's values depend on it. [...] I must die facing death, my adversary or my brother, up to the last hour. [...] It will be a great injury for me, a great irremediable injury, if I die in torpor, passively, helplessly sliding down.[102]

And:

> My last battlefield: poems against physical suffering. Or: intelligence against suffering? *Kto kogo*?[103]

What did he mean by this last statement? *Kto kogo*: who whom – who can do what to whom – was a statement of power in politics favoured by Lenin: a justification of the moral acceptability of revolution; of what needed to be done, whether by merciless subjugation or incitement to terror. Was Wat acknowledging, again and finally, communist's role in his suffering? In his death?

Ola's diary records his last months sparingly: 'A terrible day. A terrible evening. Suffering.' 'Listening to Bach. ... Relief.' 'A good walk. He feels well.' 'Great suffering.... Grief. Hopelessness. And the spring in its very bloom.'[104]

Two photographs were taken at this time.[105] In one, he sits stiffly on his bed, in a short-sleeved shirt and dark trousers, on top of the covers. Ola, face patient, beautiful in her late fifties, kneels alongside. Wat looks at her. His hand reaches towards her. The image speaks of shared suffering.

In the second photograph, taken just a month before he died, he's outdoors, pulling a funny face, acting to camera, gambolling with his grandson, dissembling his pain persona. As ever, he's immaculately clad.

At Berkeley, writes Richard Lourie in his introduction to *My Century*, he had also stepped out, 'utterly dapper – his moustache silvery, his dark fedora cocked at an alert, amused angle, [an] umbrella nonchalant on his forearm'.[106] As he had in Alma-Ata, where he'd paraded in the street in a handsome cheviot suit supplied by an American aid post, his sense of flair to the fore. 'I was the embodiment of the West and Christianity,' he says of his stylish appearance in the Kazakhstan capital. 'I walked about that barbarous land, that world of poverty and Eastern barbarity, [...] and I was an embodiment, an image, an imago.'[107]

Back in Warsaw, winter is setting in.

At the well-heated National Museum, researching *The Fountain of Tears*, I study a painting of the rescue of Poles captured during slave raids by Tatars at the Battle of Martynow in 1624 by the winged horsemen of the Polish cavalry.

All but 5,000 of the works seized by Germany during World War II have been repatriated.

The large canvas recalls the Tatar retreat at a ford on the Dniester River in the south-eastern Polish Ukraine. 'The Tatars are taken by surprise,' I write in my notebook. 'Cloud breaks over the silver helmets, lances and red-and-white ensigns of the *husaria*. Wagons are smashed. Hobbled men, women and children, and wild-eyed stock are lifted from the mud.'

Aleksander Wat died on the evening of 29 July 1967, after taking forty Nembutal tablets. Ola found him in bed, turned to one side as if sleeping. She lifted him in her arms, saying, 'Ol, wake up!'[108] but he was cold to her touch. At his feet, his notebook and two pieces of paper. On one sheet, the plea, 'Do not save me.' On the other, a letter to Ola – 'my life, my everything'.

His 'last notebook', started in May, contained memories of his life and troubled century, sometimes in streams-of-consciousness reminiscent of *Pug Iron Stove*. He remembers his Jewish ancestors, his perception of Christianity as the belief of Judaism, his loss of faith as he approaches death.

He tells of his love for Ola with her 'extraordinary strength of soul'.

He farewells Ola and Andrzej, over and over. Asks their forgiveness. Writes of torturous nights, of 'vegetation in hell'. He confesses that suicide had been on his mind for eleven years, but his love for Ola and Andrzej had prevented it. He pleads with them not to despair – he will live on in them, he promises, free of pain. He expresses the depth of his pain – pain, he says, not even Ola understood.[109]

In July, in his last poem – untitled, found among his papers – he wrote of Ola as the only word he had left:

> I clad myself in the armour of silence:
> All the words are already taken away except for one.
>
> Perhaps they were only on loan?
> Perhaps they were only displayed
>
> to tempt the eyes of a passerby?
> And now is night, the dead of night?[110]

*

A clash of seasons. The house shook, the couch shuddered, the pine rocked – its crown scratching the sky, convulsions running the length of its visible trunk. On nearby Mt Kaukau (445 metres), the wind reached 200 kilometres an hour. In the city centre, where a gust of 143 km/h was recorded, fire services raced to secure scaffolding. On the Internet, photos of windows exploding under pressure and satellite dishes lifting were posted. Local radio warned against walking in woods and near stands of old macrocarpas and pines. National Radio announced that thousands of households were without power. I toasted a sandwich and boiled the kettle; watched the cats, sensitive to barometric variations, rush up and down the hall. Wellington, the world's southernmost capital, is also the world's only capital city in the path of the Roaring Forties. An hour later, I sensed a vibration – not an earthquake, more a tearing, as if of air and tin. I checked the garden, but found no guttering or roofing iron. The next morning, when the storm had blown itself out and easterly sun burnished the pine, I saw the tree's two companions were missing.

*

9 How does it hurt?[1]

An epilogue

At the margins

2013. I wrote my dissertation lying on my back, using the bed as a desk, storing the files and books on a table and chest in the same room (John soon became accustomed to the sight of pain-related cover titles and images upon waking!). My supervisors thoughtfully offered to meet at my house, opposite Victoria University, so I could lie on a couch; and during the six-weekly three-hour PhD workshops I rested on a portable lounger close to the floor, from which I rolled and scrambled to my feet to speak because I was uneasy in what I perceived to be a diminished position.

In the beginning, I was buoyed by the prospect of raising common understanding of chronic pain. I saw, in pain's containment and interrogation, not only a means by which I could interpret the direction my life had taken, but also of lessening the isolation of others as Alphonse Daudet, Harriet Martineau and Aleksander Wat had lessened mine. In *The Wounded Storyteller* (1997), Arthur W. Frank writes of the 'the shared condition of being bodies [as] a basis of empathetic relations among living beings', and quotes Albert Schweitzer, who spoke of the 'brotherhood of those who bear the mark of pain':

> Whoever among us has learned through personal experience what pain and anxiety really are must help ensure that those out there who are in physical need obtain the same help that once came to him.[2]

In a sense, I supposed, I was reclaiming the role of a nurse.

However, I had underestimated the challenge of sustained thinking and writing about pain while living within it. On tolerable days I could believe, despite my limitations, that I was on a mission of discovery and opportunity, and was able to take a position outside my physical self, like a pathologist, above the necessary dissection. But beyond the baseline and during the too-frequent flares, I struggled to bestow detachment and balance upon the intense reality of a body in pain. Whereas writing creatively offered a degree of imaginative distraction, arguing for or against the behaviours and meanings of pain within the rigour of scholarship only served to engage and re-engage the overloaded parts of the brain marked 'pain'. The subject, actual and academic, became a double bombardment.

Less than a year into the project, my mental stamina and emotional resilience started to fluctuate. I moved unevenly between creative and critical thinking, struggling to make research part of the journey, settle on tonal balance, find a voice within the conflicting calls of memoir and aetiology. When the pain roared and I had to put the work aside, I lost my sense of rhythm, pace, narrative, thread. Moreover, oddly for a memoirist, I had a tendency to 'go missing' in the text – to pull back from revealing myself in pain and rely instead on the world views and insights of the other writers in pain. Did this cloaking and distancing extend a natural inclination to write sparingly – and, if so, why? Had the connections that pain disconnected splintered my self-awareness? Was I wary of being defined by pain? Heading off questions of veracity and victimhood? Afraid, in some psychogenic way, of making the pain worse? Maybe I was reluctant to engulf readers with pain, knowing there would be few compensating moments of lightness and humour? I had to keep reminding myself that 'Memoir', as William Zinsser writes, 'is how we try to make sense of who we are, who we once were, and what values and heritage shaped us. If a writer seriously embarks on that quest, readers will be nourished by the journey, bringing along many associations with quests of their own.'[3]

At the two-year mark I was circumventing analysis and resisting an inclination to revert to the core thoughts and bare bones of poetry; to defy deliberate evaluation with less-literal triangulations. I wanted to put pain 'through its full range of motions' in 'a gentle sweep', as the physician-poet Rafael Campo does during his examination of a patient's knee in 'On Doctoring', where he explains, in spare lines on one page, how 'like any other/my patient gives the gift of how we suffer'.[4]

And I was querying the undertaking's worth: so much of the clinical opinion and rationalisation of pain were supposition, so much of received sensation and perception was individual. For Daudet, 'the vendor of happiness', and Martineau, the 'consolator', pain might, ultimately, have been described as ennobling; for Aleksander Wat, the pain 'imago', *la maladie douleur* had been undeniably destructive; for myself, there was no avoiding the thought that, after a decade of pain, I was immersed in a narrative without a conclusion. Increasingly, I was of a mind that, as long as intractable pain remains a mystery, most sufferers – reluctant to draw family and friends into their circle, preferring solitude to social misapprehension, wary, like injured animals, of revealing their weakness to predators – will play down bodily distress; and onlookers, for reasons, perhaps, of self-preservation, will evade the domain. To what extent, I wondered, will a more active literature of physical pain reprogramme the ancient conditioning of the brain (in the way that chronic pain is said to sensitise, and rewire, the nervous system)? Can pain on the page ever be as accessible as that expressed through the primal emotional cues of sound and sight: through music, drama and art, the cries of the hypnotised man reliving the acute (and fatal) agony of his shattered leg, the pinned visual suffering of Frida Kahlo? I had been moved at contemplative and empathetic levels by the words of the writers I had studied, but which was the greater influence: their language and storytelling, or the fact that I too was in pain? If we cannot feel another's pain, is it possible to imagine or understand it?

The more I wrote, the further I felt from a conclusion. I told my supervisors, 'I've fiddled at the margins.'

'What *haven't* you said?'

I was unable to answer.

With the end of the thesis in sight, and as the physical debilitation that had kept me housebound showed signs of waning, I considered making a trip to Lourdes (lying down on the plane to Paris and taking a sleeper train south). I held no thoughts of a cure; rather, I hoped to gain a sense of a larger whole – a reorientation before my outlook became irretrievably changed. 'Nowhere,' Joris-Karl Huysmans writes of the Sanctuary in *Les Foules de Lourdes* (1906), 'have I seen such appalling illnesses, so much charity and so much good grace. From the point of view of human mercy, Lourdes is a wonder.'[5]

But increased mobility intensified the vexations of movement. Pain tightened its grip. Fentanyl was offered, but caused nausea. From France, Professor Robert put forward the option of neurostimulation (of the posterior tracts of the spinal cord).

I raised the dose of oxycodone, applied for three months' suspension from study and cancelled the trip. That summer, we reopened the house. The floorboards blocking the top of the main staircase were removed and the balustrading was reinstated. The front door opened into the garden, where the white magnolia and orange spraxias were in bloom and the coppiced stumps of the laurel bay and holly were rapidly making new growth. At the edge of the lower lawn the grass, which had turned to moss, was thick with pine needles. I set up a study facing the warm north, and bought a Chinese opium couch. The conversion of the house into two flats had taken a year; making it whole again took a couple of weeks.

Mushroom free

2014. A year after I submitted my dissertation, I stood at the top of the bank between our lower lawn and our neighbour's hillside garden, gripped a branch and cautiously tested my weight. John slid down the steep slope and balanced on a clump of vegetation at the base of the pine. A month had passed since the wild, tree-felling storm and I wanted to be sure the pine's roots were firm in the earth.

'Come on down.' John held out his hand, and stomped on a mound.

'I can't. I'll slip.'

'I'll catch you.'

'Your foothold might give way. I'll ring Irene and ask if we can use her path. I could bring my camera and get a shot of the fallen trees in close-up at the same time.'

Irene was sure the uprooted trees were macrocarpas.

'I thought they were pines,' I said over the phone.

'Oh no, definitely macrocarpas. We think they were part of a windbreak planted around 1898.' She'd been looking at options for having the trunks removed. Helicopters and cranes had been ruled out on account of the steep, bush-clad terrain. Instead, there was talk of cutting tracks and using chainsaws and motorised wheelbarrows – and the sound of teeth chewing timber for weeks. Meanwhile, the scale of the storm's clean-up meant contractors were in short supply. Of the few who'd inspected the job, the last had left, saying, 'I prune camellias.'

I negotiated the gravel downslope to the pine, holding John's shoulder. To our right: terraced flowerbeds and shrubs, a fishpond and ferns, a honeysuckle hedge. To our left: the pine, precariously rising out of our boundary bank.

'It can't be a macrocarpa,' I said. 'The crown's too imposing.'

'It's a pine, without doubt.'

'But Irene owns it and she was adamant.'

'It's a pine!' John pocketed a cone and a three-fingered needle. 'Look, I'll take these for analysis. Someone in the office has a flatmate who works at Zealandia.'

We inspected the base of the tree. The lower third of the trunk was submerged in foliage, but the bark entering the earth, which was visible and faced north, was firm and mushroom free. I unfolded my Internet checklist for conifers at risk of wind-throw.

'Does the tree lean? Has the lean increased in recent years? Are there cracks in the trunk or between its buttress roots? Do paths, pipes, walls, buildings or roads compress or entrap its root system?'

Later, we stood on Irene's balcony and surveyed the full extent of the storm's damage.

John estimated the length of each of the fallen trees to be between twenty-eight and thirty metres.

'The same height as the survivor – they were giants!'

'They seemed shorter because of their positioning further down the hill.'

One had crashed backwards into the town belt and was straddling the gulley above the Kumutoto Stream. The other had pitched forward, taking out a corrugated tin fence and a couple of trees that bloomed spectacularly in spring.

I pointed to the 'hero' pine. 'Is it hazardous? Do you worry about it?'

Irene nodded, her arms folded.

'Will the city council remove it?'

'I hope so. I've come to loathe it – looming over the garden.'

'It's strange,' I said, 'the way it dominates the landscape from our place, but from here it seems unremarkable.'

Nonchalant strolling

2018. Today, nearly fifteen years since my fall in Warsaw, with four surgeries and any number of remedies in between, pain insistently defines me. Firmly stated, this means that the nerve and its six branches fire pain signals persistently, in response to physical activity's aggravation of the dysfunctional tissue; and randomly, as a result of (pathophysiological) changes in my nervous system caused by the pain's constancy. The pain becomes intolerable if I sit, or stand for long (I continue to eat, write and entertain lying down, and I rarely travel by car); as well, and intermittently, if the pain is not promptly regulated (relief of neuropathic pain is rarely complete) the nerve 'goes berserk', in the words of my pain specialist, tipping an eviscerating tempest into the Comparative Pain Scale's Unimaginable, Unspeakable Ten. Such constraints mean that when the sun or a fresh breeze won't be ignored, the walk must be short and taken slowly (hands in pockets to indicate nonchalant strolling); and that planning, brevity and the proviso 'pain permitting' underpin appointments and occasional social events.

Daily life is not possible without oxycodone: the only potent opioid I tolerate. Taken as an elixir, the fast-acting drug masks the pain for short periods; I potentiate its performance by angling the measuring glass so that the straw-coloured sweetness catches my soft palate with what I convince myself is the magic of a placebo effect. Medical marijuana promised much, but hampered by New Zealand's restrictive cannabis laws and my medication sensitivities proved disappointing. With the aid of 'back garden' growers and suppliers ('Green Fairies') and a hay-scented fridge, I have trialled legal, non-psychoactive, THC[6]-free, CBD[7] oil, dropped onto the tongue; and illegal oral cannabis containing psychoactive THC. The former brought on vertigo without measurable relief. The latter cut the pain cleanly, as if with secateurs, at its root; however, the resultant dizziness, tinnitus, feverishness and insomnia, together with memory loss, irrational thinking and a disturbing sense of disassociation at a fundamental level were unsustainable. There was also the (still-vivid, oddly familiar) silver and gold spider glistening with droplets that entered the room, sucked itself into itself, slid under the non-existent sideboard from the dining room at the foot of the bed, re-inflated and sat blinking beneath a brilliant aureate light. (Later, I recognised the similarity between the hallucination and the Chagall-like cascade on the front cover of my novel, *The Fountain of Tears*.)

With the milestones of recovery unmet, I rarely write up a diary. And I am no closer to answering my thesis supervisors' question: 'What *haven't* you said?' apart from observing, in the manner of Alphonse Daudet, that, while for the bystander pain becomes mundane, for the sufferer pain is always new – and newly inexplicable.

Asked by those on the outside, 'How can I help, what should I say?' I'm reminded that my pain specialist's gentle 'How have you been?', his murmured 'Yes' and sympathetic awareness, are all the assistance I require.

Asked, 'What of the future, do you imagine a cure?' I speak of coping as I await enduring relief, which might mean stem-cell intervention; a failsafe micro-spinal or peripheral nerve stimulator; a failsafe pain pump; infusions without potential for hallucinations, and side-effect-free medications. At the same time, I'm aware that not all chronic and intractable pain is created equal and finding ways of dealing with pain can be confusing. The overly general strategies currently promoted are not for me. The view that ongoing pain, per se, is not harmful and can be moderated by exercise or 'worked through' is misleading and potentially injurious. I am also wary of the broad-brush assumption that pain can be integrated into a sufferer's identity as but a minor part of their being, replacing the search for relief with whatever gives 'real' satisfaction and pleasure. Such incentives are held to be beneficial for many. But for many others, the failure to consider individual pathologies causes further harm. I personally know, and have heard of, sufferers not seen in statistics for whom the outcomes have been increased pain, a dispiriting sense of their lack of resilience when their aims cannot be met, and a downplaying of their physical distress by healthcare professionals in favour of scrutiny of their mental state.[8]

For me, the most beneficial means of negotiating my new 'normal' is to be solitary. Aloneness – honed not only by physical limitations but also by a general misunderstanding of permanent pain – eludes the need to excuse, the obligation to explain, the juggling of straight talking with avoiding intimations of exaggeration or self-absorption. As a writer, I am suited to aloneness. My everyday routines – drinking coffee, revising drafts, fine-tuning poems – have not altered in the captured experience; moreover, the page is a place I can visit without provoking pain. I may be isolated, and even think of myself as exiled at times, but I don't necessarily feel lonely – I have family, friends, books, access to the Internet. I live minutes from the city centre, above the hum of the urban motorway meeting The Terrace Tunnel, kerbside to a road busy with all manner of vehicles and students of all ages on their way to and from a university. Best of all, I overlook a green town belt. In the early morning, I listen to birdsong and watch dawn dance on millions of leaves. And because our house is tall I can see into the upper reaches and crowns of the trees: karo, kowhai, ngaio, makomako – the local beauty of their names; ghost gums, common oaks and conifers from abroad – no less impressive, and enduring in exile.

Palliative care[9]

And yet – there's a space where my sentinel pine should be.

Thirty, perhaps forty, metres high and more than a hundred years old, the tree's demise was inevitable after its two shelter belt companions were uprooted in 2014.

Anticipating its end – whether by safety clearance, windfall or wavering age – I wrote a memorial while the tree was still before me.

> By day, you reach
> sylvan high distance.

> At night, your outline
> whitens the moon.

> And when turbulence
> roars through your riggings

and rips blue and green
through your crown,

and you pitch and roll
like a stand-alone ship

on a perpendicular sea
ejecting nests

and drawing cones
into the eye-locking whirl,

your habit of dancing
while rocking yourself

into a trance
invites orchestration,

choreography,
a flutter of butterflies

like clouds above
the long grass.

'Flute or violin?' I muse,
air-conducting your trunk's

unassailable rise
from the earth,

your branches' unequivocal
impressions of movement

and spread,
the erratic tempo

of rain and dust
on your scattered

understories of ferns
and small shrubs.

'The grace of long, gliding strides?
Or a clicking of light, rapid steps?'

Irene had already decided. 'I know you're fond of that tree,' she said on the phone in 2016. 'But I can't sleep at night waiting for it to collapse or crash in a gale and take out the house. Either way, an undirected fall will demolish the garden and could be fatal.'

Oh no! – the pine will go, and soon. I clutch the phone.

'I completely understand. The ending must be safely managed. Have you booked the tree surgeon?'

'Not yet. I'm having difficulty finding someone to do the work. As you know, a tree of that height overhanging a gulley is a tricky proposition – and can only be removed in pieces. I'm waiting to hear if some duck-shooting friends of my son's will do the job as a favour.'

*

A darkish afternoon. Lamps glow in the lounge. I chat with friends who examine the doomed outline from the window and pronounce it 'Sad, but not sinister.' Fifteen gulls circle the pine in a loose formation, squawking loudly. I date a notebook and scribble 'Unsettled weather. A reprieve.'

I imagine my immobile self as the tree, feet tight in the earth, body leaning and swaying, stems waving. Birds make nests in my foliage; barefooted children shinny up my trunk and swing from my branches; family and friends scoop up needles, gather cones, picnic in my shade.

The hedger comes by. 'Years ago,' he says lifting shears from his van, 'I felled a pine that big on my property – one of the first imported conifers in the country. Had a tremendous girth despite a suggestion of die back.' He closes the van door. 'There were three winters' worth of firewood in just one of its branches.'

I line up my camera, focus its telescopic lens and study the length and breadth of the tree for signs of an obvious, or discreet, wish to die: blight, rust, reddening needles.

Over the next two weeks, a prelude to winter: the nights colder, the sun less giving.

'They're on standby for a calm patch,' Irene says of the wood choppers.

As I hang up the phone, I hear a rifle-sharp crack from the opium room. I rush to the window. The tree is intact. But I can see, on the glass, the smudged reduction of a bird's bulky body and wings in what appears to have been a reflective embrace with the pane; while, below on the lawn, a kereru (wood pigeon) – drunk on fermented berries or threatened by the suggestion of an intruder in the kowhai – nods, and wobbles on short legs, its disproportionate wings hitting the ground, as if energised by a deadline. Why the disturbance? I lift the sash window and listen. Is the prescient pine communicating pain?

The waiting, the waiting.

I rise slowly, having slept late. When I open the blinds, the familiar form – stone still, as intense and impressive against the sky as I have ever seen it – is secured by Guantanamo orange ropes to fence posts and minor trees.

'Where are you?' shouts a feller from the foot of the tree to a co-worker up high, precariously looping a noose below the wind-shaped crown.

'I'm here, trying to talk myself into this!'

I put on a Mozart CD and turn up the volume: the soothing Andante from Piano Concerto No. 21 in C Major, K.467, drifts from the Opium Room to the balcony, and beyond.

An email arrives from a friend: 'I'm lighting my white, pine-scented candle.' I wonder, in reply, if in the 'wisdom of crowds' there is knowledge of the solace of candles?

A correspondent in Auckland, who has also been captured by the pine's resilience, writes 'I believe the tree watches you as closely as you watch the tree.'

Over the next three days, fellers wearing hard hats, manipulating chainsaws and a system of pulleys and ropes, reduce the pine to a ten-metre 'stump'.

The crown is dismantled in stages, within hours, without struggle or outrage, the ropes jerking to sounds of splitting and crashing. At around lunchtime, the climber descends and the men break for pies, packed sandwiches and cans of fruit juice or fizz, on the lawn. Softening clouds drift towards the tree's starkness, and the air stirs, bringing work for the afternoon to a halt. That night: showers. By daybreak: settled conditions and the pine rigid, vulnerable.

The demolition continues. With each piece of trunk thrown to the ground, the men whistle and yell. A chainsaw dangles and swings after each severance. The machine behind Irene's house chewing the incidentally damaged cypresses and other minor trees, shudders and chugs. There's a rhythm going now. In the still air: plumes of sawdust, sun-sprung atoms, particles of energy dancing into the atmosphere for dispersal and return to the universe. I lean against the stone wall in the fernery and watch the final dispatch; a gecko runs for cover, and a weta with spiked legs, rarely seen in daylight, climbs down from the black heart of the ponga (tree fern) and crawls slowly over the bark chips of its threshold.

*

Today, the northern side of the stump, and the half branch that was left on the western side, are all but covered with creepers.

Sun. Birdsong. Dandelions. I shade my eyes and search the sea of foliage for a tenacious replacement. Tui swoop between blooms – curved bills agape, thin tongues imaginable – sipping nectar and accosting the air with staccato trilling. Ladybirds – tiny wings black and vermillion vivid, but unencumbered by colour – land and flit.

Is the busy young fir laden with limbs, gaining height on the opposite bank of the stream, a tree for all seasons?

I need the clarity of a ground report.

John puts on his boots and slides down the bank. He returns with surprising news. The trunk is split at its base, but with its roots seemingly intact in the earth, it looks healthy, and the remaining branch – the sole recipient of the soil's nutrition – thrives: lengthening and producing cones, vibrant with fresh needles.

10 White train

A narrative poem

Pain, reflect in my eyes the places you will not let me visit.

Alphonse Daudet[1]

We are on the platform talking.[2]
'The couchettes are too basic.'
'We cannot sleep in a six-person berth.'
'This is what we get for booking online,
in haste,
in French.'
'We should change to a two-person sleeper
with an attendant to convert
the seats into beds, and bring us
coffee and rolls in the morning.'

A long train jolts in from a siding
flying flags fore and aft –
a white train,
reserved for the most afflicted,
the most loved by the Virgin,
the ones she has chosen
for the most miraculous cures –
the first of fourteen transportations
(grey, green, pink, yellow and blue),
timed to leave for Lourdes from midday.
Pilgrims, apparently in good health,
drinking beer and lemonade
in the refreshment room,
vacate their small tables.
At the goods entrance, bearers
clear paths for stretchers and hand carts;
mid platform, porters tidy a heap
of pillows and pallets

beside a lamppost,
and hand out bottles
for filling with preternatural water.
Cups and bowls,
trays of bread
and containers of broth,
oil stoves
and medicine chests
shuttle past on trolleys;
piles of blue, devotional books
follow in barrows.
'Don't block up the platform, please.
Keep the way open for the speedy
passage of patients.'

We stand back from the lines.
The train clanks into position.
Organisers, wearing the scarlet
cross of the pilgrimage,
direct the wild rush into ticketed squares.
A young man,
pale and shivering,
is carried past on a stretcher,
white card of hospitalisation
around his neck.
'Chalk. My tablets taste like chalk.'
An elderly woman
trundles by in a hand cart
wrapped in a rug,
leaning on an elbow,
a basin at her feet,
'Where is the carriage?
Why should I travel like this?
Why risk the sick headache
the journey brings on?'
A gentleman, otherwise in his prime,
wipes his brow and clutches
the attendant pushing his chair.
'Please, gently lift my leg to the left.'
He turns to a fellow traveller.
'My hip is being torn from me,
pain penetrates my whole being,
it's as natural as breathing.'
'Is this your first trip?'

'My third. And you?'
'My second.
I accompany my uncle who has ulcers
and will bathe in the pools.[3]
I myself have attacks
of coughing and vomiting,
I was the last of a large family.'
'Where will you shelter?'
'A hotel,
a private home,
a hut,
a tent, if the fields are dry,
wherever the Sisters suggest.'
Queues form.
Auxiliaries distribute sputum mugs
and folding stools,
cover suppurations,
adjust pillows.
From the step of a third-class carriage, a call:
'Can someone pass us our youngster?'
The child lies in a narrow,
shallow, box –
a gutter on wheels –
her eyes closed,
her hair, spared by the illness,
a halo,
barely aware of the priest
and white-bibbed Sister of Assumption
who carry her
to a crowded compartment
and place her,
between parcels and cases,
at her parents' feet.
'She's been living like this for seven years, Sister,
wasting,
weak to the point of exhaustion.'
'Do you have food for the journey –
would she eat a few grapes?'
'She cannot eat.
She drinks only milk.'
Bernadette appears,
held aloft in a dark dress,
kneeling.
'It's the only portrait taken from real life.

She had beautiful feet,
they spoke for her purity.'
'You are?'
'Elodie,
I sketched the first train as it came in.
Tomorrow I will add the colours.
White takes a long time to dry.
This is my neighbour.
She has forgotten how to see and speak.'
'Can she hear?'
'Only music.
She stays in a musty room
with a towel over her head.
I am bringing her into the open.'

Whistles blow.
A last minute physician,
black bag in hand,
accompanies the stationmaster
to the front of the train.
'So, Ferrand, we meet again.
Did you hear about last season's cure –
the first for years?
I am writing a pamphlet about it.'
'Lourdes has caught on well, sir.
The question is, will it last?'
'Healing takes time, Ferrand.
Everyone who visits the Sanctuary
carries seeds of relief home with them.'

Bells ring.
Signals work.

A night-blue sleeper
slides into the station.
'Should we board,
and surrender our passports
until disembarkation?'
'Count down the stops?'
'Listen assiduously to each
arrival announcement
as we near our destination,
prepared to leave promptly
because Lourdes is not the end of the journey?'

Steam gathers.
Iron rattles and grinds.
The white train disappears into the tawny
heat of high summer
windows closed against the breeze.[4]

Appendix

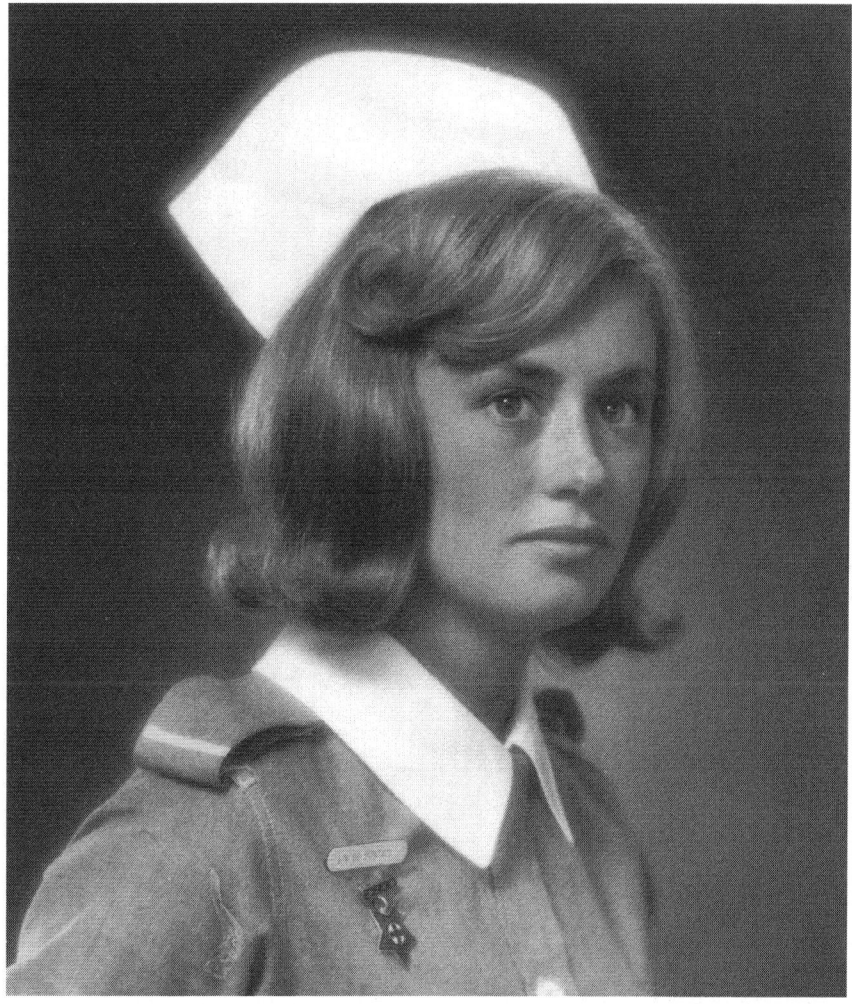

Figure A.1 Staff Nurse, Wellington Hospital, 1966.

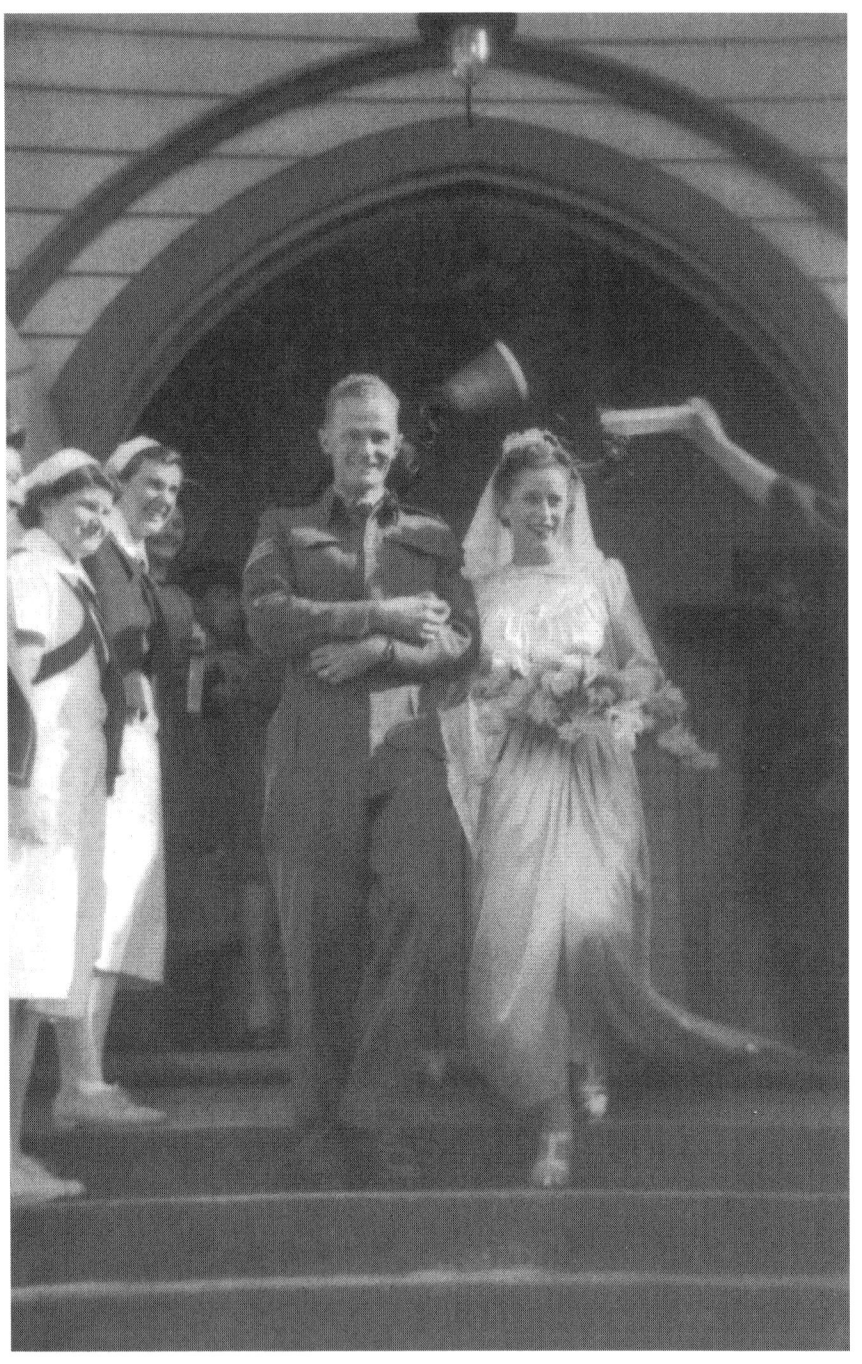

Figure A.2 My parents, Kenneth William de Montalk and Margaret Jessie Wilson.

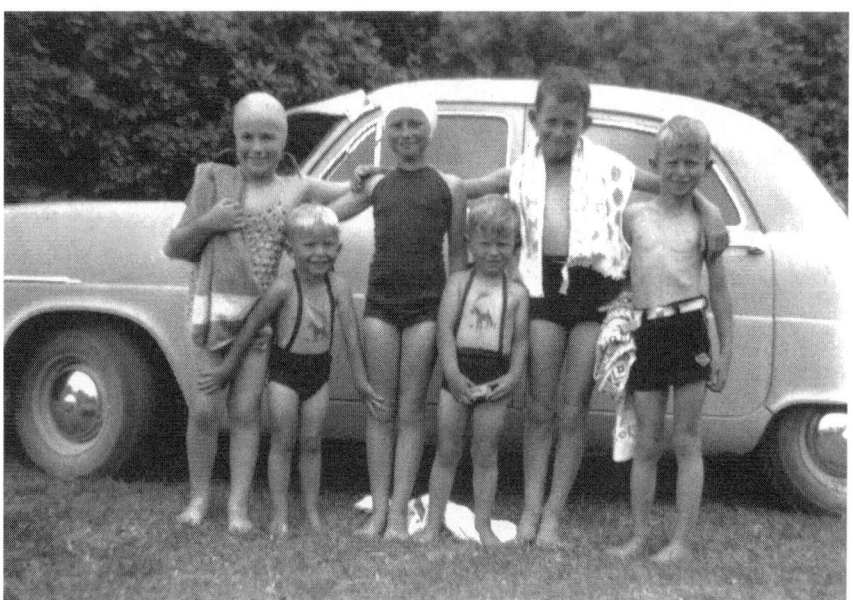

Figure A.3 'Summer of Childhood', the Bay of Islands, New Zealand; David far right, me centre, and twins Philip and Brian (with friends), 'in front of a Zephyr Six'.

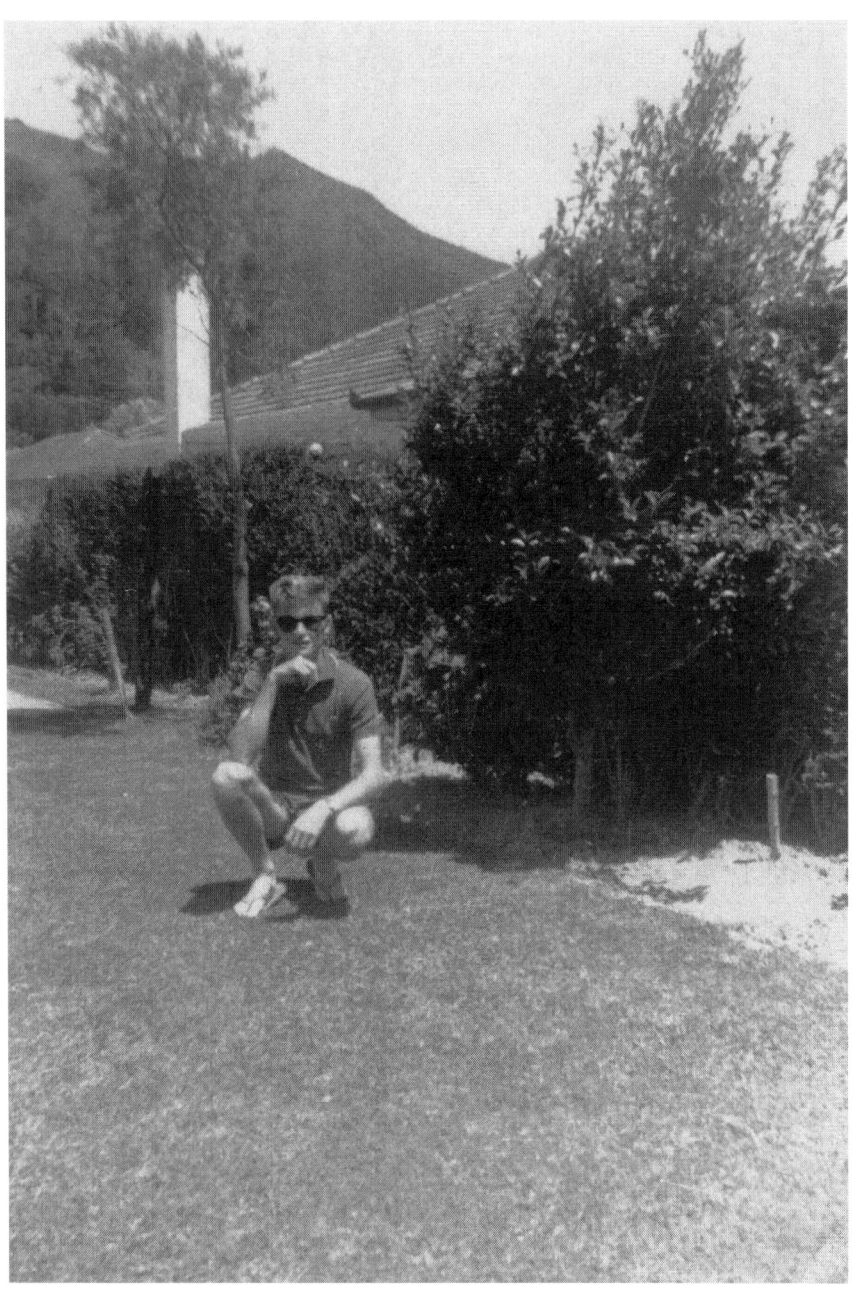

Figure A.4 My brother, David, shortly before his accident.

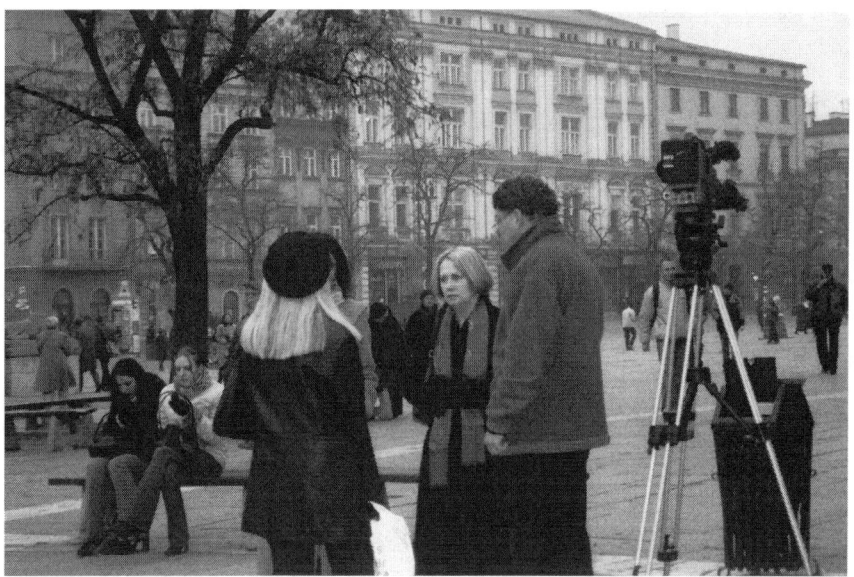

Figure A.5 Filming for Polish TV in the Market Square, Kraków, following my fall in Warsaw, 2003.

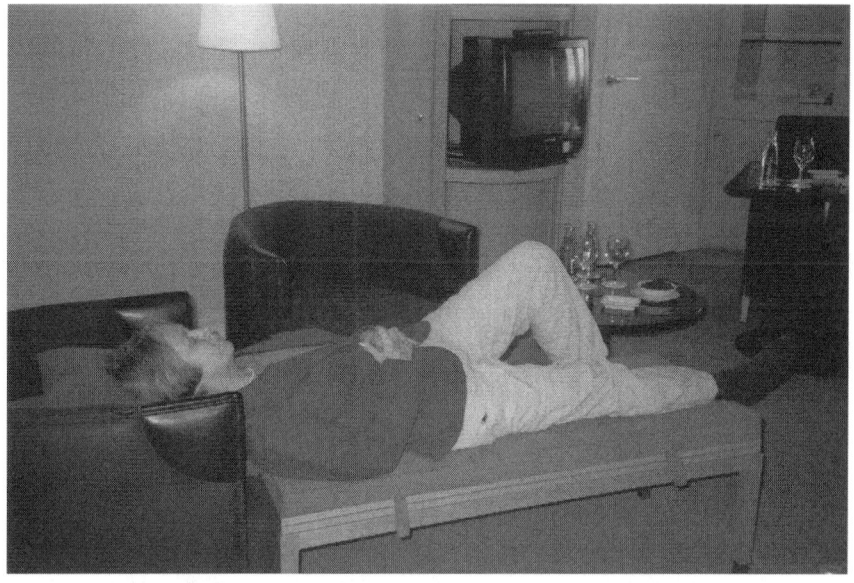

Figure A.6 The Sheraton Hotel Club Room, Paris, en route to Nantes, 2004.

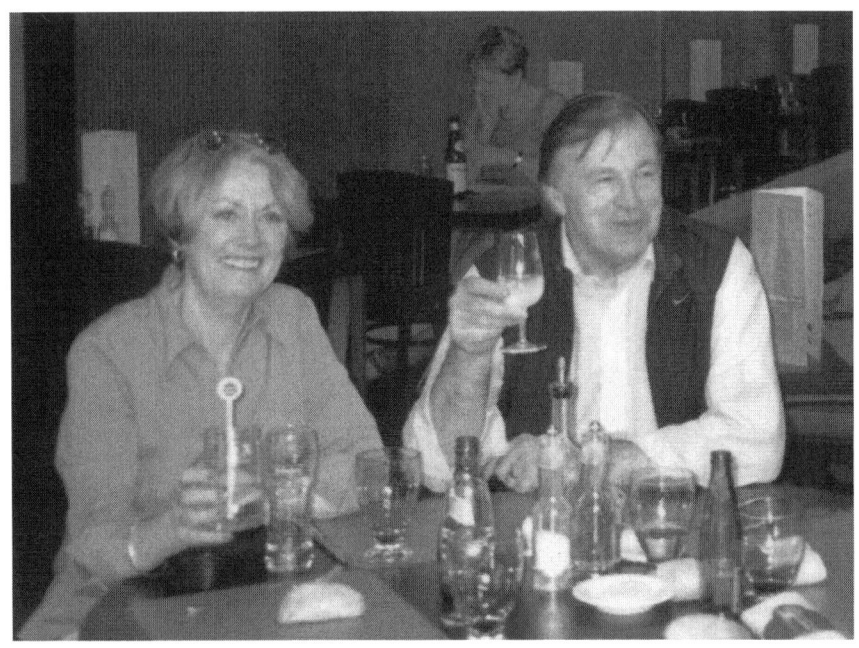

Figure A.7 Sitting, calling in pain; with John in Nantes, 2004.

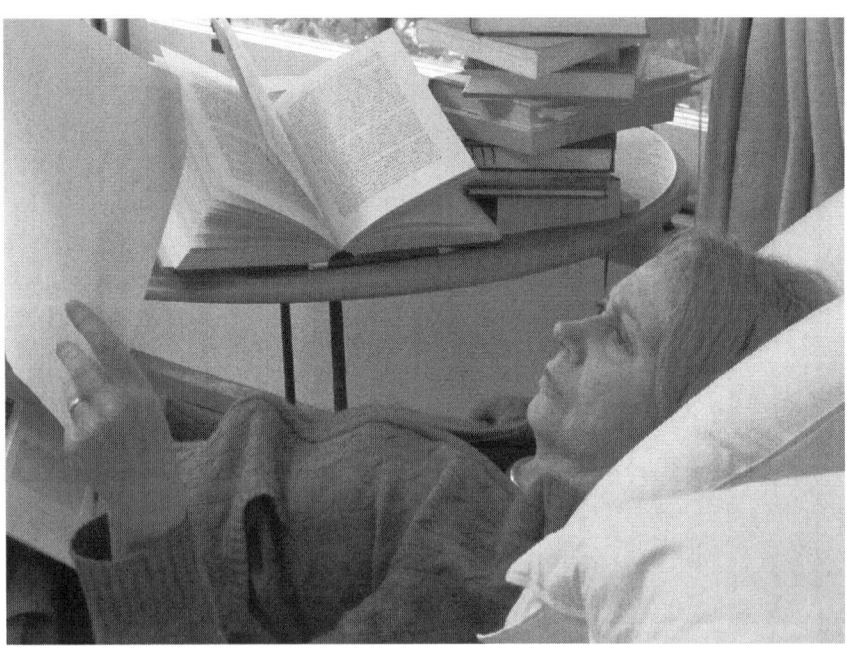

Figure A.8 Communicating pain, PhD, Wellington 2013.

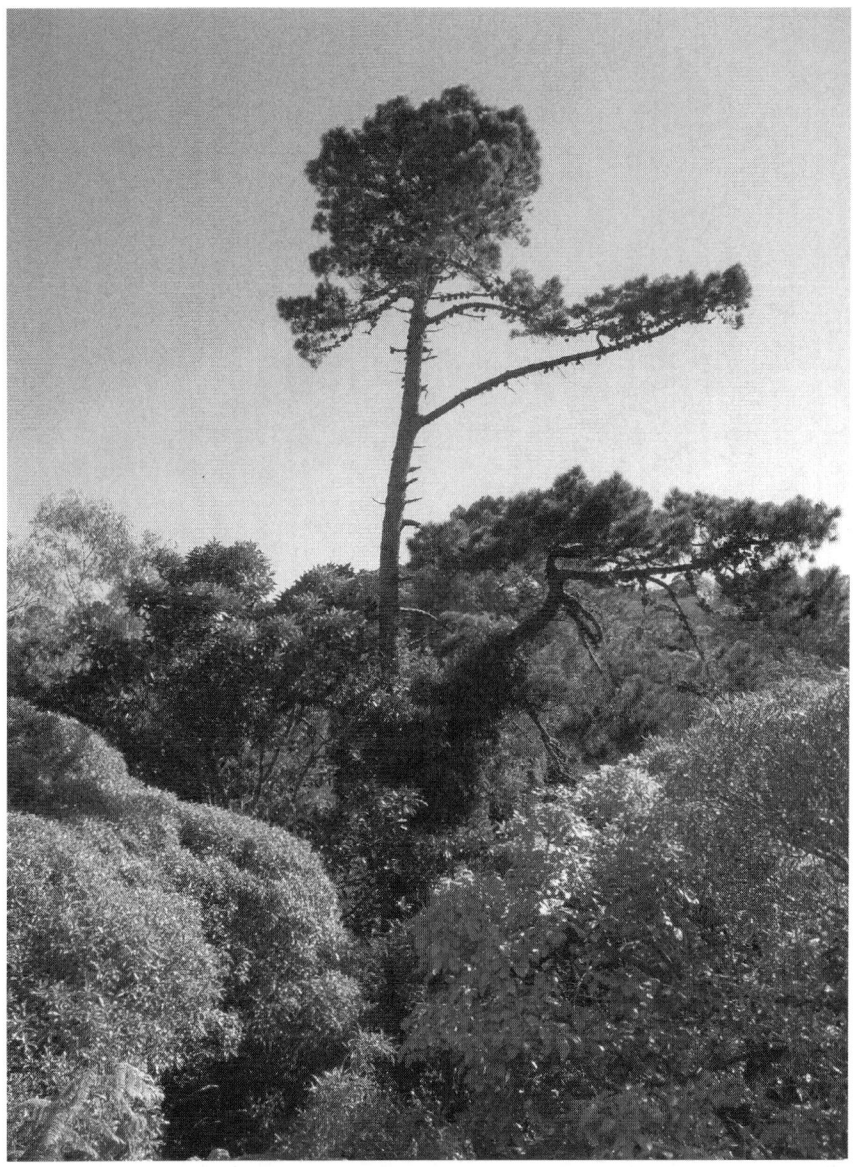

Figure A.9 The 'hero' pine, from my bedroom window.

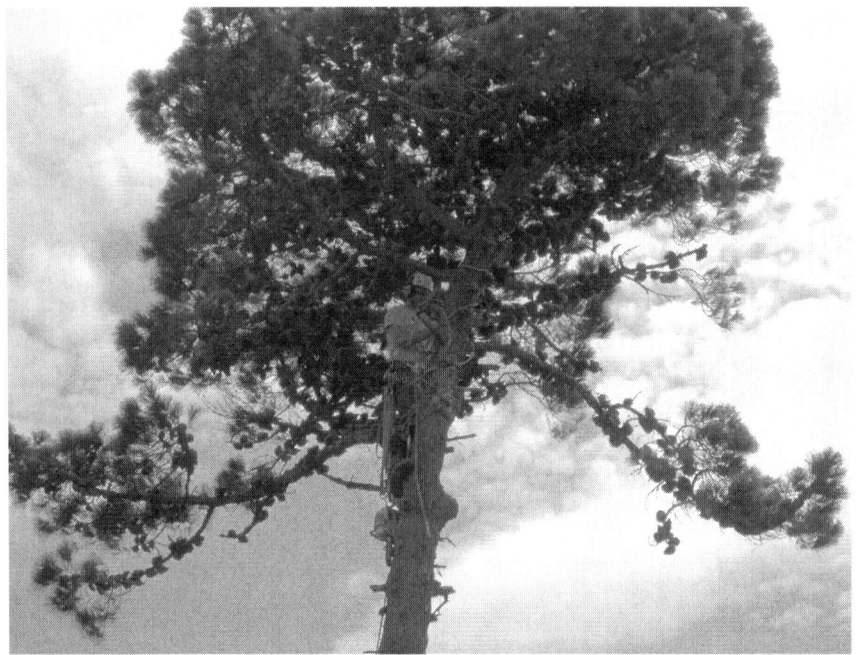

Figure A.10 The crown is dismantled, 2016.

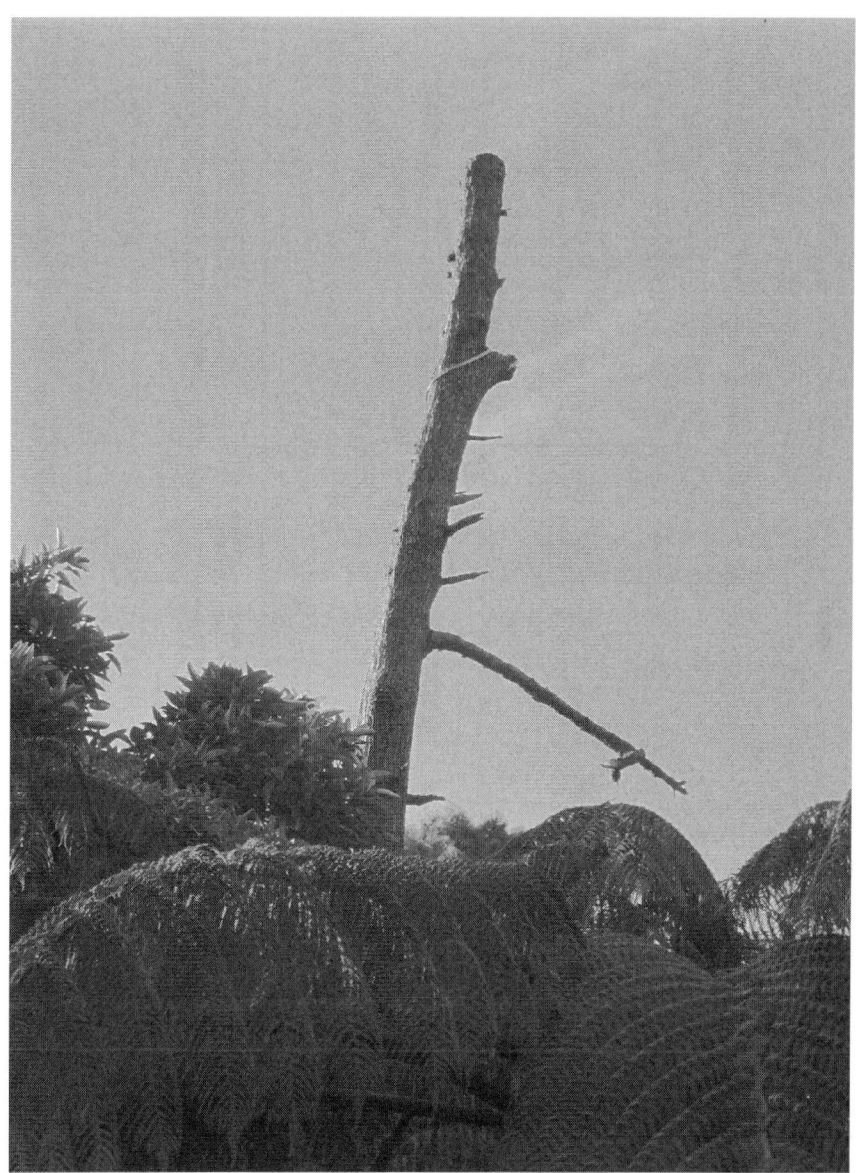

Figure A.11 'Without struggle or outrage'.

Notes

1 The shirt of Nessos

1 The title of this chapter relates to the story of Herakles, Nessos and Deianira in Greek mythology, in which the chiton of the dying Thessalian centaur, Nessos, tainted with his poisoned blood and unwittingly gifted to Herakles by his wife Deianira, caused such an unbearable burning pain that Herakles threw himself on a funeral pyre.

2 A widely used definition of pain published in the 'IASP Subcommittee on Taxonomy, Pain Terms: A List with Definitions and Notes on Usage', which first appeared in the journal *Pain* 6 (1979), 249–52.

3 'Pain Beyond Words and an Impulse Just to Endure', *New York Times*, 21 September 2009.

4 Andrew Jack, 'An End to the Agony', *Financial Times*, 20 November 2012.

5 Pain that results from injury to the peripheral sensory nerves or the brain and spinal cord of the central nervous system – to which networks it can cause lasting changes. Of neuropathic pain, Dr Clifford Woolf, Harvard professor and leading researcher of neuropathic pain, observes: 'There's tremendous ignorance about neuropathic pain. Most doctors don't know how to look for it.' Quoted in Melanie Thernstrom, *The Pain Chronicles: Cures, Myths, Mysteries, Prayers, Diaries, Brain Scans, Healing, and the Science of Suffering* (2010), 141.

6 Poem 1049, *Poems by Emily Dickinson: The Original* (2007), 1168.

7 Elaine Scarry, *The Body in Pain: The Making and Unmaking of the World* (1987), 9.

8 John Berryman interviewed by Peter A. Stitt, 'The Art of Poetry No. 16', *Paris Review*, October 1970.

9 Scott Fishman, the head of pain services at UC Davis, quoted in Melanie Thernstrom, *The Pain Chronicles*. As Fishman reminds us, fMRI views only the brain, not the mind – 'a virtual organ [without] a physical address that we know of' (328).

10 Thernstrom, *The Pain Chronicles*, 328.

11 Michel de Montaigne, *The Complete Essays of Montaigne*, trans. Donald M. Frame (1958), 577.

12 Paraphrased from Stephen Pender, 'Seeing, Feeling, Judging: Pain in the Early Modern Imagination', in *The Sense of Suffering: Constructions of Physical Pain in Early Modern Culture*, ed. Jan Frans van Dijkhuizen and Karl A.E. Enenkel (2009), 477.

13 'Only by actual sensation'; Montaigne, 577 and 840.

14 Of significance is the Birkbeck Pain Project (2012), led by Professor Joanna Bourke of the Department of History, Classics and Archaeology, which has facilitated papers, seminars and conferences on physical pain.

15 David Morris, *The Culture of Pain* (1993), 70.

16 Thernstrom, *The Pain Chronicles*, 189.

17 Morris, *The Culture of Pain*, 73.

18 'The Need for Knowledge Translation in Chronic Pain', *Pain Research and Management* 3, no. 6 (2008), 468, as cited by Lous Heshusius in her memoir *Inside Chronic Pain: An Intimate and Critical Account* (2009), 3. Henry is scientific director of the Michael G. de Groot Institute for Pain Research and Care at McMaster University.

19 Until the early twentieth century, the leading cause of death, worldwide, was infectious disease, and childbirth represented almost half of all deaths among young women. In the US, tuberculosis, pneumonia and diarrhoeal disease caused 30 per cent of all deaths ('Centres for Disease Control and Prevention', *1994 Fact Book*, 7, 1974). By the end of the twentieth century, in most of the developed world, owing to advancements in sanitation, nutrition, education, medicine and economic well being, the leading causes of death were chronic illnesses such as heart disease, stroke and cancer (M.L. Cohen, 'Changing Patterns of Infectious Disease', *Nature*, 2000: 406, 762–67). The aforementioned sources are cited in 'Incidence and Prevalence of Chronic Disease' on the website of The Marshall Protocol Knowledge Base Autoimmunity Research Foundation (neither author nor date noted).

20 Heshusius's work is a meticulously documented account of thirteen years' constant, severe spinal (neck) pain, sustained in a car accident in 1996. It is at once a narrative of her fruitless search for relief and the absence of sympathetic medical and social awareness, and a stinging critique of Canada's healthcare system with regard to chronic pain. Practitioners, notes Heshusius, who are still geared, and receptive to, the model of acute pain, are only adding to the suffering of patients living in an 'inexpressible, misunderstood' state – in which 'doctors, employers, friends and even family members […] can't believe [their pain] can be all that bad' (17). In commenting on the growing number of chronic pain patients, Heshusius cites Russell Portenoy, chair of Pain Medicine at New York's Beth Israel Medical Centre, who concludes: 'The problem is absolutely enormous. It rivals every serious public-health issue, whether you're talking about disease, cancer, obesity or anything else' (xxv–xxvi).

21 Professor Ted Shipton, Clinical Director of the Pain Management Centre for the Canterbury District Health Board, quoted in Margo White, 'Breaking the Pain Barrier', *New Zealand Listener*, 2–8 March 2013. The figure itself, also quoted by White, comes from the New Zealand Health Survey, 2006/07.

22 This line is from Czesław Miłosz's poem 'The Fall', *Bells in Winter* (1978), 15. The poem concludes: 'Its land once bringing harvest is overgrown with thistles,/Its mission forgotten, its language lost,/The dialect of a village high upon inaccessible mountains.'

23 William Carlos Williams, quoted in Louis Simpson, *The Character of the Poet* (1986), 5.

24 An article on the online Accident Compensation Corporation (ACC) Forum, discussing the use of cannabis for chronic pain (25 November 2012), is indicative of the thinking often applied to chronic pain and the confusion that still exists between the acute and chronic forms: 'One of the issues rarely mentioned on accforum is not the miserable lives that chronic pain sufferers suffer (this is posted about regularly) but what miseries those sufferers can. [*sic*] be.' The writer then suggests that if one is a 'friendly and socially well balanced "get up and go" type well used to facing adversity', the effect of chronic pain will be less than that experienced by someone who is 'depressed' or 'socially isolated', and urges the latter 'to grab what is left of life – where there's life there's hope – and make the best of it on your own'.

25 Scott M. Fishman M.D., 'Clinical Commentary' in Lous Heshusius, *Inside Chronic Pain*, 23.

26 Roselyne Rey, *The History of Pain*, trans. Louise Elliott Wallace, J.A. Cadden and S.W. Cadden (1993), 10.

27 Ibid. 14.

28 Ibid. 14.

29 Ibid. 16.

30 Ibid. 15.
31 Philoctetes' foot was bitten by a snake in a sacred grove on the island of Lemnos during an interlude en route by ship to the Trojan War, following which he was abandoned on the island by his compatriots because they could tolerate neither the sight and stench of his wound, nor his expressions of pain. The play takes place a decade after Philoctetes' suffering began.
32 *Philoctetes* (c. 409), trans. Ian Johnston, Vancouver Island University (2012). '... I looked everywhere,/but all I found around me was my pain' (ll. 282–83).
33 '... no one there/to answer him with sympathy/when he cried out against the plague/ that ate at his flesh and made him bleed' (ll. 695–98).
34 *Selected Poetry of W.H. Auden* (1971), 45.
35 Miroslav Holub, trans. Ewald Osers, *Intensive Care: Selected and New Poems* (1996), 157.
36 Ludwig Wittgenstein, *Philosophical Investigations*, 2nd ed., trans. G.E.M. Anscombe (1958), 88, section 243.
37 Wittgenstein, 89 (sections 244, 246), 92 (section 257).
38 The essay, which takes its title from William Hazlitt's essay 'On Going a Journey' (1882), is published as *On Being Ill* with an introduction by Hermione Lee (2002). It first appeared as an essay commissioned by T.S. Eliot in the *New Criterion* (January 1926); was reprinted with revisions in the New York magazine *The Forum* (April 1926) as 'Illness: An Unexplored Mine'; and was published as a separate edition typeset by Woolf herself for Hogarth Press (1930).
39 Woolf's essay is less a personal illness narrative than a wry manifesto on bodily illness and pain as topics for creative exploration, but lacking as such in literature. Although Woolf herself was not subject to chronic bodily distress (refer to Hilary Mantel's comments on Woolf's credentials for commenting on the absence of a language of pain, later in this chapter), it could be said that Woolf's struggle with the physical illnesses (including fatigue, palpitations and severe headaches) collectively known as neurasthenia, that accompanied the episodes of mental pain that were prevalent throughout her life, equipped Woolf to write with insight about the contracted language of physical illness and pain.
40 The timing of Woolf's essay, written against a lessening of invalid writing as society and literature moved in a more secular direction, is significant. Since the Reformation and science's increasing presence, there had been a gradual erosion of religious faith and the metaphoric belief in pain as a precious metal forged and refined by fire. In 'Languages of Pain' (*The Lancet* 379, 2420–21), Joanna Burke reminds us that the 'rich narratives of suffering supplied by the Bible' were 'a world away from the secular metaphors of later periods, with the emphasis not on submission to physical agony, but on precisely the opposite: fighting, and ultimately conquering pain'. The nature of tribulation as of moral benefit would continue to diminish as medical progression, previously measured in centuries, advanced in decades and visibility of pain rose in the face of World Wars I and II and other twentieth and twenty-first century global and national tragedies.
41 *On Being Ill*, 3–4.
42 Ibid. 4.
43 Ibid. 6–7.
44 Ibid. 7.
45 Ibid. 5.
46 Ibid. 12.
47 Ibid. 12.
48 Elaine Scarry, *The Body in Pain: The Making and Unmaking of the World* (1985), 4.
49 Ibid. 4.
50 Ibid. 5.
51 Ibid. 4–5.

52 Ibid. 5.

53 Ibid. 162. Scarry's comment in this paragraph about the pain's non-linkage to objects, reminds me of the response to pain by a man with a phenomenal memory and capacity for visualisation, who was a research subject of the Russian neurologist, A.R. Luria. The (anonymous) man, once able to visualise and understand something, never forgot it, including volumes of text. Regarding the word ' "pain" ', he said that he saw ' "bands – little round objects, and fog. It's the fog," ' he responded, 'that has to do with the abstractness of the word." ' A.R. Luria, *The Mind of a Mnemonist* (1968), 134.

54 Louise Hide, Joanna Burke and Carmen Mangion (eds.), 'Perspectives on Pain: Introduction', *19: Interdisciplinary Studies in the Nineteenth Century*, no. 15 (2012), 1.

55 Vincent Crapanzano, *Imaginative Horizons: An Essay in Literary-Philosophical Anthropology* (2010), 81.

56 Hilary Mantel, 'Diary', *London Review of Books* 32, no. 21 (4 November 2010), 41–42. This essay was subsequently published as the memoir *Ink in the Blood: A Hospital Diary* (2010).

57 Hilary Mantel describes her experience of long-misdiagnosed endometriosis in her memoir *Giving Up the Ghost: A Memoir* (2004).

58 Lucy Bending, *The Representation of Bodily Pain in Late Nineteenth-Century English Culture* (2000), 3.

59 Ibid. 86.

60 Ibid. 89.

61 'underpinned human existence' – *A Tale of Two Cities*: ibid. 89–90.

62 Ibid. 100.

63 Arne Johan Vetlesen, *A Philosophy of Pain*, trans. John Irons (2009), 157.

64 *The Language of Pain: Finding Words, Compassion, and Relief* (2010) was prompted by Biro's experience of illness and pain ten years earlier, documented in his memoir *One Hundred Days: My Unexpected Journey from Doctor to Patient* (2000). The latter recalls the onset and (successful) treatment, including a bone marrow transplant, of the rare and potentially fatal blood disorder, paroxysmal nocturnal haemoglobinuria. Biro, aged thirty-one, a young 'doctor with too much information', was lastingly affected by his ordeal. *Days* details his fears, phobias, panic attacks and 'paroxysms of pain', and the emotional isolation of being unable to describe, and share, his suffering. He wrote his memoir for purposes of ordering the experience, and providing insights for members of the medical community and others who have not experienced significant illness and pain.

65 Biro, *The Language of Pain*, 39.

66 Ibid. 42–43. It is worth noting that the focus of Biro's *Language of Pain* is, as so often, acute pain, in line with his own experience of pain, within which framework he also examines emotional and mental distress. Chronic pain appears as but a part of the general pattern of pain.

67 Ibid. 84. As an example, I offer my own instinctive, visually imagined linking of the pain of the scalpel during a Caesarean section under failed general anaesthesia, with the jagged neck of a broken bottle (refer to Chapter 2). It occurs to me that, in terms of authenticated awareness, the attachment of the metaphoric bottle to the scalpel as the pain-giving instrument was more powerful than the attachment of my body in pain.

68 I also note Aleksander Wat's view (refer to Chapter 8) that metonymy's associations of the senses and memory based on a contiguity of common experience was more enduring than the limited similarities of metaphor. In this regard, I wonder if the specificity and direct comparison of metaphor might be suited to description of acute pain; and the more subtle and broadly imagined association (or contiguity) of metonymy, which brings language's wider attributes into play, to chronic pain and, in particular, to the storytelling of that pain: as David Morris observes in *Illness and Culture in the Postmodern Age* (1998), chronic pain is 'saturated in emotion, memory, and consciousness' (144).

69 Biro, *The Language of Pain*, 10.
70 Susan Sontag, *Illness as Metaphor and AIDS and Its Metaphors* (1989), 3.
71 Anne Hunsaker Hawkins, *Reconstructing Illness: Studies in Pathography* 393 (1999), 23.
72 Martha Stoddard Holmes, 'After Sontag: Reclaiming Metaphor', *Genre: Forms of Discourse and Culture* 44, no. 3 (Autumn 2011), 274.
73 Ibid. 267–68.
74 Arthur Kleinman: presently Professor of Medical Anthropology and Cross-Cultural Psychology at Harvard University.
75 David B. Morris: presently Emeritus Professor of Literature at the University of Virginia.
76 Arthur Kleinman, M.D., *The Illness Narratives: Suffering, Healing and the Human Condition* (1988), 181.
77 Ibid. xii.
78 Morris reminds us that for the last 100, science has viewed pain in strictly medical terms: as a message sent from a site of injury to the brain, a straightforward separation of disease as objectively verifiable. But exploration of the 'historical, cultural and psychosocial construction of pain' shows that pain 'is always more than a matter of nerves and neurotransmitters' *The Culture of Pain* (1991), 2.
79 Morris writes widely about chronic pain and the place of pain in literature, and does so with unusual perception and empathy. There is no indication he expresses a personal standpoint. He does, however, acknowledge the influence of his physician father, who demonstrated that 'medicine, literature and the arts need not belong to separate worlds' (*The Culture of Pain*, xi). He also refers to his own teaching of medicine in literature, and to the chronic pain patients he met while carrying out research in pain clinics.
80 Morris, *The Culture of Pain*, 2.
81 Virginia Woolf, *On Being Ill*, 2.
82 Arthur Frank, *The Wounded Storyteller: Body, Illness and Ethics* (1997), xi. Frank first wrote about his illnesses in *At the Will of the Body: Reflections on Illness* (1991).
83 Frank, *The Wounded Storyteller*, ii.
84 Ibid. 75–96; 'the "chaos" narrative': 97–114; 'the "quest" narrative': 115–37.
85 Guest editors Louise Hide, Joanna Bourke and Carmen Mangion, 'Introduction: Perspectives on Pain', *19: Interdisciplinary Studies in the Long Nineteenth Century*, no. 15 (2012).
86 In this regard, I remember US writer, poet and 'painter of words', Kenneth Patchen (1911–1972), who became bed-bound with the pain of the spinal arthritis that developed as the result of first one accident, and then another. Patchen was the subject of Henry Miller's pamphlet 'Patchen: Man of Anger and Light' – collected in Miller's *Stand Still Like the Hummingbird* (1962) – in which Miller writes that Patchen 'labours in a state of almost unremitting pain' (33). Patchen, who describes himself as 'rigid inside with the constant pressure of illness', the pain 'almost a natural part of me now' (29), was given to limiting his medications so that his mind could remain clear.
87 William Zinsser (ed.), *Inventing the Truth: The Art and Craft of Memoir* (1998), 6, 12.
88 Lous Heshusius, *Inside Chronic Pain*, xxiii.
89 In 'Narrative and Pain: An Integrative Model', *Handbook of Pain and Palliative Care: Behavioural Approaches for the Life Course*, ed. Rhonda J. Moore (2012), David B. Morris accepts that 'core uncertainties make fully objective knowledge of pain a pipedream' (734). He continues: 'Uncertainty is constitutive of pain – especially chronic pain – much as it is a constitutive principle in quantum mechanics' (734).
90 In *Reconstructing Illness: Studies in Pathography* (1999), Anne Hunsaker Hawkins characterises pathography as a 'subgenre of autobiography' (3), that takes the form of

'an autobiographical or biographical narrative about an experience of illness' (229). 'In some sense,' Hawkins says, 'the pathography is our modern adventure story [...] as the ill person is transported out of the familiar everyday world [...] into essential experience – the deeper realities of life' (1). It might be said that blogging fulfils a similar, albeit less considered, objective.

91 John Berger and Jean Mohr, *A Fortunate Man: The Story of a Country Doctor* (1967), 158: 'It is to reasoning that the poetic gives its most famous license.'

2 Going nursing

1 From a letter written 8 February 1860, *Life in the Sick-Room*, 'Appendix E: Harriet Martineau and Florence Nightingale', ed. Maria H. Frawley (2003), 217. This edition reproduces Harriet Martineau's memoir, *Life in the Sick-Room: Essays by an Invalid* (1844). In *Florence Nightingale, the Woman and Her Legend* (2008), Mark Bostridge writes that Nightingale contracted Crimean Fever at Scutari and returned to England in 1856 in poor health. She remained ill, at times seriously so and bedridden, until the early 1880s, with what is now thought to have been a severe form of chronic brucellosis – a condition of partial improvement and relapse, the latter marked by extreme physical exhaustion, 'crippling depression' (326) jokingly referred to by Nightingale as 'a compound fracture of the intellect' (281–82), tachycardia, insomnia, muscle spasms and 'excruciating' spondylitis (inflammation of the spinal cord) (325) necessitating the use of opium, bromide and morphine.

2 'It is the consummate surface and bloom of all things', Percy Bysshe Shelley, 'A Defence of Poetry', essay published posthumously in *Essays: Letters from Abroad, Translations and Fragments, Volume One* (1840), 47.

3 'What were our consolations on this side of the grave – and what were our aspirations beyond it, if poetry did not ascend to the light and fire from those eternal regions where the owl-winged faculty of calculation dare not ever soar?' ibid. 56.

4 John Cairney (1961), 237.

5 *The Birdsville Track* first screened in 1954.

6 Julia Hallam, *Nursing the Image: Media, Culture and Professional Identity* (2000), 81.

7 Ann Bradshaw, *The Nurse Apprentice 1860–1997* (2001), 122.

8 Barbara Gay Williams, Victoria University of Wellington PhD thesis, *The Primacy of the Nurse in New Zealand 1960s–1990s: Attitudes, Beliefs and Responses Over Time* (2000), 91.

9 Bradshaw, *Apprentice*, 2.

10 Jackie Crisp and Catherine Taylor (eds.), 'Science and Art of Nursing Practice' in *Potter & Perry's Fundamentals of Nursing* (3rd ed., 2008), 8.

11 Bradshaw, *Apprentice*, 236.

12 I noted these remarks, as a patient, during informal conversations with registered nurses, Wellington, 2011.

13 Ann Bradshaw, 'Measuring Nursing Care and Compassion: the McDonalised Nurse?', *Journal of Medical Ethics* 35, no. 8 (2009), 465–68.

14 Helen Garner refers to Australian nurse, novelist, essayist and playwright Elizabeth Jolley in the interview 'Helen Garner's Return to Fiction with *The Spare Room*', The Book Show, Radio National (8 April 2008).

15 Helen Garner quotes Elizabeth Jolley on The Book Show, Radio National; and in the epigraph to Garner's *The Spare Room* (2008).

16 *The Collected Works of Florence Nightingale.* ed. Lynn McDonald, vol. 6, *Florence Nightingale on Public Health Care* (2004), 215.

17 Boris Pasternak's words about nurses are recorded by Olga Ivinskaya in *A Captive of Time: My Years with Pasternak* (1978), 345. Pasternak (1890–1960) died of lung cancer.

3 At the end of the mind, the body

1 Paul Valéry, *Monsieur Teste*; in *The Collected Works of Paul Valéry* (1973), 68. Monsieur Teste, the subject of Valéry's novel, was a rationalist. When in pain, he observed that 'Pain was searching for the mechanism that might have converted pain into knowledge – something the mystics glimpsed and disapproved' (68). He further noted: 'I feel zones of pain … rings, poles, plumes of pain. Do you see these living forms, this geometry of my suffering? […] When *it* is coming on, I find something confused or diffused inside of myself' (165).

2 Letter from Robert Louis Stevenson to Dr Japp, 1 April 1882. In *Robert Louis Stevenson: A Record, an Estimate, and a Memorial*, A.H. Japp (1905), 29.

3 Alphonse Daudet, *In the Land of Pain* (2002), 9.

4 Aleksander Wat, 'Diary Without Vowels' (essay, from *Diary Without Vowels*), in *Polish Writers on Writing* (ed. Adam Zagajewski, 2007), 74.

5 Harriet Martineau, *Life in the Sick-Room* (ed. Maria H. Frawley, 2003), 39.

6 Arthur Schopenhauer's rendering of Aristotle's dictum from the *Nichomachean Ethics*, vii. In *Counsels and Maxims*, Chapter 1, 'General Rules' (2007), 7. '[N]ot pleasure, but freedom from pain, is what the wise man will aim at.'

7 '*Treatise of Man*, René Descartes: Harvard Monographs in the History of Science' (1972), 34.

8 The GCT presumed that special spinal nerve cells, or 'gates', in the dorsal horn at each segmental level of the spinal cord, admitted and intensified or reduced pain impulses before either transmitting them to pain centres in the brain, or blocking transmission altogether; pain was experienced when the arrival of signals at the pain centres in the brain exceeded certain levels. The GCT also presumed that nerves recording pain, touch and pressure deposited separate sensations into the spinal cord, and that the balancing of, or competition between, these sensations dictated the extent to which pain was admitted to the cord and registered by the brain – an explanation for the efficacy of pain-inhibiting mechanisms such as heat, cold, rubbing and acupuncture. The GCT further suggested that admittance of pain could be influenced by interpretative responses to pain – by expectation, attitude, memory – thus introducing a mind-body hypothesis. With regard to chronic pain, the theory held that if the pain gate changed or became damaged as a result of unrelieved pain, it stayed open, even after the pain-producing tissue had been treated or controlled. In such instances, pain, often out of proportion to the original injury and level of harm diagnosed, continued, at which stage pain itself became the diagnosis or disease. Indeed, the GCT proposed, for the first time, that pain was not only a symptom, but also a distinct disease with a neurobiological foundation. See *Pain Management: An Interdisciplinary Approach*, ed. Chris J. Main and Chris C. Spanswick (2000), 8–10.

   In 1983, Clifford Woolf demonstrated that overstimulation of neurons (nerve cells) within the central nervous system (CNS, brain and spinal cord) could cause normally non-provocative stimulation to start producing pain (the touch of clothing, for instance, during shingles). And that a persistent state of severe pain could result in pain-sensitising neurons in the dorsal horn of the spinal cord rewiring the CNS into an over-reactive state of sensitivity, known as 'central sensitization'.

   In 1997, Ronald Dubner suggested that the CNS, in altering its sensitivity, could give rise to nervous system plasticity, and the occurrence of peripheral, as well as central nervous system, sensitisation. Today, the sensitisation theory dictates that pain be relieved as quickly and as completely as possible – in order to avoid a state of chronic pain in which constant impulses from the original pain site can rewire the brain to believe pain is a normal state, even if the original pain source has been resolved. The sensitisation findings endorse the modern concept of pre-emptive surgical anaesthesia: prior to 1983, anaesthetics included negligible, if any, analgesia; this meant the unconscious patient's brain received, in full, pain signals from the surgical site. Today, narcotics, nerve blocks or local anaesthesia administered before and during surgery, block the possibility of sensitisation and ensure less pain for patients in the post-operative period.

Prior to the GCT, says Dubner, 'clinicians [...] tended to avoid patients who complained of chronic pain. [...] Clinicians assumed that their chronic pain must be due to an underlying psychological condition [...] Our understanding of pain was so rudimentary back then and, in some cases, dead wrong. [...] We certainly knew nothing – NOTHING – about the changes in the nervous system that result from the barrages of information that emanate from the periphery after injury.' Reference: 'Pain Research: Past, Present and Future', an article in which Dubner (Professor, Neural Pain Sciences, University of Maryland, Baltimore) was interviewed by the *National Institute of Dental and Cranial Research* (National Institutes of Health, Bethesda, Maryland), October 2003.

9 Restriction of pelvic size can cause non-rotation of the foetus necessary for delivery.

10 '[I]ntense pain creates extraordinarily clear awareness of surroundings,' writes Melanie Thernstrom in *The Pain Chronicles* (2010) of surgery before anaesthesia, 'as people sense mortal danger they become hyperalert, fixing details in memory' (94).

11 *Silenced Screams – Surviving Anesthetic Awareness During Surgery: A True-life Account* (2002), 15, 106. Dr Liska experienced this event in 1990. She found the key to overcoming her subsequent post-traumatic stress disorder lay in advocacy for other victims of sustained 'anaesthetic awareness with implicit recall' and, twelve years later, publishing her memoir of the medical misadventure.

12 *Chronic Pelvic Pain: A Patient Education Booklet*, Michael Wenof, C. Paul Perry, The International Pelvic Pain Society (1999).

13 The pudendal nerve crosses the boundaries of many medical specialties, including neurology, orthopaedics, urology and gynaecology. 'The reason [PNE] is not commonly diagnosed is that it is the mother of all masqueraders,' writes Jerome M. Weiss, M.D. in 'Pudendal Nerve Entrapment', a paper presented at the International Pelvic Pain Society 10th Scientific Meeting on Chronic Pelvic Pain, Alberta, Canada, August 2003. 'I believe that this diagnostic deception, in the eyes of most medical practitioners, stems from two causes. The first is that it is a relatively new diagnosis [...] and therefore is a relatively unfamiliar entity. And secondly, the symptoms it produces fall into the domain of many medical specialists who falsely recognize them as more familiar problems and therefore give them a knee jerk diagnosis-treatment response.' The condition – which is similar to carpal tunnel syndrome, but is complicated by its occurrence deep in the pelvis amidst muscles, vessels and other structures such as organs – arises when the nerve is compressed and becomes aggravated by pressure. Neuralgia (nerve pain) without entrapment is not uncommon, although often misdiagnosed, and usually settles. Some cases of sub-acute entrapment may be managed without surgery. However, entrapment of the nerve necessitating surgical decompression is 'very rare [...] I don't know of any studies that have addressed the actual incidence of it' (specialist PNE neurosurgeon, Lee V. Ansell, Houston, Texas, in email correspondence with me, 2010).

14 R. Robert *et al.*, 'Anatomic Basis of Chronic Perineal Pain: Role of the Pudendal Nerve', *Surgical and Radiologic Anatomy* 20 (1988), 93–98.

15 Richard Selzer, *The Wilson Quarterly* 18, no. 4 (Autumn 1994), 28.

16 This is not to diminish the suffering and fortitude of our pain-familiar predecessors. Take novelist Fanny Burney D'Arblay, who in 1811 underwent a mastectomy for breast cancer (a not uncommon surgery) without anaesthesia, in France, and summoned the additional courage to document her experience in the earliest recorded account of a mastectomy from the patient's point of view. Burney had 'felt the instrument – describing a curve – cutting against the grain', at which time she 'began a scream that lasted intermittently during the whole time of the incision – & I marvel that it rings not in my Ears [*sic*] still': *Fanny Burney: Selected Letters and Journals*

(1986), 139. So traumatised was Burney by the operation that for six months she could not mention her 'utterly speechless torture' (139). Nonetheless, in time, over a three-month period, experiencing nausea and headaches as she relived the ordeal, she completed a 3,000-word letter/memoir, addressed to her sister, Esther.

17 Established by Jack Harich, 14 July 2002. Reproduced in 'A Review of the Evaluation of Pain Using a Variety of Pain Scales' (undated), 2.

18 *Prison Notebooks*, vol. 1 (2011), 12.

19 *The Meditations of Marcus Aurelius Antonius: And a Selection from the Letters of Marcus and Fronto* (1989), 61.

20 *The Complete Works of Michael de Montaigne* (1842), 505.

21 Nietzsche, *The Gay Science* (1982), quoted in *Nietzsche, Theories of Knowledge, and Critical Theory: Nietzsche and the Sciences* (1999), 187.

22 Essay 152, 'Doctrine of Suffering of the World', *Parerga and Paralipomena: Short Philosophical Essays, Volume 2* (2000), 293.

23 John Milton, 'Samson Agonistes, A Dramatice Poem', *The Poetical Works of John Milton Volume 3*: 'Samson Agonistes, A Dramatic Poem' (1851), 32, lines 652 and 653, 661 and 662.

24 Philippus Aureolus Theophrastus Bombastus von Hohenheim (1493–1541). I originally found this phrase during random reading; it is formally cited in *An Encyclopaedia of Occultism*: *Cosimo Classics Metaphysics*, Lewis Spence (2006), 261.

25 The potential of amitriptyline and other tricyclic anti-depressants for reducing chronic pain was discovered in the mid-1960s, when patients with severe chronic pain who were medicated for depression with amitriptyline coincidentally experienced a lessening of pain. These drugs, in addition to regulating mood by increasing levels of naturally occurring CNS-regulating chemicals including serotonin and norepinephrine, were found to stabilise changed or damaged pain receptors and calm overactive pain pathways and abnormal signalling systems. Anti-convulsant, or epileptic, medications, such as gabapentin (Neurontin), which dampen down and decrease generation and conduction of impulses, reduce the uncontrollable firing of pain nerves in a similar way.

26 This term applies to opiates derived naturally from the opium poppy, and also to synthetic or semi-synthetic opiates known as opioids.

27 *The Analects of Confucius, or The Conversations of Confucius with His Disciples and Certain Others* (1958), 97, 98 and 195 respectively.

28 Jalal al-Din Rumi, *The Essential Rumi*, trans. Coleman Barks (1995), 20.

29 *The Fountain of Tears* (2006), 16.

30 William Wordsworth, 'Intimations of Immortality from Recollections of Early Childhood' (1807). 'What though the radiance which was once so bright/Be now forever taken from my sight, […] In the faith that looks through death/In years that bring the philosophic mind', lines 180, 181, 190, 191.

31 Louis Simpson recalls William Carlos Williams who said 'No ideas but in things', in *The Character of the Poet* (1989), 14.

32 Richard Burton, quoted in Bryon Farwell, *Burton: A Biography of Sir Richard Francis Burton* (1998), 145.

33 Ibid. 341.

34 'Poems Grow', Marina Tsvetayeva, in *Selected Poems* (1988), 107: 'We sleep, and suddenly, moving through flagstones,/The celestial, four-petalled guest appears.'

35 Refers to Ivan Sergeyevich Turgenev's short story 'The Living Relic' (1874).

36 This reference adapts Boris Pasternak's 'A Definition of Poetry' ('It is a fully ripe whistle/It is ice, shard on shard') in *Second Nature: New Translations of Poems by Boris Pasternak* (1990), 28.

37 John le Carré, introduction to Bruce Page, David Leitch and Phillip Knightley, *Philby: The Spy Who Betrayed a Generation* (1977), 39.

38 'Warsaw', de Montalk, *Cover Stories* (2005), 27.

39 'Working Days', ibid. 11.
40 'Cracked Pots Last Longest', ibid. 47.
41 'Last Stand', ibid. 16.
42 'Working Days', ibid. 12.
43 'Camping Beside the Axeinous Sea', ibid. 49.
44 'Talking Pictures', ibid. 40.
45 'Waxing and Salting', ibid. 71.
46 André Breton quoted, unsourced, in *Nantes Maps and Visitor Information* (2004); also France Guide site *official du tourisme en France*, franceguide.com.
47 His Holiness Tenzin Gyatso, the Fourteenth Dalai Lama, and Howard C. Cutler, M.D., *The Essence of Happiness: A Guidebook for Living* (2003), 61.
48 Dinah Hawken, *Oh There You Are Tui! New and Selected Poems* (2001), 106.
49 *Cover Stories*, 73.
50 Boris Pasternak, *Doctor Zhivago* (1958), 131.
51 *The Selected Poetry of Rainer Maria Rilke* (1987), 273.
52 'Enhancement', *Cover Stories*, ibid. 44.
53 John Cairney, (1961), 59–61.
54 'What is grief compared': *A Grief Observed*, C.S. Lewis (1973), 46, 34.
55 Arthur Koestler, *The Roots of Coincidence* (1972), 110.
56 Arthur Schopenhauer, *On The Basis of Morality* (1915), 170.
57 Maxim Gorky, *My Childhood* (1967), 34.
58 Marco Iacoboni, neuroscientist, University of California, quoted in Eric Falkenstein, *Finding Alpha: The Search for Alpha When Risk and Return Break Down* (2009), 145. Iacoboni continues, 'To understand myself I must recognize myself in other people.'
59 Voltaire, *Candide* (1947), 23.
60 René Guy Cadou, quoted in Nantes tourism brochure, unsourced; jotting made by me in Nantes, 2004.
61 André Breton, *Manifestos of Surrealism* (1969), 117.
62 'old wives, gypsies, sorcerers': Paracelsus, quoted in Richard Morris, *The Last Sorcerers: The Path from Alchemy to the Periodic Table* (2003), 31.

4 But at the end of the body, the mind

1 Paul Valéry, *Monsieur Teste*, in *The Collected Works of Paul Valéry* (1973), 68.
2 'There is certainly data that suggest that just being in the healing situation accomplishes something': Dr Walter A. Brown, M.D., Clinical Professor of Psychiatry at Brown University and Tufts University School of Medicine, quoted in Margaret Talbot, 'The Placebo Prescription', *New York Times*, 9 January 2000.
3 René Lerich, foreword to *La Philosophie de la Chirurgie* (1951), trans. Roberta Hurwitz.
4 'Enhancement', de Montalk, *Cover Stories* (2005), 46.
5 Nelda Wray, placebo researcher, quoted in Talbot, 'The Placebo Prescription'.
6 Aleš Šteger, *The Book of Things* (2010), 11. Excerpt: 'You remember how your mother, Jocasta,/Returned from the pigsty with a gaping palm. // Inside the madness of pain a window opened./She stepped out and stepped out of her body.'
7 Jennifer Schneider, *Living With Chronic Pain: The Complete Health Guide to the Causes and Treatment of Chronic Pain* (2004), ix.
8 Claudia Wallis, 'The Right (and Wrong) Way to Treat Pain', 20 February 2005.
9 The description of the approach to the cave recalls Czesław Miłosz's lines in 'Notes', from *Bells in Winter* (1978), 34. Miłosz writes: 'Mountains//Wet grass to the knees, in the clearing, raspberry bushes taller than a man, a cloud on the slope, in the cloud a black forest.'

10 Lesley Blanch, *The Sabres of Paradise* (1978), 19.
11 Ovid, 'Tereus, Procne, and Philomela' (1987), 134–42.
12 de Montalk, *The Fountain of Tears* (2006), 64.
13 Ibid. 62.
14 Ibid. 65.
15 Ibid. 64.
16 Ibid. 109.
17 Alphonse Daudet, *In the Land of Pain*, trans. Julian Barnes (2002), 15.
18 Ibid. 24–25.
19 Ibid. 15.
20 'His Warmth as Always', de Montalk, *Cover Stories* (2005), 77–79.
21 See also Gate Control Theory (GCT), previous chapter. 'Wind-up' refers to the increased excitability of neurons within the central nervous system (specifically the dorsal horn of the spinal cord) as a result of changes occurring following repeated nerve stimulation by pain. The phenomenon, or 'neural memory' of pain, mimics and shares some of the features and mechanisms of central sensitisation.
22 By Pieter Breughel the Elder (1555). In Ovid's *Metamorphoses*, Daedalus fashioned wings from feathers and wax for himself and his son Icarus, so that they might escape exile on Crete. On account of the wings' flimsy construction, Daedalus, who would lead in flight, warned Icarus to fly neither too close to the spray of the sea, nor too close to the melting heat of the sun.
23 *Selected Poetry of W.H. Auden* (1971), 49.
24 Daudet, *In the Land of Pain*, 19.
25 Arthur Kleinman, *The Illness Narratives: Suffering, Healing & the Human Condition* (1988), 181.
26 Florence Nightingale, *Notes on Nursing: What It Is and What It Is Not* (1992), 55.
27 Harriet Martineau, *Life in the Sick-Room*, 49.
28 William Hazlitt; essay first published as 'Table Talk 1' in *The New Monthly Magazine* (1822); see *Selected Essays of William Hazlitt 1778–1830* (2004).
29 Daudet, *In the Land of Pain*, 14.
30 Michael Ondaatje, *The English Patient* (1993).
31 Arthur Schopenhauer, *On the Suffering of the World: Essays* (2004), 7.
32 Ibid. 54.
33 Friedrich Nietzsche, 'On the Despisers of the Body', *Thus Spoke Zarathustra: A Book for All and None* (2003), 24–25.
34 Cole Porter, 1926.
35 Cole Porter to his friend, musicologist, Dr Albert Sirmay, in 'About this Recording', Richard Ouzounian re. Porter's Aladdin, DuPont Show of the Month, CBS TV, February 1958.
36 Cole Porter, 1936.
37 Cole Porter, 1932.
38 Fiona MacCarthy, *Guardian*, 15 November 2003.
39 William Carlos Williams (1984), 88.
40 Denis Glover, 'The Magpies'. 'And Quardle oodle ardle wardle doodle/The magpies said.' *An Anthology of Twentieth-Century New Zealand Poetry* (1970), 131.
41 Andrew, in an explanation to me, said, 'Myeloma is a cancer of the plasma cells, which among other things prevents the formation of full and complete antibodies. Normal antibodies have a Y shape made up from heavy and light chains in combination. In my form of myeloma, the heavy chains get dropped and so there are lots of free light chains floating about in the blood unattached. That's why they're a major measure of the presence of the disease.'
42 'Pain', de Montalk, *Sport 33: Performance Pain* (Summer 2005).
43 Zbigniew Herbert, *The Collected Poems: 1956–1998* (2007), 416.

44 Sir Sidney Webb, economist and historian, said of the Fabian Society's tolerant approach to shifting British capitalism towards socialism: 'The inevitability of gradualness cannot fail to be appreciated.'

45 'See a nail and pick it up, and all the day you'll have good luck' – old Scottish saying.

46 'Leave this military hurry and adopt the pace of nature. Her secret is patience.' Ralph Waldo Emerson, 'Nature', essay, 1836.

47 Ralph Waldo Emerson, lecture, 'Tragedy', quoted in Emerson, *The Mind on Fire: A Biography, Robert D. Richardson Jnr* (1995), 309.

48 Anne Manchester, 'Encouraging Healing Through Touch', 1 August 2003.

49 Richard Jefferies, quoted in Walter Besant, *The Eulogy of Richard Jefferies* (1888) and cited by Lucy Bending in *The Representation of Bodily Pain in Late Nineteenth-Century English Culture* (2000), 107; Jefferies, the naturalist and visionist, suffered from undiagnosed tuberculosis with an anal fistula.

50 Ryszard Kapuściński, *Imperium* (2007), 53.

51 Sora Song, 'Health: Mind over Medicine', *TIME Magazine*, 19 March 2006.

52 Selected case studies were published in Dulce Arnall Bloxham's book *Who Was Ann Ockenden?* (1958). In 1976, the BBC aired *The Bloxham Tapes* – a documentary investigation by producer Jeffrey Iverson and journalist/broadcaster Magnus Magnusson into hitherto unknown and potentially verifiable historical details in Britain and abroad. Iverson reiterated his findings in *More Lives than One? The Evidence of the Remarkable Bloxham Tapes* (1977), in which he and Magnusson (who wrote the Foreword) concluded that the tapes defied human logic and supported Bloxham's concept of reincarnation.

53 Neuro-imaging has shown that the anterior corpus callosum (attention-related area) in the brains of readily hypnotisable subjects is 'about a third larger' than that of less successful subjects. Successful subjects have been found to have 'above-average abilities, in general, to control pain, because they are better able to filter out unwanted stimuli'. Melanie Thernstrom, 'Pain as Perception', *The Pain Chronicles*, 299.

54 Andrew Mason, *Henry Cooper of Auckland Grammar School* (2005).

55 Ovid, 'Daedalus and Icarus', *Metamorphoses* (1987), 176–78.

56 'Feathers and Wax', de Montalk, *Vivid Familiar* (2000), 32.

57 Ibid. 31.

58 Ibid. 32.

59 Pain in areas of the body – principally the legs and feet, hands and fingers – provoked by, and often at some distance from, the pain of the original injury. The cause is unknown, but thought to be due to irritated and damaged nerves in the sympathetic nervous system (which controls unconscious physical functions, such as heart beat and blood flow) sending incorrect messages – including symptoms of swelling, reddening and burning – to the brain.

60 Excerpts from letters written by Ivan Turgenev, quoted in Galina S. Rylkova, 'Oyster Fever: Chekhov and Turgenev', *The Bulletin of the North American Chekhov Society* XV, no. 1 (Autumn 2007).

61 Daudet, *In the Land of Pain*, 23.

62 Aleksander Wat, *Polish Writers on Writing*, 72.

63 Harriet Martineau, *Life in the Sick-Room*, 44.

64 *A Twist of Fate: Tackling Arthritis, New Zealanders Share their Stories*, ed. Mary Ciurlionis (2003), primarily 21 and 92.

65 David B. Morris, *The Culture of Pain* (1993), 20.

66 Arthur Rosenfeld, *The Truth About Chronic Pain: Patients and Professionals on How to Face It, Understand It, Overcome It* (2004). Rosenfeld's book collects the testimonies of chronic sufferers who might not otherwise be heard, describing the work as 'an expedition that strikes out, equipped with a high-powered lantern, in search of some of our most deeply buried and closely held secrets' (xix).

67 Lous Heshusius, *Inside Chronic Pain: An Intimate and Critical Account* (2009), 8.

68 Leo Tolstoy, *The Death of Ivan Ilych* (2004), chapter 12.

69 'Sebastopol in December' by Leo Tolstoy was first published in 1855. My reference is my personal copy, *Sebastopol* by Count Tolstoy, 16. As neither publication date nor translator are noted, I also refer to *The Sebastopol Sketches* (1986), 47–48. However, I prefer the understated strength of the first translation; for example: 'he merely mutters: "There's a gnawing at my heart,"' over '"My h-heart's on fire," he gasped.'

70 Tolstoy, *Sebastopol*, as above, 19.

71 Douglas Lilburn, *A Search for Tradition & A Search for a Language* (2011), 60.

72 Ibid. 70.

73 Quoted in Elizabeth Nash, 'Veteran Saramago Reaches End of Epic Journey', *The Independent*, 8 September 2008.

74 C.S. Lewis, *The Problem of Pain* (1966), 90.

75 Ibid. 157.

76 Isak Dinesen, quoted in Aage Henriksen, *Isak Dinesen/Karen Blixen: The Life and the Work* (1988), 126.

77 Letter from Isak Dinesen to Aage Henriksen, ibid. 129.

78 Ibid. 43.

79 Isak Dinesen, quoted in Judith Thurman, *Isak Dinesen: The Life of Karen Blixen* (1986), 298.

80 Isak Dinesen, *Out of Africa and Shadows on the Grass* (1985), 176.

81 Carlos Fuentes, 'Introduction', in *The Diary of Frida Kahlo: An Intimate Self-Portrait* (1995), 13.

82 Ibid. 8.

83 Ibid. Full-page colour plate, '*Yo soy la DISINTEGRACION …*' unnumbered; small, black and white version in 'Translation of the Diary', 225.

84 Daudet, *In the Land of Pain*, 15.

85 Michel de Montaigne, quoted in Sarah Bakewell, *How to Live: A Life of Montaigne in one question and twenty attempts at an answer* (2011), 38.

86 Aleksander Wat, quoted (unsourced) in Ryszard Zajackowski, 'Aleksander Wat's Leap from Poetry into Politics', *The Polish Review* L, no. 4 (2005), 339.

87 Ruth Harris, *Lourdes: Body and Spirit in the Secular Age* (1999), 22.

88 Ibid. 282.

89 Stephen Marche, *Atlantic Magazine*, May 2012.

90 The Blue Planet Run Foundation was formed to provide safe drinking water to 200 million people by 2027. See Rick Smolan and Jennifer Erwitt, *Blue Planet Run: The Race to Provide Safe Drinking Water to the World* (2007).

91 David B. Morris, *Illness and Culture in the Postmodern Age* (1998), 129.

92 Arthur Kleinman, M.D., *The Illness Narratives: Suffering, Healing & the Human Condition*, 225.

93 Julia Magnet, 'Sickened by the Nurses Who Don't Care', 23 November 2003.

94 David B. Morris, 'Foreword', in *Inside Chronic Pain: An Intimate and Critical Account*, Lous Heshusius (2009), xv.

95 *Life Sentence: Selected Poems* (1990), 33.

96 'some sort of exhaustion': Boris Pasternak, *Dr Zhivago* (1958), 353.

97 Ibid. 354.

98 From 'Feathers and Wax', *Vivid Familiar* (2009), 36.

99 Ibid. 41.

100 Ibid. 46.

101 *Russia: a Journey with Jonathon Dimbleby*, BBC series, 2008. Dialogue not verbatim.

102 'Fourteen Thousand Miles', *Vivid Familiar*, 9.

103 'The Swan': Stephané Mallarmé in Louis Simpson (ed.), *Modern Poets of France: A Bilingual Anthology* (1997), 103. Excerpt:

> Virginal, vivid, beautiful, will this be.
> The day that shatters with a drunken wing.
> The lake beneath the frost, still mirroring.
> Flights that were never made, transparency?

104 'White Bee': Pablo Neruda, *Pablo Neruda: The Early Poems* (1969), 60. Excerpt:

> You are a white bee, drunk with honey,
> twirling through my soul in slow spirals of smoke.
> I'm desperate. I'm the word with no echoes,
> the man who lost it all, and the man who had it all.

105 This interlude references 'The Queen's Croquet-Ground' in Lewis Carroll's *Alice's Adventures in Wonderland and Through the Looking Glass*, Chapter 8.

5 The vendor of happiness

1 Alphonse Daudet's responses and the descriptions of his surroundings are both imagined and factually based. Much of his dialogue is drawn from the random notes, kept 1887–1895, that constitute his memoir, *La Doulou* (published 1930), as they have been translated into English by Milton Garver as *Suffering* (Yale University Press, 1934), and by Julian Barnes as *In the Land of Pain* (Alfred A. Knopf, New York, 2002); and from his son Léon Daudet's *Alphonse Daudet: A Memoir* (*Memoirs of Alphonse Daudet*, including 'The Daudet Family, Mon Frere et Moi' by Ernest Daudet, 1897; transl. Charles de Kay, Wildside Press, Maryland, USA, 2007). Daudet's sourced responses have been adjusted for voice and narrative purposes as my own free translations and presented selectively, at times as composite passages, without referencing and in accordance with his replies as I have imagined them.

Other significant sources include: Léon Daudet's *Devant La Douleur* (Paris 1915), and *Quand Vivait Mon Père* (Paris 1940), and Charles Mantoux's *Alphonse Daudet et la Souffrance Humaine* (Paris 1941), each of which is cited in *Neurological Disorders in Famous Artists: Frontiers of Neurology and Neuroscience* (Volume 19, ed. J. Bogousslavsky and F. Boller, 'The One-Man Band of Pain: Alphonse Daudet and His Painful Experience of Tabes Dorsalis', Sebastian Dieguez and Julien Bogousslavsky, Dept. of Neurology, University Hospital, Lausanne, 2005). I note that the editors' reference to Julian Barnes' translation as the only English translation of *La Doulou* is incorrect.

Further sources: 'Four Illustrious Neuroleutics', MacDonald Critchley, *History of Medicine* Vol. 62, July 1969; *Alphonse Daudet: A Biographical and Critical Study*, R.H. Sherard (Edward Arnold, London, 1894, Google Archive); *The Nabob*, Alphonse Daudet (Critical Introduction by Professor W.P. Trent, Biographical Note Edmund Gosse, Translation W.P. Blades, P.F. Collier & Son, 1902, digitised 28 January 2008); *French Profiles*, Edmund Gosse (first published 1898, this edition, W. Heinmann, London, 1913, digitised 26 March 2008).

2 Zbigniew Herbert, 'The Hygiene of the Soul', *The Collected Poems: 1996–1998* (2007), 215.

3 Leigh Gilmore, *The Limits of Autobiography: Trauma and Testimony* (2001), 24.

4 *Le Journal*, 27 December 1897, quoted in Appendix to Daudet, *Suffering* (1930/1934), 65.

5 'In the French Capital the Publication of Daudet's New Novel, *La Fedor*, is the Literary Event of the Day', Roland Strong, *New York Times*, 30 May 1897.

6 *Les Femmes d'artistes*, quoted in 'An Appreciation of Alphonse Daudet by André Ebner' in *Suffering*, 84.

7   *Les Romanciers Naturalistes*, quoted in J. Bogousslavsky and F. Boller (eds.), *Neurological Disorders in Famous Artists: Frontiers of Neurology and Neuroscience* 19 (2005), 19.

8   *In the Land of Pain* (2002), 4.

9   *Alphonse Daudet: A Memoir* (2007), 192.

10   Ernest Daudet, 'The Daudet Family: My Brother and I', *Alphonse Daudet: A Memoir*, 351.

11   Bernard Swift, *The New Oxford Companion to Literature in French* (ed. Peter France, 1995), 221.

12   In *Alphonse Daudet: A Memoir* (2007), Léon writes, 'My father was often wont to repeat: "When my task is finished I should like to establish myself as a Vendor of Happiness; my profits would consist in my success"' (89).

13   *Suffering*, 2.

14   *In the Land of Pain*, 68.

15   Ibid. 26.

16   *Suffering*, 19.

17   *In the Land of Pain*, 3.

18   *Suffering*, 3.

19   Richard Eder, 'Another Country', *New York Times*, 2 February 2003.

20   *Alphonse Daudet: A Memoir*, 96.

21   *Quand Vivai Mon Père*, 113, quoted in *Neurological Disorders in Famous Artists*, 24.

22   *In the Land of Pain*, 19.

23   Used as a treatment for alcoholism and range of neurological and glandular disorders, gold chloride was known to induce 'aphrodisiac effects' (Samuel Otway Lewis Potter, *Materia Medica*, 1894), to 'act as a powerful sexual stimulant' (H.A. Hare, *Text Book of Practical Therapeutics*, 1912); similarly, neurologist Charles-Édouard Brown-Séquard's hypodermic injections of testicular venous blood and other 'juices' of guinea pigs (and monkeys and dogs). Could these remedies, the responses to which are now thought to have been placebo effects, have contributed to the continuance of Daudet's famous libido despite his pain and debilitation?

24   Montaigne writes, 'The very sight of another's pain materially pains me, and I often usurp the sensations of another person.' 'Of the Force of Imagination', *The Complete Essays of Michel de Montaigne* (2009), 61.

25   Act 1, Scene 2. Benvolio to Romeo:

> Tut, man, one fire burns out another's burning,
> One pain is lessen'd by another's anguish;
> Turn giddy, and be holp by backward turning;

26   *In the Land of Pain*, 5.

27   *In the Land of Pain*, 24.

28   *Suffering*, 32.

29   Literary critic, Charles Augustin Sainte-Beuve (1802–1869), ref. *Encyclopaedia Britannica*, 9th ed.

30   Marcel Proust, from his (untitled) article in *La Presse*, 11 August 1897, as reproduced in *Suffering*, 70.

31   *Alphonse Daudet: A Memoir*, 35.

32   *Suffering*, 35.

33   *French Profiles*, 122.

34   *Alphonse Daudet: A Memoir*, 93–94.

35   Ibid. 96.

36   Ibid. 96.

37   *Suffering*, 84.

38   Ibid. 87.

39   'Daudet and his wife Julia at Champrosay, *c.* 1892', *In the Land of Pain*.

40 *Alphonse Daudet: A Memoir*, 100.
41 *Much Ado About Nothing*: Act 5, Scene 1. Leonato:

> For there was never yet philosopher.
> That could endure the toothache patiently,
> However they have writ the style of gods,
> And made a push at chance and sufferance.

42 *Suffering*, 37.
43 *Quand Vivait Mon Père*, 238, quoted in *Neurological Disorders in Famous Artists*, 38. Blaise Pascal (1623–1662), mathematician, scientist, religious philosopher, suffered severe chronic pain, possibly due to stomach cancer.
44 *Suffering*, 5, 11, 34.
45 *In the Land of Pain*, 42.
46 Ibid.
47 The Global Language Monitor (1 January 2014), in conjunction with a Google/Harvard Study, reports 1,025,109 words in the English language.
48 *Alphonse Daudet et la Souffrance Humaine* (1941), 24, and *Neurological Disorders in Famous Artists*, 39.
49 [Blaise] Pascal's *Pensées* (1958), 'Thoughts on Mind and on Style', Section 22, 7.
50 Spider Robinson, *Callahan's Crosstime Saloon* (1977).
51 *Alphonse Daudet: A Memoir*, 126.
52 In Greek mythology, the kingfisher Halcyon was given seven calm days either side of the winter solstice in which to lay her eggs in a nest on the sea.

6 The consolator

1 Unitarianism, founded on principles of rationality, individuality and democracy, was established in the late eighteenth century. The movement held that Jesus Christ, as a leader (rather than the Father, Son and Holy Ghost), should not be worshipped, and that evil in the world was the responsibility of human beings, rather than a supernatural force.
2 Harriet Martineau's obituary, written in the third person in 1855 when she again became invalided, this time permanently, and expected to die of heart disease despite medical advice to the contrary. The obituary, entitled 'An Autobiographic Memoir', is included in 'Memorials', *Autobiography*, vol. 2. *Autobiography* was written in 1855 and published in 1877 unchanged – apart from the addition, by Martineau's friend, trustee and editor Maria Weston Chapman, of the 'Memorials' and 'Notes'. Martineau's obituary was held by the *Daily News*, in which it was published in 1876. Part of the obituary appears in *Life in the Sick-Room*, Appendix D, 212–13. My references are: Harriet Martineau's *Autobiography* Volumes 1 and 2, and *Memorials of Harriet Martineau*, ed. Maria Weston Chapman (1877); page numbers are not available.
3 *Life in the Sick-Room* (first published 1844; this edition 2003), 153. *Life in the Sick-Room* was published during the 'climate of invalidism' prevalent in Britain in the nineteenth century. Acceptance of invalidism arose, as Maria H. Frawley explains in *Invalidism and Identity in Nineteenth-Century Britain* (2004), within a social and medical culture that perceived suffering as 'God-given', and as an outcome of industrialisation which gave rise to medical diagnoses associated with 'overwork'.

In terms of illness narratives, that century had seen a culmination of the increase in personal writing since the seventeenth century, in which the invalid narrator assumed a familiar identity as an immobile, socially displaced observer, who found purpose in reflecting on the daily routines of the sick-room, offering practical advice and aiming to make their surroundings places of 'cheerfulness and joy'. Even children's literature espoused the elevated identity of the Victorian invalid. (I refer to my childhood copy of Susan Coolidge's *What Katy Did*, first published in 1872. Katy Carr, bed-bound and in pain between the ages of 12 and 16 after falling from a swing, is coached in the art of invalidism by an invalid cousin, Helen. Katy is given lessons in patience and encouraged to keep herself 'as fresh and dainty as a rose' (80), and her room a sanctuary for all who visit it.) Not that the blessings of pain were necessarily readily shared, writes Frawley, citing Harriet Martineau's reference to the invalid state as one of disconnection, or exile, between 'life and death' (163).

4 Nightingale made this remark to her father in 1844, during a period of illness some twelve years before returning from the Crimean War; however, she agreed with Martineau's conclusion that 'pain is no evil' (quoted by Mark Bostridge in *Florence Nightingale, The Woman and Her Legend*, 2008, 76). In the latter regard, Martineau writes in *Sick-Room* that pain is the 'chastisement of a Father; or, at least, that it is in some way or other, ordained for, or instrumental to good' (46). Martineau, 'a prisoner to the couch', and Nightingale, 'a prisoner of the bed' (as each described herself), corresponded regularly, 1858–1868. (Re Nightingale's invalidism, see also Note 1 for Chapter 2 'Going Nursing'.)

5 *The Quarterly Review* 107 (April 1860), 336. Here, Martineau favourably reviews Nightingale's *Notes on Nursing* (1860) and takes the opportunity to heighten the profile of *Sick-Room*, now in its third edition (1849), and which has themes in common with *Notes*, without identifying herself as *Sick-Room*'s author.

6 R.K. Webb, *Harriet Martineau: A Radical Victorian* (1960), 3.

7 Ibid. 3.

8 Harriet Martineau, *Autobiography*, vol. 1, period 3, section 3.

9 *Life in the Sick-Room*, ed. Maria Frawley (2003), 111.

10 Ibid. 138.

11 Ibid. 84.

12 Quoted in Webb, *Harriet Martineau*, 196. Re the 'Socinian formula': Socinianism developed in the sixteenth and seventeenth-centuries as the forerunner of Unitarianism. Included in the movement's beliefs: rejection of the Holy Trinity and the concept of original sin, promotion of religious tolerance, and the elevation of reason in interpretation of the scriptures.

13 *Autobiography*, vol. 1, period 5, section 1.

14 Martineau's positive response to her deafness and profile as a writer resulted in a hearing trumpet that carried her name. The 'Martineau Horn or Dipper Trumpet' was described in the *Armamentarium Chirugicum* (1889) as 'a powerful instrument suitable [for] public lectures or sermons'.

15 Webb, *Harriet Martineau*, 40.

16 *Autobiography*, vol. 1, period 5, section 1, quoted in *Sick-Room*, Appendix D, 209.

17 *Dublin University Magazine* (23 May 1844), 573–82; reproduced in *Sick-Room*, Appendix B, 170–80. The reviewer closes by suggesting the anonymous author, the 'invalid', is Harriet Martineau.

18 *The Review* (no. 18, 1844), 472–81, reproduced in *Sick-Room*, Appendix B, 180–86.

19 *The Collected Letters of Thomas and Jane Welsh Carlyle* 18 (1990), 170.

20 *Sick-Room*, 42.

21 Ibid. 114.

22 Ibid. 129.

23 Ibid. 157.

24 Ibid. 78.

25 Ibid. 88.

26 Jessica Riskin, *Science in the Age of Sensibility: The Sentimental Empiricists of the French Enlightenment* (2002), 206.

27 Webb, *Harriet Martineau*, 255.

28 *Sick-Room*, Appendix C, 196. Sir Thomas Watson's observation appeared in his letter published in the *British Medical Journal*, 8 July 1876.

29 *The Quarterly Review* 107 (April 1860), 335.
30 *Autobiography*, vol. 2, Memorials, 'Self-Estimate and Other'.
31 *Autobiography*, vol. 1, period 5, section 1; also *Sick-Room*, 211.
32 Ibid. 211.
33 Maria Frawley, *Invalidism and Identity*, 234.
34 Gillian Thomas, 'Harriet Martineau', *Dictionary of Literary Biography* 55 (1987), 175.
35 *Sick-Room*, 60.
36 Webb, *Harriet Martineau*, 252.
37 *Autobiography*, vol. 2, Memorials, 'Eastern Journal'; also *Deerbrook: A Novel* (1839), 64.
38 'Letter to the Deaf', Tait's *Edinburgh Magazine* (April 1834), 174–79; quoted in *Sick-Room*, Appendix F, 234.
39 *Autobiography*, vol. 1, period 4, section 1.
40 *Autobiography*, vol. 1, period 2, section 1.
41 Ibid.
42 *Sick-Room*, 154.
43 Webb, *Harriet Martineau*, 358.
44 *Sick-Room*, 122.
45 Thomas M. Greenhow, M.D. (Martineau's physician and brother-in-law) examines Martineau's health history in his article 'Termination of the Case of Miss Harriet Martineau', *British Medical Journal* (14 April 1877), 449–50; his article also appears in *Sick-Room*, Appendix C, 195–99.
46 The ingredients of this sausage were obtained during my phone call to the proprietress of Martineau House, Tynemouth, May 2011.
47 'Māori plugged up their wounds with its leaves during the Land Wars': The Land Wars were nineteenth-century New Zealand battles involving land disputes between some Māori tribes and British government troops and their Māori allies. The major engagements took place in the 1840s and the 1860s.

7 Observatory

1 This poem is both factually based and imagined.
2 Harriet Martineau, *Autobiography* (1877), vol. 1, period 6, section 1.
3 Letter from Martineau to Mrs Romilly, 9 March 1844, cited by Maria H. Frawley in *Invalidism and Identity in Nineteenth-Century Britain* (2004), 200.
4 Harriet Martineau, *Deerbrook* (1839), 64–65.
5 Maria Weston Chapman, American anti-slavery campaigner, friend of Harriet Martineau and editor of Martineau's two-volume *Autobiography*.
6 The painting (6 × 8 feet), the work of Ary Scheffer, France, was completed in 1836 and widely circulated in Europe and America in both engraved and lithographic reproduction. A reduced painting of the same name, by Scheffer, appeared in 1851. The image was inspired by Luke 4:18: 'The spirit of the Lord is upon me, because he hath anointed me to preach the gospel to the poor; he hath sent me to heal the broken-hearted, to preach deliverance to the captives, and recovering of sight to the blind, to set at liberty them that are bruised.' (Authorised King James Version.)
7 A reference to the failed Polish insurrection against Russia, 1830–1831.
8 Lines 138 and 139, from *Paradise Lost*, John Milton, Book IV (with Elijah Fenton and Samuel Johnson, printed for John Bumpus, Holborn-Bars, London, 1821, digitised by Google 7 September 2007), 103.
9 I have presumed that a Henry Martineau (1794–1844) identified on 'An Alphabetical List of the Founders of the British Colony of New Zealand commencing January 1840, ending December 1845', http://shadowsoftime.co.nz/settlers.html, and listed as

a cabin passenger on the *Arab* settler ship which sailed from England 5 June 1841, who arrived at Port Nicholson 16 October 1841, http://freepages.genealogy.rootsweb. ancestry.com/, was Harriet Martineau's brother. It would appear that this is the same Henry Martineau who, as a merchant and storekeeper on Lambton Quay, Port Nicholson, gave evidence, August 1842, at the trial of a tent-dweller charged with stealing items of clothing from two establishments, one of which was Martineau's store. The jury found the 'prisoner' guilty, and the judge awarded the 'severest penalty the law allowed' for crimes of this sort: transportation for seven years.

10 In *Sick-Room*, 58.

11 Although the Carlyles visited Martineau at Tynemouth in September 1841, their visit in 1843, as recorded in the poem, is fictitious. A number of details, however, are factually based, including Thomas's painful stomach ailment, which was lifelong, caused him to be crotchety, and although likely to have been due to hyperactivity or gastric ulcers, was attributed to a crisis of faith; Jane's intermittently low spirits and adoration of her father; the accidental burning, by John Stuart Mill's maid of Thomas's manuscript of Volume One of his three-volume *The French Revolution: A History* (1837), the work that first brought him to prominence; Thomas's comment regarding Martineau as a 'female Christ'; Thomas's comment about their house at Kirkcaldy, Scotland. Regarding Harriet's 'flutter' upon her guest's arrival, I note that despite Carlyle's sometime criticisms of Martineau he confessed to Ralph Waldo Emerson, in 1839, that he missed her 'blithe, friendly presence' when she became invalided at Tynemouth (Webb, 3), and I also note that Jane Carlyle's comment that Harriet presented her husband 'her ear trumpet with a pretty blushing air of coquetry which would almost convince one out of belief in her identity' (Jane Carlyle to John Stirling, 1 February 1837, *The Collected Letters of Thomas and Jane Welsh Carlyle*, Volume 9, 132–36, The Carlyle Letters Online: A Victorian Cultural Reference, carlyleletters. dukejournals.org/).

12 Thomas Carlyle's comment – as related by Lucretia Mott (American proponent of social reform, abolition and women's rights) to Maria Weston Chapman – is quoted by R.K. Webb in *Harriet Martineau: A Radical Victorian*, 199.

13 Thomas Carlyle to Margaret A. Carlyle, 7 September 1843, The Collected Letters of Thomas and Jane Welsh Carlyle, Volume 17, 117–19. carlyleletters.dukejournals.org/.

14 Old Scottish saying (Sir Walter Scott, *Rob Roy*).

15 François de Salignac de la Mothe-Fénelon (1651–1715). The doctrine of Quietism holds, in a broad sense, that human perfection is achieved, even in everyday life, by remaining passive in will and thought, enabling absorption of the soul into the 'Divine Essence'.

16 In *Sick-Room*, 116.

8 An imago

1 Aleksander Wat's italicised dialogue is imagined, apart from occasional thoughts sourced from his writing. His words as they appear in Tomas Venclova's *Aleksander Wat: Life and Art of an Iconoclast* (1996) have been translated by Venclova, unless otherwise stated.

2 'Has Anyone Seen Pigeon Street?', *Lucifer Unemployed* (1990), 43.

3 Ed. Adam Zagajewski (2007).

4 Julia Hartwig, 'Long Vigil', *In Praise of the Unfinished* (2008), 105.

5 *Polish Writers on Writing*, 70–77.

6 Ibid. 70.

7 Ibid. 70.

8 Georg Philipp Friedrich Freiherr von Hadenberg (1772–1801), pseudonym Novalis, was a German Romantic poet, novelist and philosopher noted for his use of

'magical substitution', or magic realism, and of dreams as symbols. His witness of the suffering and death, from tuberculosis, of his beloved fifteen-year-old fiancée, Sophie von Kühn, two years after they became engaged, closely followed by the death of his much loved younger brother, Erasmus, had a profound effect on his thinking in this respect. In *Storied Revelation: Parables, Imagination, and George MacDonald's Christian Fiction* (2013), Gisela H. Kreglinger explains Novalis's use of dreams as 'a poetic device to open up one's vision to the divine'. Kreglinger continues: 'The highest form of dreams happens in a synthesis of dreaming and waking. In this synthesis the experience of the individual is brought into the spiritual world created by the imagination' (67). This view is, perhaps, consistent with Wat's statement that his own life 'had been a constant search for an enormous dream [...]' as expressed on page 283. Novalis's thinking in this regard influenced poet and theologian George MacDonald, who in turn influenced C.S. Lewis. Novalis died of tuberculosis.

9 Ibid. 72.
10 Ibid. 74.
11 Ibid. 74.
12 Ibid. 74–75.
13 Ibid. 76.
14 'Dialogue on Wat Between Czesław Miłosz and Leonard Nathan', *With the Skin* (1989), x.
15 Wat, *My Century: The Odyssey of a Polish Intellectual* (2003), 12.
16 Wat, *Kartki na wietrze* (*Scraps of Paper in the Wind*), in *Pisma wybrane* (1986), 173, quoted in Tomas Venclova, *Aleksander Wat: Life and Art of an Iconoclast* (1996), 213.
17 'Has Anyone Seen Pigeon Street?', *Lucifer Unemployed*, 50.
18 Aleksandr Solzhenitsyn, *Cancer Ward* (1973), 86.
19 Aleksandr Solzhenitsyn, *One Day in the Life of Ivan Denisovich* (1963), 31.
20 Venclova, *Iconoclast*, 174.
21 Wat, *Mediterranean Poems* (1977), 45–46.
22 Anna Świrszczyńska, *Building the Barricade and other Poems of Anna Swir* (2011), 33. The scale of the razing of Warsaw has been compared to that of the destruction of Hiroshima.
23 *Polish Writers on Writing*, 75.
24 'Lucifer Unemployed', *Lucifer Unemployed*, 98.
25 *My Century*, 115.
26 Anatol Stern, *Bruno Jasieński* (1969), 15, quoted in Marci Shore, *Caviar and Ashes: Ashes: A Warsaw Generation's Life and Death in Marxism, 1918–1968* (2006), 23.
27 Władysław Daszewski (set designer and caricaturist), quoted in Shore, *Caviar and Ashes*, 153–54.
28 Ibid. 4.
29 *My Century*, 12.
30 Venclova, *Iconoclast*, 45.
31 Ibid. 46.
32 Ibid. 62.
33 Ibid. 50.
34 Mayakovsky, quoted by Czesław Miłosz in Wat, *With the Skin*, 102. Futurism in Poland meant rejecting Poland's cultural heritage and values. This included moving away from artistic tradition in favour of innovation and spontaneity, the liberation of vocabulary and grammar, the simplification of Polish spelling, and the idea that as life continues without repeating itself, so too should art.
35 Irena Krzywicka, *Wyznania gorszycielki* (1992), 274, quoted in Shore, *Caviar and Ashes*, 15.
36 *Scraps of Paper in the Wind*, quoted by Venclova, *Iconoclast*, 78.

37 Marci Shore, 'Love in the Time of Revolution: The Polish Poets of Café Ziemianska', in *New Dangerous Liaisons: Discourses on Europe and Love in the Twentieth Century*, ed. Luisa Passerini and Liliana Ellena, Alexander C.T. Geppert (2010), 131.

38 *My Century*, 15.

39 Ibid. 89.

40 de Montalk, *Unquiet World: The Life of Count Geoffrey Potocki de Montalk* (2001), 231.

41 Leigh Gilmore, *The Limits of Autobiography: Trauma and Testimony* (2001), 31.

42 *My Century*, 96–97.

43 Ibid. 21.

44 'Polskiesovetskie pisateli', *Literaturnaia Gazeta* (1939), 4, quoted in Shore, *Caviar and Ashes*, 162.

45 *My Century*, 112.

46 *Czerwony Sztandar* (27 January 1940), 104, quoted in Shore, *Caviar and Ashes*, 170.

47 Venclova, *Iconoclast*, 179.

48 Ibid. 179.

49 *My Century*, 329.

50 Ola Watowa, *Wszystko co najwazniejsze* (*All That Is Most Important*, 1990), 83, quoted in Venclova, *Iconoclast*, 144.

51 Watowa, *All That Is*, 88–89, quoted in Venclova, *Iconoclast*, 147.

52 *My Century*, 370.

53 Ibid. 374.

54 Neil Ascherson, *The Polish August: The Self-Limiting Revolution* (1981), 41.

55 Watowa, *All That Is*, 129, quoted in Shore, *Caviar and Ashes*, 274.

56 *My Century*, 4.

57 'Has Anyone Seen Pigeon Street?', *Lucifer Unemployed*, 41.

58 Czesław Miłosz to Leonard Nathan, *With the Skin*, 106.

59 *Dziennik bez samoglosek* (*Diary Without Vowels*, 1986), 92, quoted in Venclova, *Iconoclast*, 210. Venclova notes that Wat's words were 'echoed by Miłosz' in his own poem 'Ars Poetrica?' in which Miłosz writes: 'a thing is brought forth which we didn't know we had in us' (*Bells in Winter*, 30).

60 Elaine Scarry, *The Body in Pain*, 171.

61 *With the Skin*, 106.

62 *My Century*, 209.

63 Ibid. 209; also 234, relating St Augustine's definition 'to love or to God or to poetry', and its changing of the 'mind's orientation'.

64 Ibid. 209.

65 *Polish Writers on Writing*, 72.

66 Venclova, *Iconoclast*, 177.

67 *Mediterranean Poems*, 3.

68 Tomas Venclova, *Forms of Hope: Essays* (1999), 133.

69 Trans. Ryszard Reisner, *Ars Interpres: An International Journal of Poetry, Translation and Art* no. 9 (September 2007). Venclova's translation 'In the Four Walls of My Pain' is found in *Iconoclast*, 213.

70 Trans. Ryszard Reisner, as above.

71 Alissa Valles, *Brick: A Literary Journal*, no. 87 (Summer 2011), 92–95.

72 Venclova, *Iconoclast*, 212.

73 Ibid. 212. Venclova refers to Roman Jakobson's *Selected Writings*, vol. 5 (1979).

74 First published as *Twórczość* (1956), 11, quoted in Venclova, *Iconoclast*, 216, trans. Stanisław Baranczak.

75 Venclova, *Iconoclast*, 217–18.

76 'Has Anyone Seen Pigeon Street?', *Lucifer Unemployed*, 42.

77 Wat, *Scraps of Paper in the Wind*, 181, quoted in Venclova, *Iconoclast*, 180.

78 *Mediterranean Poems*, 42–53.

79 *With the Skin*, 105.

80 *My Century*, xix.

81 *Mediterranean Poems* (this poem jointly translated by Czesław Miłosz, David Brodsky and Stephen Grad), 26–41.

82 Aleksander Wat papers, Uncat MS Vault 526, Beinecke Rare Book and Manuscript Library, Yale University, New Haven, quoted in Shore, *Caviar and Ashes*, 341.

83 Ibid. quoted in Shore, *Caviar and Ashes*, 342.

84 *Diary Without Vowels*, 111, quoted in Venclova, *Iconoclast*, 249.

85 *My Century*, xxiii.

86 *Polish Writers on Writing*, 75.

87 Ibid. 71–72.

88 Ola quoted in Alissa Valles, 'A Wound Like a Mouth', *Brick: A Literary Journal*, no. 87 (Summer 2011), 94.

89 *My Century*, 12.

90 Ibid. xxiii.

91 Ibid. xxix.

92 Ibid. 11.

93 Ibid. 12.

94 Ibid. 13.

95 Ibid. 16.

96 'Lucifer Unemployed', *Lucifer Unemployed*, 106.

97 Venclova, *Iconoclast*, 250.

98 *Kultura* (1966), 3, quoted in Venclova, *Iconoclast*, 251.

99 *Polish Writers on Writing*, 72.

100 First stanza, trans. Richard Lourie, *My Century*, 5.

101 Watowa, *All That Is*, quoted in Shore, *Caviar and Ashes*, 216.

102 *Diary Without Vowels*, 152, quoted in Venclova, *Iconoclast*, 251.

103 *Scraps of Paper in the Wind*, 220, quoted in Venclova, *Iconoclast*, 251.

104 Wat archive, file 67, quoted in Venclova, *Iconoclast*, 253.

105 Shore, *Caviar and Ashes*, 352; *My Century*, 164–65.

106 Richard Lourie, introduction to *My Century*, xxx.

107 *My Century*, 355.

108 Ola Wat to her sister-in-law Seweryna Broniszówna, in Toulon 20 August 1967, in *All That Is*, quoted in Shore, *Caviar and Ashes*, 350.

109 *Zezsyt ostatni* (*Final Notebook*), 1967, 14, Aleksander Wat Papers, Beinecke Rare Book and Manuscript Library, Yale University, letter trans. Gail Glickman, quoted in Shore, *Caviar and Ashes*, 350–54.

110 Wat, *Poezje zebrine*, compiled by Anna Micinska and Jan Zielinski (1992), trans. Venclova, *Iconoclast*, 253.

9 How does it hurt?

1 This title adapts Michael Foucault's phrase 'Where does it hurt?' as it appears in *The Birth of the Clinic: An Archaeology of Medical Perception* (2003), xviii. In *Clinic*, Foucault examines the expansion in medical knowledge from the eighteenth century, and the exactitude and mappability of the body that followed. Rather than ask a patient 'What is wrong with you?' Foucalt suggests, ask 'Where does it hurt?' thereby bringing into focus the patient's biology. At *Clinic*'s centre is the concept of the 'medical gaze', as it distances the body from the patient as a person: as, in essence, it renders the patient as a separate and distanced category of person.

2 Arthur Frank, *The Wounded Storyteller* (1997), 35. The passage by Albert Schweitzer appears in his autobiography *Out of My Life and Thought* (1933), translated by Antje Bultmann Lemke.

3   William Zinsser (ed.), *Inventing the Truth: The Art and Craft of Memoir* (1998), 6.

4   Rafael Campo, 'On Doctoring', *The Enemy* (2007), 98.

5   *Les Foules de Lourdes*, Joris-Karl Huysmans, 105, quoted in Ruth Harris, *Lourdes: Body and Spirit in the Secular Age*, 339. In 1858, the 14-year-old peasant girl Bernadette Soubirous saw the first of eighteen apparitions of a girl in white in a Grotto beside the Gave du Pau river outside the town of Lourdes; at a subsequent appearance, a day after the Annunciation, the apparition introduced herself saying, 'I am the Immaculate Conception.' Pilgrims flocked to the shrine for healing and forgiveness. In 1866 a railway line, carrying the sick and suffering in special 'white trains', opened; in 1908 over one and a half million pilgrims commemorated the fiftieth anniversary of the apparitions – a number that rose to five million or more annually from the early 1990s, and is sustained today.

6   Tetrahydrocannabinol is an active cannabinoid responsible for most of the cannabis plant's psychoactive effects. Although cannabis is widely grown in New Zealand, it is not legally available. An imported, pharmaceutically regulated and costly product is supplied, with Ministry of Health permission, to a limited number of chronic pain and other condition-specific patients.

7   Cannabidiol, or CBD, found in cannabis and hemp, is a non-psychoactive cannabinoid containing low or trace amounts of THC. An imported, pharmaceutically regulated extraction of CBD oil (dropped onto the tongue) recently became a controlled drug in New Zealand and legally available, at considerable cost, as a prescription medicine.

8   'scrutiny of their mental state': In this regard, I note the landmark decision of Judge M.J. Beattie in *Bryan v Accident Compensation Commission Corporation*, January 2013, which rejected the ACC's long-held view that a claim for compensation of chronic pain caused by an injury sustained in an accident should succeed only by way of a claim for a mental injury. ACC thus required that Andrew Bryan show that his 'extreme chronic pain syndrome', which was 'separate from but associated with' the back injury for which he had already been compensated, had caused a deterioration in his mental state, to be confirmed by psychiatric assessment. Bryan, however, like many ACC claimants before him, was 'wholly opposed to being required to be identified as having a mental injury'. John (Miller), who was counsel for Andrew Bryan, took this case as a result of both the insights he gained into chronic pain through my experience and the research I undertook for my dissertation. John argued that Bryan's ACC 'impairment assessment had taken no account' of his continuing pain; and that as this was a pain that went beyond the 'usual or normal pain associated with a physical injury', it was a serious condition worthy of compensation in its own right, without the need for a mental injury assessment.

9   'Palliative Care': I think of palliative care and remember Walt Whitman, and his role as a voluntary carer in Washington hospitals during the American Civil War. Late each afternoon, and for the duration of the war, Whitman, having finished his remunerative odd jobs for the day, began his compassionate work in the wards: sitting with the dying, and nursing and comforting the injured – to whom he would bring sustenance, often paid for from his own pocket, and, as befitted his poetic self, the solace of words for men unable to read or pen letters home. For Whitman, 'To sit by the wounded and soothe them', as he wrote in his poem, 'The Wound Dresser', was to emanate relief through empathetic fellow feeling and support.

Thankfully, that same sense of compassion is the bedrock of the care that sustains patients through protracted and terminal illnesses, today.

However, for many sufferers, despite more than a century of medical advancement and decades of professionally managed palliative kindness, there is still no adequate response to intractable and unbearable distress. Indeed, in the life-extending twenty-first century, the incidence of long-term suffering that cannot be rendered tolerable or cast in an ultimately hopeful light, only increases.

Over the last fifteen years, pain – burrowing within, deepening my understanding of the resilience and limitations of the body and mind – has reframed the way in which I think about dying. Formerly, I viewed death – especially the medically sufficient endings thought to embody its mythical kindness and easement – with a secular sense of justification of the uninterrupted status quo. Now, fully aware of the constraints of palliative care, I believe the humane option of a legally steadfast, physician-assisted death should be the right of anyone who is terminally ill and suffering unbearably, and wants only to die 'as we all want to live: free from pain, connected to people we love, with agency and dignity' ('End-of-Life Choice Society of New Zealand Inc', Issue 50, May 2018).

10 White train

1 An adaptation of Alphonse Daudet, 'Pain, you must be everything for me. Let me find in you all those foreign lands you will not let me visit. Be my philosophy, be my science', *In the Land of Pain*, 42.
2 The tone of the poem's opening recalls Vijay Sheshadri's poem 'Visiting Paris' (*The New Yorker*, 1 February 2010). I composed the poem after reading Émile Zola's novel *Lourdes* (1894). Zola's novel was written as a result of a fifteen-day visit to Lourdes in the early autumn of 1891, and a three-day visit the following summer, during which he joined the National Pilgrimage. Zola says, in the Preface to *Lourdes*, that he 'came across some instances of real cure'. He continues: 'Many cases of nervous disorders have undoubtedly been cured, and there have also been other cures which may, perhaps be attributed to errors of diagnosis.' He notes: many of the pilgrims came from 'the country', where doctors were not necessarily 'men of either great skill or great expertise'; 'all doctors make mistakes'; there will inevitably 'be cures out of so large a number of cases'; 'Nature often cures without medical aid'. He also speaks of the 'necessity for credulity, which is a characteristic of human nature.' Lourdes eventuated, he believes, 'just as the Christian religion did, because suffering humanity in its despair must cling to something, must have some hope; and, on the other hand, because humanity thirsts after illusions'. Based on interviews he conducted regarding apparently miraculous cures at the time of his visit, he finds that 'The Lourdes miracles can neither be proved nor denied.'

   Historian Ruth Harris writes of her own visit to Lourdes, ninety years later, in the 1980s, when she assisted a mother travelling with her blind, paralysed, incontinent adult son, that on previous visits she had been 'appalled by the pious commerce'. Now, writes Harris in *Lourdes: Body and Spirit in the Secular Age*, '[w]orking with the hospital pilgrims […] these judgements melted away; it was hard even to remember that such trading existed when their more pressing needs took over' (xv).
3 Unsanitary conditions prevailed in the Sanctuary, in the pools in particular. Of the *piscines*, Zola recalls in *Lourdes*, as quoted by Harris in *Lourdes: Body and Spirit in the Secular Age*, 'threads of blood, sloughed-off skin, scabs, bits of cloth and bandage, an abominable soup of ills' (338).
4 Nineteenth-century trains to Lourdes, in which windows tended to be closed to protect the consumptives, were considered a breeding ground for tuberculosis.

Bibliography

American Medical Association. *Module 1 – Pain Management: Pathophysiology of Pain and Pain Management*. AMA Continuing Medical Education (CME) Paper. Original release 2003, updated 2013, expiration 2016. Available at www.ama-cmeonline.com/pain_mgmt/printversion/ama_painmgmt_m1.pdf. [Accessed April 2013].

Ascherson, Neil. *The Polish August: The Self-Limiting Revolution*. London: Penguin Books, 1981.

Auden, W.H. *Selected Poetry of W.H. Auden*. New York: Vintage Books, 1971.

Aurelius, Marcus. *The Meditations of Marcus Aurelius Antonius: And a Selection from the Letters of Marcus and Fronto*. Translated by A.S.L. Farquharson. New York: Oxford University Press, 1989.

Babich, Babette, and Robert S. Cohen, eds. *Nietzsche, Theories of Knowledge, and Critical Theory: Nietzsche and the Sciences*. Dordrecht, The Netherlands: Kluwer Academic Publishers, 1999.

Bakewell, Sarah. *How to Live: A Life of Montaigne in One Question and Twenty Attempts at an Answer*. London: Vintage, 2011.

Bending, Lucy. *The Representation of Bodily Pain in Late Nineteenth-Century English Culture*. Oxford: Clarendon Press, 2000.

Berger, John, and Jean Mohr. *A Fortunate Man*. Cambridge: Granta, 1989. First published 1967 by Penguin.

Biro, David. *One Hundred Days: My Unexpected Journey from Doctor to Patient*. New York: Pantheon Books, 2000.

Biro, David. *The Language of Pain: Finding Words, Compassion, and Relief*. New York and London: W.W. Norton and Company, 2010.

Blanch, Lesley. *The Sabres of Paradise*. London: Quartet Books, 1978.

Bloxham, Dulce Arnall. *Who Was Ann Ockenden?* London: Neville Spearman Publishers, 1958.

Bostridge, Mark. *Florence Nightingale, the Woman and Her Legend*. London: Viking, 2008.

Bourke, Joanna. 'Languages of Pain'. *The Lancet* 379, no. 9835 (June 2012), 2420–21.

Bradshaw, Ann. *The Nurse Apprentice 1860–1997*. Farnham, UK: Ashgate Publishing, 2001.

Bradshaw, Ann. 'Measuring Nursing Care and Compassion: The McDonalised Nurse?' *Journal of Medical Ethics* 35, no. 8 (2009), 465–68.

Brennan, Bernadette. 'Frameworks of Grief: Narrative as an Act of Healing in Contemporary Memoir'. *TEXT* 16, no. 1 (April 2012), 1–23. Available at www.textjournal.com.au/april12/brennan.htm. [Accessed April 2012].

Breton, André. *Manifestos of Surrealism*. Translated by Richard Seaver and Helen R. Lane. Ann Arbor, MI: University of Michigan Press, 1969.

Bunyan, John. *The Pilgrim's Progress*. London: J.M. Dent and Sons Ltd, 1954.

Burney, Fanny. *Fanny Burney: Selected Letters and Journals*. Edited by Joyce Hemlow. Oxford: Clarendon Press, 1986.

Cairney, John. F.R.A.C.S., *Surgery for Students of Nursing*. 4th ed. Christchurch: N.M. Peryer Ltd, 1961.

Campo, Rafael. *The Enemy*. Durham, NC: Duke University Press, 2007.

Carlyle, Thomas. *Reminiscences*. 1881. Edited by K.J. Fielding and Ian Campbell. New York: Oxford University Press, 2000.

Carlyle, Thomas, and Jane Welsh Carlyle. *The Carlyle Letters Online* [*CLO*]. Edited by Brent E. Kinser. Vols. 9 (July 1836–December 1837), 17 (August 1843–March 1844), 18 (April–December 1844). Duke University Press, 14 September 2007. Available at carlyleletters.dukejournals.org/. [Page temporarily unavailable August 2018; last accessed May 2011].

Cartagena, Teresa de. *The Writings of Teresa de Cartagena. Comprising Grove of the Infirm and Wonder at the Works of God*. Translated by Dale Speidenspinner Núñez. Cambridge, UK: D.S. Brewer, 1998.

Cassell, Eric J. *The Nature of Suffering and the Goals of Medicine*. New York: Oxford University Press, 2004.

Cassian, Nina. *Life Sentence: Selected Poems*. Edited by William Jay Smith. London: Anvil Press Poetry Ltd, 1990.

Ciurlionis, Mary, ed. *A Twist of Fate: Tackling Arthritis, New Zealanders Share their Stories*. Wellington: Trio Books Ltd, 2003.

Claxton, Eve, ed. *The Book of Life: A Compendium of the Best Autobiographical and Memoir Writing*. London: Ebury Press: 2008.

Cohen, Esther. *The Modulated Scream: Pain in Late Medieval Culture*. Chicago, IL and London: The University of Chicago Press, 2010.

Confucius. *The Analects of Confucius, or The Conversations of Confucius with His Disciples and Certain Others*. 1910. Translated by W.E. Soothill and edited by Lady Hosie. London: Oxford University Press, 1958.

Coolidge, Susan. *What Katy Did*. 1872. London: Dean and Son Ltd, 1964.

Crapanzano, Vincent. *Imaginative Horizons: An Essay in Literary-Philosophical Anthropology*. Chicago: University of Chicago Press, 2010.

Crisp, Jackie and Taylor Catherine, eds. *Potter and Perry's Fundamentals of Nursing*. 3rd ed. Chatswood, NSW: Elsevier, 2008.

Critchley, MacDonald. 'Four Illustrious Neuroluetics: (Heinrich Heine, Jules de Goncourt, Alphonse Daudet, Guy de Maupassant)'. *Proceedings of the Royal Society of Medicine* 62, no. 7 (July 1969): 669–73.

Cuming, Angela. 'Cannabis Stops the Pain'. *ACC Forum*, 24 November 2012. Available at https://accforum.org/forums/index.php?/topic/13829-cannabis-stops-the-pain/. [Accessed November 2012].

Daudet, Alphonse. *The Nabob*. Translated by W. Blaydes, introduction by Prof. W.P. Trent. New York: P.F. Collier and Son, 1902.

Daudet, Alphonse. *Suffering*. Translated by Milton Garver. New Haven, CT: Yale University Press, 1934.

Daudet, Alphonse. *In the Land of Pain*. 1930. Translated and edited by Julian Barnes. New York: Alfred A. Knopf, 2002.

Daudet, Léon. *Alphonse Daudet: A Memoir*. 1897. Translated by Charles de Kay. Rockville, MD: 2007.

Descartes, René. *Treatise of Man, Harvard Monographs in the History of Science*. Translated by Thomas Steel Hall. Cambridge, MA: Harvard University Press, 1972.

Dickinson, Emily. *Poems by Emily Dickinson: The Original*. 1890. Edited by Mabel Loomis Todd and T.W. Higginson. Raleigh, NC: Hayes Barton Press, 2007.

Dieguez, Sebastian, and Julien Bogousslavsky. 'The One-Man Band of Pain: Alphonse Daudet and His Painful Experience of Tabes Dorsalis'. *Neurological Disorders in Famous Artists: Frontiers of Neurology and Neuroscience* 19 (2005): 17–45.

Dinesen, Isak. *Out of Africa and Shadows on the Grass*. Harmondsworth, Middlesex: Penguin: 1985.

Dubner, Ronald. 'Pain Research: Past, Present and Future'. *National Business Institute of Dental and Cranial Research*. Bethesda, MD: National Institutes of Health, October 2003. Available at www.nidcr.nih.gov/Research/ResearchResults/InterviewsOHR/TIS102003.htm. [Accessed February 2011].

Eder, Richard. 'Another Country'. *New York Times*, 2 February 2003.

Emerson, Ralph Waldo. *Nature*. 1836. Corvallis, OR: Oregon State University. Available at https://oregonstate.edu/instruct/phl302/texts/emerson/nature-contents.html. [Accessed October 2011].

Falkenstein, Eric. *Finding Alpha: The Search for Alpha When Risk and Return Break Down*. New Jersey: John Wiley and Sons Inc, 2009.

Farwell, Byron. *Burton: A Biography of Sir Richard Francis Burton*. London: Viking, 1998.

Foucault, Michael. *The Birth of the Clinic: An Archaeology of Medical Perception*. Translated by A.M. Sheridan. London: Routledge, 1973.

France, Peter, ed. *The New Oxford Companion to Literature in French*. Oxford: Clarendon Press, 1995.

Frank, Arthur W. *The Wounded Storyteller: Body, Illness and Ethics*. Chicago and London: University of Chicago Press, 1997.

Frawley, Maria. *Invalidism and Identity in Nineteenth-Century Britain*. Chicago: The University of Chicago Press, 2004.

Freeman, John, ed. *Granta 120: Medicine*. Granta: The New Magazine of New Writing. London: Grove Press/Granta, 2012.

Garner, Helen. *The Spare Room*. Melbourne: The Text Publishing Company, 2008.

Gilmore, Leigh. *The Limits of Autobiography: Trauma and Testimony*. New York: Cornell University Press, 2001.

Global Language Monitor. 'Number of Words in the English Language: 1,025,109.8'. *No. of Words*, 1 January 2014. Available at www.languagemonitor.com/number-of-words/number-of-words-in-the-english-language-1008879/. [Accessed January 2014].

Greenlaw, Lavinia, ed. *Signs and Humours: The Poetry of Medicine*. London: Calouste Gulbenkian Foundation, 2007.

Gorky, Maxim. *My Childhood*. 1913–14. Translated by Ronald Wilks. Hammondsworth, Middlesex: Penguin Books, 1967.

Goss, Edmund. *French Profiles*. 1898. London: W. Heinmann, 1913.

Gramsci, Antonio. *Prison Notebooks*. Vol. 1. Edited by Joseph A. Buttigieg. New York: Columbia University Press, 2011.

Greenhow, Thomas M. 'Termination of the Case of Miss Harriet Martineau'. *British Medical Journal* 1 (14 April 1877): 449–50.

Gyatso, Tenzin, The Fourteenth Dalai Lama, and Howard C. Cutler. *The Essence of Happiness: A Guidebook for Living*. Sydney: Hodder, 2001.

Hall, Michael R., and Susan Hoecker-Drysdale, eds. *Harriet Martineau: Theoretical and Methodological Perspectives*. New York: Routledge Chapman & Hall, 2002.

Hallam, Julia. *Nursing the Image: Media, Culture and Professional Identity*. London: Routledge, 2000.

Harich, Jack. 'The Comparative Pain Scale'. In Michael L. Whitworth, 'A Review of the Evaluation of Pain Using a Variety of Pain Scales'. San Antonio, TX: Danne Miller Education Center, 6 January 2011. Available at https://cme.dannemiller.com/articles/activity.cfm?id=318. [Accessed January 2011].

Harris, Ruth. *Lourdes: Body and Spirit in the Secular Age*. London: Penguin Books, 1999.

Hartwig, Julia. *In Praise of the Unfinished: Selected Poems*. Translated by John and Bogdana Carpenter. New York: Alfred A. Knopf, 2008.

Hawken, Dinah. *Oh There You Are Tui! New and Selected Poems*. Wellington: Victoria University Press, 2001.

Hawkins, Anne Hunsaker. *Reconstructing Illness: Studies in Pathography* 393. 2nd ed. West Lafayette: Purdue University Press, 1999.

Hazlitt, William. *Selected Essays of William Hazlitt 1778–1830*. Edited by Geoffrey Keynes. Whitefish, Montana: Kessinger Publishing, 2004.

Henriksen, Aage. *Isak Dinesen/Karen Blixen: The Life and the Work*. Translated by William Mishler with an introduction by Paul Houe. New York: St Martin's Press, 1988.

Herbert, Zbigniew. *Zbigniew Herbert, The Collected Poems 1956–1998*. Translated by Alissa Valles, Czesław Miłosz and Peter Dale Scott, with an introduction by Adam Zagajewski. New York: Ecco, 2007.

Heshusius, Lous. *Inside Chronic Pain: An Intimate and Critical Account*. Foreword by David B. Morris, Clinical Commentary by Scott M. Fishman, M.D. New York: Cornell University Press, 2009.

Hide, Louise, Joanna Burke and Carmen Mangion. 'Perspectives on Pain: Introduction'. *19: Interdisciplinary Studies in the Long Nineteenth Century*, no. 15 (2012). Available at www.19.bbk.ac.uk/85/volume/0/issue/15/. [Accessed August 2018].

Holmes, Martha Stoddard. 'After Sontag: Reclaiming Metaphor'. *Genre: Forms of Discourse and Culture* 44, no. 3 (Autumn 2011): 263–76. Guest edited by Michael Hanne.

Holub, Miroslav. *Intensive Care: Selected and New Poems*. Oberlin, OH: Oberlin College Press, 1996.

Hustvedt, Siri. *The Shaking Woman or a History of My Nerves*. London: Sceptre, 2010.

Iverson, Jeffrey. *More Lives than One? The Evidence of the Remarkable Bloxham Tapes*. Foreword by Magnus Magnusson. New York: Warner Books, 1977.

Ivinskaya, Olga. *A Captive of Time: My Years with Pasternak*. Translated by Max Hawyard. London: Collins and Harvill Press, 1978.

Jack, Andrew. 'An End to the Agony'. *Financial Times*, 20 November 2012.

Japp, A.H. *Robert Louis Stevenson: A Record, an Estimate, and a Memorial*. 1905. Available at www.gutenberg.org/files/590/590-h/590-h.htm. [Accessed May 2011].

Jennings, Dana. 'Pain Beyond Words and an Impulse Just to Endure'. *New York Times*, 21 September 2009.

Kahlo, Frida. *The Diary of Frida Kahlo: An Intimate Self-Portrait*. Translated by Barbara Crowe de Toledo and Rickardo Pohlenz, with an introduction by Carlos Fuentes, and essays and commentary by Sarah M. Lowe. New York: Harry M. Abrams; Mexico: La Vaca Independiente, S.A. de C.V., 1995.

Kapuściński, Ryszard. *Imperium*. Translated by Klara Glowczewska, with an afterword by Margaret Atwood. London: Granta Books, 2007. First published (Polish) 1993 by Czytelnik.

Klaus, Carl H., and Ned Stuckey-French, eds. *Essayists on the Essay: Montaigne to Our Time.* Iowa City, IA: University of Iowa Press, 2012.

Kleinman, Arthur. *The Illness Narratives: Suffering, Healing and the Human Condition.* New York: Basic Books, 1988.

Koestler, Arthur. *The Roots of Coincidence.* New York: Random House, 1972.

Leriche, René. *La Philosophie de la Chirurgie.* Paris: Flammarion, 1951.

Lewis, C.S. *A Grief Observed.* London: Faber and Faber, 1973. First published 1961 by Seabury Press.

Lewis, C.S. *The Problem of Pain.* New York: The Macmillan Company, 1966. First published 1940 by Centenary Press.

Lilburn, Douglas. *A Search for Tradition and A Search for Language.* Afterword by Jack Body. Wellington: Lilburn Residence Trust in association with Victoria University Press, 2011.

Lindop, Grevel. *The Opium-Eater: A Life of Thomas de Quincey.* London: J. M. Dent & Sons Ltd, 1981.

Liska, Jeanette. *Silenced Screams: Surviving Anesthetic Awareness During Surgery: A True Account.* Park Ridge, IL: American Association of Nurse Anesthetists Publishing Inc. and the Council for Public Interest in Anesthesia, 2002.

Lopate, Phillip. *The Art of the Personal Essay: An Anthology from the Classical Era to the Present.* Anchor Books, 1995.

Luria, A.R. *The Mind of a Mnemonist.* Translated by Lynn Solotoroff. New York: Basic Books, 1968.

MacCarthy, Fiona. 'The Curse of Byron'. *Guardian Review*, 15 November 2003.

Magnet, Julia. 'Sickened By the Nurses Who Don't Care'. *The Sunday Times*, 23 November 2003.

Main, Chris J., and Chris C. Spanswick, eds. *Pain Management: An Interdisciplinary Approach.* Edinburgh, London, New York: Churchill Livingston/Harcourt Publishers Ltd, 2000.

Manchester, Anne. 'Encouraging Healing Through Touch'. *Kai Tiaki: Nursing New Zealand* 9, no. 7 (1 August 2003): 12–13.

Mantel, Hilary. *Giving Up the Ghost: A Memoir.* London: Picador, 2004.

Mantel, Hilary. 'Diary'. *London Review of Books* 32, no. 21 (4 November 2010): 41–42.

Marche, Stephen. 'Is Facebook Making Us Lonely?' *Atlantic Magazine*, 2 April 2012.

The Marshall Protocol Knowledge Base: Autoimmunity Research Foundation. 'Incidence and Prevalence of Chronic Disease'. Available at https://mpkb.org/home/pathogenesis/epidemiology. [Accessed November 2011].

Martineau, Harriet. *Harriet Martineau's Autobiography.* Vol. 1. Edited by Maria Weston Chapman. Boston: James R. Osgood and Co, 1877.

Martineau, Harriet. *Deerbrook: A Novel.* London: Edward Moxon, 1839.

Martineau, Harriet. *Life in the Sick-Room: Essays by an Invalid.* 1844. Edited by Maria H. Frawley. Peterborough, ON: Broadview Literary Texts, Broadview Press Ltd, 2003.

Martineau, Harriet. 'Letter to the Deaf'. *Tait's Edinburgh Magazine* 1 (1834): 174–79.

Martineau, Harriet. 'Miss Nightingale's *Notes on Nursing*'. *The Quarterly Review* 1, no. 107 (1860): 392–422.

Miller, Henry. *Stand Still Like the Hummingbird: Essays.* New York: New Directions, 1962.

Miłosz, Czesław. *Bells in Winter.* Translated by Czesław Miłosz and Lillian Vallee. New Jersey: The Ecco Press, 1978.

Milton, John. *Paradise Lost*. 1667. With essays by Elijah Fenton and Samuel Johnson. London: John Bumpus, 1821.

Milton, John. 'Samson Agonistes, A Dramatic Poem'. In *The Poetical Works of John Milton* 3, 78–73. London: William Pickering, 1851.

Montaigne, Michel de. *The Complete Works of Michael de Montaigne*. Translated by Charles Cotton, edited by William Hazlitt. London: J Templeman, 1842.

Montaigne, Michel de. *The Complete Essays of Montaigne*. Translated by Donald M. Frame. Stanford, CA: Stanford University Press, 1958.

Montaigne, Michel de. *The Complete Essays of Michel de Montaigne*. 1877. Translated by Charles Cotton, edited by William Carew Hazlitt. Digireads.com Publishing, 2009.

Montalk, Stephanie de. *Unquiet World: The Life of Count Geoffrey Potocki de Montalk*. Wellington: Victoria University Press, 2001. Published in Polish translation as *Niespokojny świat*. Kraków: Jagiellonian University Press, 2003.

Montalk, Stephanie de. *Cover Stories*. Wellington: Victoria University Press, 2005.

Montalk, Stephanie de. 'Pain'. In *Sport 33: Performance Pain, New Zealand New Writing*, 3–30. Edited by Fergus Barrowman. Wellington: Victoria University Press, 2005.

Montalk, Stephanie de. *The Fountain of Tears*. Wellington: Victoria University Press, 2006.

Montalk, Stephanie de. *Vivid Familiar*. Wellington: Victoria University Press, 2009.

Morris, David B. *Illness and Culture in the Postmodern Age*. Berkeley and Los Angeles, CA: University of California Press, 1998.

Morris, David B. *The Culture of Pain*. Berkeley and Los Angeles, CA: University of California Press, 1993.

Morris, David B. 'Narrative and Pain: An Integrative Model'. In *Handbook of Pain and Palliative Care: Behavioural Approaches for the Life Course*, 733–51. Edited by R.J. Moor. New York: Springer, 2012.

Morris, Richard. *The Last Sorcerers: The Path from Alchemy to the Periodic Table*. Washington DC: Joseph Henry Press, 2003.

Nash, Elizabeth. 'Veteran Saramago Reaches End of Epic Journey'. *The Independent*, 8 September 2008.

Neruda, Pablo. *Pablo Neruda: The Early Poems*. New York: New Rivers Press, 1969.

New Zealand Colonist and Port Nicholson Advertiser 1, no. 5 (16 August 1842). Available by searching on https://paperspast.natlib.govt.nz/.

New Zealand Gazette and Wellington Spectator 4, no. 318 (27 January 1844). Available by searching on https://paperspast.natlib.govt.nz/.

Nietzsche, Friedrich. *Thus Spoke Zarathustra: A Book for All and None*. 1892. Translated by Thomas Wayne. New York: Algora Publishing, 2003.

Nightingale, Florence. *Notes on Nursing: What It Is and What It Is Not*. 1859. Philadelphia: Lippincott, Williams and Wilkins, 1992.

Nightingale, Florence. *Florence Nightingale on Public Health Care*. The Collected Works of Florence Nightingale, vol. 6. Edited by Lynn McDonald. Waterloo, ON: Wilfrid Laurier University Press, 2004.

Ondaatje, Michael. *The English Patient*. London: Picador, 1993. First published 1992 by McClelland and Stewart.

O'Sullivan, Vincent, ed. *An Anthology of Twentieth-Century New Zealand Poetry*. London: Oxford University Press, 1970.

Ouzounian, Richard, 'About this Recording', DuPont Show of the Month, CBS TV, February 1958.

Ovid. *Metamorphoses.* Translated by A.D. Melville with an introduction and notes by E.J. Kennedy. Oxford: Oxford University Press, 1987.

Page, Bruce, David Leitch and Phillip Knightley. *Philby: The Spy Who Betrayed a Generation.* Introduction by John le Carré. London: Sphere Books/Andre Deutsch Ltd, 1977.

Parris, Winston C.V. 'The History of Pain Medicine'. In *Practical Management of Pain*, 3rd ed. 529–43. Edited by P. Prithvi Raj. St Louis, MI: Mosby, 2000.

Pascal, Blaise. *Pascal's Pensées.* Introduction by T.S. Eliot. New York: E.P. Dutton and Co Inc., 1958.

Pasternak, Boris. *Doctor Zhivago.* Translated by Max Haywood and Manya Harai. London: Collins and Harvill Press, 1958.

Pasternak, Boris. *Second Nature: New Translations of Poems by Boris Pasternak.* Translated by Andrei Navrozov. London: Peter Owen Publishers, 1990.

Pender, Stephen. 'Seeing, Feeling, Judging: Pain in the Early Modern Imagination'. In *The Sense of Suffering: Construction of Physical Pain in Early Modern Culture*, 469–96. Edited by Jan Frans van Dijkhuizen and Karl A.E. Enenkel. Leiden and Boston: Brill, 2009.

Read, Christopher. *Lenin: A Revolutionary Life.* Abington, Oxon: Routledge, 2005.

Rey, Roselyne. *The History of Pain.* Translated by Louise Elliott Wallace, J.A. Cadden and S.W. Cadden. Cambridge, MA and London: Harvard University Press, 1995.

Richardson, Robert D. Jnr. *Emerson, the Mind on Fire: A Biography.* Berkeley, CA: University of California Press, 1995.

Rilke, Rainer Maria. *The Selected Poetry of Rainer Maria Rilke.* Translated and edited by Stephen Mitchell. London: Picador/Pan Books, 1987.

Riskin, Jessica. *Science in the Age of Sensibility: The Sentimental Empiricists of the French Enlightenment.* Chicago, IL and London: The University of Chicago Press, 2002.

Robert, R., D. Prat-Pradal, J.J. Labat, M. Bensignor, S. Raoul, R. Rebai and J. Leborgne. 'Anatomic Basis of Chronic Perineal Pain: Role of the Pudendal Nerve'. *Surgical and Radiologic Anatomy* 20, no. 2 (1988): 93–98.

Robinson, Spider. *Callahan's Crosstime Saloon.* New York: Ace Books, 1977.

Rosenfeld, Arthur. *The Truth About Chronic Pain: Patients and Professionals on How to Face it, Understand It, Overcome It.* New York: Basic Books, 2004.

Rumi, Jalal al-Din. *The Essential Rumi.* Translated by Coleman Barks with John Moyne, A.J. Arberry and Reynold Nicholson. London: Penguin, 1995.

Rylkova, Glina, S. 'Oyster Fever: Chekhov and Turgenev'. *The Bulletin of the North American Chekhov Society* XV, no. 1 (Autumn 2007): 1–6.

Scarry, Elaine. *The Body in Pain: The Making and Unmaking of the World.* New York: Oxford University Press, 1987.

Schneider, Jennifer. *Living with Chronic Pain: The Complete Health Guide to the Causes and Treatment of Chronic Pain.* New York: Healthy Living Books, 2004.

Schoenfeldt, Michael. 'Aesthetics and Anesthetics: The Art of Pain Management in Early Modern England'. In *The Sense of Suffering: Constructions of Physical Pain in Early Modern Culture*, 19–38. Edited by Jan Frans van Dijkhluizen and Karl A.E. Enekel. Leiden and Boston: Brill, 2009.

Schopenhauer, Arthur. *On The Basis of Mortality.* 2nd ed. Translated by Arthur Brodrick Bullock. London: Allen and Unwin, London, 1915.

Schopenhauer, Arthur. *Parerga and Paralipomena: Short Philosophical Essays. Vol. 2.* Translated and edited by E.F.J. Payne. Oxford: Oxford University Press, 2000.

Schopenhauer, Arthur. *On the Suffering of the World: Essays.* 1850. Translated by R.J. Hollingdale. London: Penguin, 2004.

Schopenhauer, Arthur. *Counsels and Maxims.* 1890. Translated by T. Bailey Saunders. New York: Cosimo Inc, 2007.

Selzer, Richard. 'The Language of Pain'. *The Wilson Quarterly* 18, no. 4 (Autumn 1994): 28.

Shadows of Time: Genealogical Services and Information. *Early NZ Settlers.* Extracted from R.A.A. Sherrin and L.H. Wallace, *Early History of New Zealand* H. Brett: Auckland, 1890.

Shakespeare, William. 'Much Ado About Nothing' and 'Romeo and Juliet'. *The Works of William Shakespeare Gathered into One Volume.* London: Studio Editions Ltd, 1993.

Shelley, Percy Bysshe. 'A Defence of Poetry'. In *Essays: Letters from Abroad, Translations and Fragments*, vol. 1, 1–57. London: Edward Moxon, 1840.

Sherard, R.H. *Alphonse Daudet: A Biographical and Critical Study.* London: Edward Arnold, 1894.

Shore, Marci. *Caviar and Ashes: A Warsaw Generation's Life and Death in Marxism, 1918–1968.* New Haven, CT and London: Yale University Press, 2006.

Shore, Marci. 'Love in the Time of Revolution: The Polish Poets of Café Ziemianska'. In *New Dangerous Liaisons: Discourses on Europe and Love in the Twentieth Century*, 117–36. Edited by Louisa Passerini, Liliana Ellena and Alexander C.T. Geppert. New York: Berghahn Books, 2010.

Simpson, Louis. *The Character of the Poet.* Ann Arbor, MI: The University of Michigan Press, 1989.

Simpson, Louis and Aston Marantz, ed., trans. *Modern Poets of France: A Bilingual Anthology.* Brownsville, OR: Story Line Press, 1997.

Smolen, Rick and Jennifer Erwitt. *The Blue Planet Run: The Race to Provide Safe Drinking Water to the World.* Foreword by Robert Redford. San Rafael: Earth Aware Editions, 2007.

Smolen, Kazimierz. *Auschwitz Birkenau Guide-Book.* Translated by Stephen Lee. Oświęcim: Publishing House of the State Museum, 2002.

Solzhenitsyn, Alexander. *One Day in the Life of Ivan Denisovich.* Translated by Ralph Parker, introduction by Marvin Kalb, foreword by Alexander Tvardovsky. New York: Signet/E.P. Dutton and Co, 1963.

Solzhenitsyn, Alexander. *Cancer Ward.* Translated by Nicholas Bethell and David Burg. Harmondsworth, Middlesex: Penguin, 1973.

Song, Sora. 'Health: Mind Over Medicine'. *TIME Magazine*, 19 March 2006.

Sontag, Susan. *Illness as Metaphor and AIDS and Its Metaphors.* New York: Picador and Farrar, Straus and Giroux, 1989. *Illness as Metaphor* first published 1978 in the *New York Review of Books.*

Sophocles. *Philoctetes. c.* 409BC. Translated by Ian Johnston. Nanaimo, BC: Vancouver Island University, 2012. Available at https://records.viu.ca/~johnstoi/sophocles/philoctetesrtf.rtf. [Accessed August 2018].

Spence, Lewis. *An Encyclopaedia of Occultism: Cosimo Classics Metaphysics.* 1920. New York, Cosimo Inc, 2006.

Šteger, Aleš. *The Book of Things.* Translated by Brian Henry. Rochester, NY: BOA Editions Ltd, 2010.

Strachey, Lytton. *Eminent Victorians: Cardinal Manning, Florence Nightingale, Dr Arnold, General Gordon.* Introduction by Noel Annan. London and Glasgow: Collins, 1965.

Strong, Rowland. 'In the French Capital the Publication of Daudet's New Novel, *La Fedor*, is the Literary Event of the Day'. *The New York Times*, 30 May 1897. Available at www. nytimes.com/1897/05/30/archives/in-the-french-capital-the-publication-of-daudets-new-novel-la-fedor.html. [Accessed September 2012].

Swir (Świrszczyńska), Anna. *Building the Barricade and other poems of Anna Swir*. Translated by Piotr Florczyk, foreword by Jericho Brown. Philadelphia, PA: Calypso Editions, 2011.

Talbot, Margaret. 'The Placebo Prescription'. *New York Times*, 9 January 2002.

Thernstrom, Melanie. *The Pain Chronicles: Cures, Myths, Mysteries, Prayers, Diaries, Brain Scans, Healing, and the Science of Suffering*. New York: Farrar, Straus and Giroux, 2010.

Thomas, Gillian. 'Harriet Martineau'. In *Dictionary of Literary Biography* vol. 55, 168–75. Edited by William B. Thesing. Farmington Hill, MI: Gale Research Company, 1987.

Thurman, Judith. *Isak Dinesen: The Life of Karen Blixen*. Harmondsworth, Middlesex: Penguin, 1986. First published 1982 by St. Martin's Press.

Tolstoy, Leo. *Sebastopol*. Edited by Ivan Lipinski. London: The Lotus Library, Greening and Co. Neither translator nor publication date noted.

Tolstoy, Leo. *The Sebastopol Sketches*. Translated by David McDuff. London: Penguin, 1986.

Tolstoy, Leo. *The Death of Ivan Ilych*. 1886. Translated by Louise and Aylmer Maude, edited by D. Bannon. Raleigh, NZ: Bilingual Library, Lulu Enterprises Inc., 2010.

Tsvetayeva, Marina. *Selected Poems*. Translated by David McDuff. Tarset, Northumberland: Bloodaxe Books, 1988.

Turgenev, Ivan Sergeyevich. 'The Living Relic'. 1874. In *Sketches from a Hunter's Album*, 354–67. Translated by Richard Freeborn. London: Penguin Classics, 1990.

Valéry, Paul. *The Collected Works of Paul Valéry*. 1896. Translated and edited by Jackson Mathews. London: Routledge and Keegan Paul, 1973.

Valles, Alissa. 'A Wound Like a Mouth'. *Brick: A Literary Journal*, no. 87 (June 2011): 92.

Venclova, Tomas. *Aleksander Wat: Life and Art of an Iconoclast*. New Haven and London: Yale University Press, 1996.

Venclova, Tomas. *Forms of Hope: Essays*. New York: The Sheep Meadow Press, 1999.

Vetlesen, Arne Johan. *A Philosophy of Pain*. Translated by John Irons. London: Reaktion Books Ltd, 2009.

Voltaire. *Candide*. 1759. Translated by John Butt. West Drayton, Middlesex: Penguin 1947.

Wallis, Claudia. 'The Right (and Wrong) Way to Treat Pain'. *TIME Magazine*, 20 February 2005.

Wat, Aleksander. *Mediterranean Poems*. Translated and edited by Czesław Miłosz. Ann Arbor, MI: Ardis, 1977.

Wat, Aleksander. *With the Skin: Poems of Aleksander Wat*. Translated and edited by Czesław Miłosz and Leonard Nathan. New York: Ecco Press, 1989.

Wat, Aleksander. *Lucifer Unemployed*. Translated by Lillian Vallee with a foreword by Czesław Miłosz. Evanston, IL: Northwestern University Press, 1990.

Wat, Aleksander. *My Century: The Odyssey of a Polish Intellectual*. Translated and edited by Richard Lourie with a foreword by Czesław Miłosz. New York: New York Review of Books, 2003.

Wat, Aleksander. 'Diary Without Vowels'. Translated by Alissa Valles. In *Polish Writers on Writing*, 71–78. Edited by Adam Zagajewski. San Antonio, TX: Trinity University Press, 2007.

Wat, Aleksander. 'The Four Walls of My Pain', 'Here There is No Space No Will'. Translated by Ryszard Reisner. *Ars Interpres: An International Journal of Poetry, Translation and Art*, no. 8–9 (September 2007).

Webb, R.K. *Harriet Martineau: A Radical Victorian*. New York: Columbia University Press, 1960.

Weiss, Jerome. 'Pudendal Nerve Entrapment'. Paper presented at the International Pelvic Pain Society 10th Scientific Meeting on Chronic Pelvic Pain, Alberta, August 2003. Available at pudendalhope.info/sites/default/files/JeromeWeiss.pdf. [Accessed 2005].

Welch, Denton. *A Voice Through a Cloud*. Boston, MA: Exact Change, 1996.

Wenof, Michael and C. Paul Perry. *Chronic Pelvic Pain: A Patient Education Booklet*. Chicago, IL: The International Pelvic Pain Society, 1999. Available at hermanwallace.com/download/IPPS_chronic_pelvic_pain_booklet.pdf. [Accessed March 2004].

Wheeler, Lesley. 'Illness and Poetic Language'. *Literature and Medicine* 29, no. 1 (Spring 2011), 197–212.

White, Margo. 'Breaking the Pain Barrier'. *New Zealand Listener*, 2–8 March 2013.

Williams, Barbara Gay. *The Primacy of the Nurse in New Zealand 1960s–1990s: Attitudes, Beliefs and Responses Over Time*. PhD thesis, Victoria University of Wellington, 2000. Available at researcharchive.vuw.ac.nz/handle/10063/65. [Accessed January 2010].

Williams, William Carlos. *The Doctor Stories*. 1948. Compiled by Robert Coles, M.D. with an afterword by William Eric Williams, M.D. New York: New Directions Publishing Corp, 1984.

Wittgenstein, Ludwig. *Philosophical Investigations*. 2nd ed. Translated by G.E.M Anscombe. Oxford: Basil Blackwell, 1958.

Woolf, Virginia. *On Being Ill*. 1926. Introduction by Hermione Lee. Ashfield, MA: Paris Press, 2002.

Wordsworth, William. 'Intimations of Immortality from Recollections of Early Childhood'. 1807. In *The Oxford Book of English Verse 1250–1900*, 609–16. Edited by A.T. Quiller-Couch. Oxford: Clarendon Press, 1906.

Zagajewski, Adam, ed. *Polish Writers on Writing*. San Antonio, TX: Trinity University Press, 2007.

Zajaczkowski, Ryszard. 'Alexander Wat's "Leap from Poetry into Politics"'. *The Polish Review* L, no. 4 (2005), 399–424.

Zinsser, William, ed. *Inventing the Truth: The Art and Craft of Memoir*. Boston and New York: Houghton Mifflin Company, 1998.

Zola, Émile. *Lourdes: Of the 'Three Cities'*. 1894. Translated by Ernest A. Viztelly, 1894.

Index

Page numbers in *italics* denote photographs; n denotes notes.